The
Hands-on Guide
for Junior Doctors

The
Hands-on Guide
for Junior Doctors

Fourth Edition

ANNA DONALD
BA (Sydney), BM, BCh (Oxon), MPP (Harvard)
Late of Bazian Ltd, London

MICHAEL STEIN
MB ChB, BSc (Hons) (UCT), DPhil (Oxon)
Chief Medical Officer, Map of Medicine, London
and Medical Advisor, Hearst Business Media,
Hearst Corporation, New York

CIARAN SCOTT HILL
BSc (Hons) MSc (Clin. Neuro.) MBBS MCSP MRCS MRCP
Speciality Trainee in Neurosurgery, London

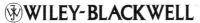

⟨W⟩WILEY-BLACKWELL

A John Wiley & Sons, Ltd., Publication

Blackwell Publishing was acquired by John Wiley & Sons in February 2007. Blackwell's publishing program has
been merged with Wiley's global Scientific, Technical and Medical business to form Wiley-Blackwell.

Registered Office
John Wiley & Sons Ltd, The Atrium, Southern Gate, Chichester, West Sussex, PO19 8SQ, UK

Editorial Offices
9600 Garsington Road, Oxford, OX4 2DQ, UK
The Atrium, Southern Gate, Chichester, West Sussex, PO19 8SQ, UK
111 River Street, Hoboken, NJ 07030-5774, USA

For details of our global editorial offices, for customer services and for information about how to
apply for permission to reuse the copyright material in this book please see our website at
www.wiley.com/wiley-blackwell

Library of Congress Cataloging-in-Publication Data

Donald, Anna.
    The hands-on guide for junior doctors / Anna Donald, Michael Stein, Ciaran Scott Hill. – 4th ed.
        p. ; cm.
    Includes bibliographical references and index.
    ISBN 978-1-4443-3466-1 (hardcover : alk. paper)
    1. Residents (Medicine)–Handbooks, manuals, etc. 2. Medicine–Handbooks, manuals, etc.
I. Stein, Michael.   II. Hill, Ciaran.   III. Title.
    [DNLM: 1. Medical Staff, Hospital–organization & administration–Great Britain–Handbooks.
2. Clinical Competence–Great Britain–Handbooks.   3. Internship and Residency–organization &
administration–Great Britain–Handbooks.   4. Medicine–Great Britain–Handbooks. WX 203]
    RA972.D66 2006
    610.92–dc22
                                            2010039148

A catalogue record for this book is available from the British Library.

Set in 8/10pt Humanist by SPi Publisher Services, Pondicherry, India
Printed and bound in Malaysia by Vivar Printing Sdn Bhd

Contents

Introduction

Your junior doctor years are guaranteed to be one of the big experiences of your life. Free at last from rote learning and endless exams, your first job is intensely practical. The trouble is that the theoretical training in medical school does not usually prepare you for the physical and emotional rigours of hundreds of tasks being thrust upon you around the clock. Similarly, medical textbooks rarely deal with the practical know-how which makes all the difference between clumsy and elegant doctoring.

This book is based on the collective experience of junior doctors who remember only too well the highs and lows of their first year. It contains information not readily available in standard texts that will help you to feel competent and confident despite sleepless nights and low blood sugars. It assumes minimal practical know-how. Subjects are listed in alphabetical order within each chapter. A detailed index is also provided for rapid reference.

Whatever you do, keep your head up and keep smiling. Hospitals are funny places. Lots of people love their first job; we hope you are one of them. Take care and good luck!

A.K.D.
C.S.H.
M.L.S.
J.T.H.T.

How to use this book

This book is designed as a user-friendly manual. We recommend skimming through it when you first buy it, and then referring to relevant sections for particular problems that you come across.

This book provides standard algorithms for diagnosis and management of clinical problems that worked for us and our colleagues, in different settings throughout Britain. Please don't follow our instructions slavishly. We realize that every firm has its own way of doing things and that there may be more appropriate algorithms for specialist wards or unusual situations. Like a recipe book, feel free to scrawl in the margins to make it more usable for you. We have included some blank pages at the back for extra notes.

We want to emphasize that this book is not the *Oxford Textbook of Medicine*, so please don't expect to find the 337 causes of tropical swollen legs here!

To keep the book compact and maximally relevant to what you need, we have not attempted to replicate the *British National Formulary*. While we do suggest drugs where relevant, we realized from our own experience that the safest and most efficient way to prescribe drugs is to use the *BNF* in conjunction with your hospital's drug formulary.

Finally, if you discover a better way of doing something, please let us know. If we can use your suggestion, you will be acknowledged in the next edition of the book.

Acknowledgements

This book is dedicated to Uncle Ivan Harris and to Bruce, Janet and Tom Donald, for the support and love that made writing this book possible.

Fifty per cent of the authors' royalties for this book are donated to the University of Cape Town Medical School.

Dedication

The wonderful Anna Donald died during the preparation of this fourth edition of *Hands-on Guide for Junior Doctors*. For those who never had the privilege of meeting Anna, here is a little bit about an extraordinary friend and colleague (also see her obituary in the BMJ – 4 February 2009 – by Richard Smith and Sir Muir Gray):

Anna had a brilliant and inquisitive mind, receiving degrees from not one but three top-flight universities:

■ University of Sydney: Bachelor of Arts, majoring in history and preclinical medicine
■ University of Oxford: Bachelor of Medicine and Surgery degree (Rhodes Scholar)
■ Harvard University: Master's degree in Public Policy

Anna worked as a doctor and lecturer in epidemiology and public policy at University College London, and was founding editor of the British Medical Journal's *Clinical Evidence*, the journal of evidence-based health care and evidence-based health policy. Anna's professional passion was the delivery of high-quality health care for everyone. Indeed, in 1998, as a pioneer in evidence-based health care, Anna founded Bazian, one of the first companies in the world to provide specialist evidence-based consulting and analysis to support the delivery of health care.

In 2007, Anna learned that her breast cancer, first diagnosed in 2003, had metastasized. Anna remained incredibly positive and said this: 'When you discover you have metastatic cancer you think you've picked a black ball in the lottery. But I've discovered it's a luminescent ball. I'm becoming the person I want to be. I'm not putting it off until I retire'.

Anna died two years later on 1 February 2009 having become the person she wanted to be. And she was always a person that everyone who met her, loved.

For more about Anna Donald, see her entry in Wikipedia.

Abbreviations

We include a long list of abbreviations to aid reading medical notes and for reference throughout this book.

μg	micrograms
−ve	negative
+ve	positive
A&E	accident and emergency
ABC	airway, breathing, circulation
ABG	arterial blood gases
ac	*ante cibum* (before food)
ACE	angiotensin-converting enzyme
ACTH	adrenocorticotrophic hormone
ADH	antidiuretic hormone
AF	atrial fibrillation
AFB	acid-fast bacillus
AIDS	acquired immunodeficiency syndrome
ALP (alkphos)	alkaline phosphatase
ALS	Advanced Life Support
ALT	alanine aminotransferase
ANA	antinuclear antigen
ANCA	antineutrophil cytoplasmic antigen
ANF	antinuclear factor
APTT	activated partial thromboplastin time
ARC	AIDS-related complex
ARDS	adult respiratory distress syndrome
ARF	acute renal failure
ASAP	as soon as possible
ASD	atrial septal defect
ASOT	antistreptolysin O titre
AST	aspartate transaminase
ATN	acute tubular necrosis
AV	atrioventricular
AVCs	additional voluntary contributions
AXR	abdominal X-ray (plain)
Ba	barium
BBB	bundle branch block
bd	*bis die* (twice per day)
bHCG	beta-human chorionic gonadotrophin
BMA	British Medical Association
BMJ	*British Medical Journal*
BNF	*British National Formulary*
BP	blood pressure
bpm	beats/minute
Ca	carcinoma
Ca	calcium
CABG	coronary artery bypass graft
CBD	common bile duct
CCF	congestive cardiac failure
CCU	coronary care unit
CEA	carcino-embryonic antigen
CFC	complement fixation test
Cl	contraindications
CK	creatinine kinase
CK-MB	creatine kinase cardiac isoenzyme
CLL	chronic lymphocytic leukaemia
CML	chronic myeloid leukaemia
CMV	cytomegalovirus
CNS	central nervous system
COAD	chronic obstructive airways disease
COPD	Chronic Obstructive Pulmonary Disease
CPR	cardiopulmonary resuscitation
CRF	chronic renal failure
CRP	C-reactive protein
CSF	cerebrospinal fluid
CT	computed tomography

CTG	cardiotocography	FVC	forced vital capacity
CV	curriculum vitae	Fx	family
CVA	cerebrovascular accident	FY1	Foundation Year 1
CVP	central venous pressure	FY2	Foundation Year 2
CVS	cardiovascular system	g	gram(s)
CXR	chest X-ray	G&S	group and save
D&V	diarrhoea and vomiting	G6PD	glucose-6-phosphate dehydrogenase
DDAVP	desmopressin		
DIC	disseminated intravascular coagulation	GBM	glomerular basement membrane
DIP	distal interphalangeal	GCS	Glasgow Coma Scale
DKA	diabetic ketoacidosis	GFR	glomerular filtration rate
dl	decilitre(s)	GGT	gamma-glutamyl transferase
DM	diabetes mellitus	GH	growth hormone
DNR	do not resuscitate	GI (GIT)	gastrointestinal
DOA	date of admission	GKI	glucose, potassium and insulin
DOB	date of birth		
DOD	date of death	GMC	General Medical Council
DoH	Department of Health	GN	glomerulonephritis
DVLC	Driver and Vehicle Licensing Centre	GP	general practitioner
		GT	glutamyl transferase
DVT	deep venous thrombosis	GTN	glyceryl trinitrate
DXT	radiotherapy	GTT	glucose tolerance test
EBV	Epstein–Barr virus	GU	genito-urinary
ECG	electrocardiogram	HB	heart block
ECHO	echocardiography	Hb	haemoglobin
EDTA	ethylene diamine tetra-acetic acid	HBsAg	hepatitis B surface antigen
		Hct	haematocrit
EEG	electroencephalogram	HDL	high density lipoprotein
ELISA	enzyme-linked immuno-sorbent assay	HDU	high dependency unit
		Hep	hepatitis
EM	electron microscope	HiB	*Haemophilus influenzae* B vaccine
ENT	ear, nose and throat		
EPC	early pregnancy clinic	HIV	human immunodeficiency virus
ERCP	endoscopic retrograde cholangiopancreatography		
		HLA	human leukocyte antigen
ESR	erythrocyte sedimentation rate	HO	House Officer
		HOCM	hypertrophic obstructive cardiomyopathy
FBC	full blood count		
FDP	fibrin degradation product	HPC	history of presenting complaint
FEV₁	forced expiratory volume in first second		
		HS	heart sounds
FFP	fresh frozen plasma	HT	hypertension
FOB	faecal occult blood	IBD	inflammatory bowel disease
FSH	follicle stimulating hormone	IBS	irritable bowel syndrome

ICP	intracranial pressure	*mane*	in the morning
ID	identification	MC&S	microscopy, culture and
IDDM	insulin-dependent diabetes		sensitivity
	mellitus	MCV	mean cell volume
Ig	immunoglobulin	MDU	Medical Defence Union
IHD	ischaemic heart disease	Mg	magnesium
IM	intramuscular	mg	milligrams
INR	international normalized	MI	myocardial infarction
	ratio (prothrombin ratio)	ml	millilitres
IPPV	intermittent positive	mmHg	millimetres of mercury
	pressure ventilation	MND	motor neurone disease
ISDN	isosorbide di-nitrate	MPS	Medical Protection Society
ITP	idiopathic thrombocyto-	MRI	magnetic resonance imaging
	penic purpura	MRSA	methicillin resistant
ITU	intensive therapy unit		*Staphylococcus aureus*
iu (IU)	international unit	MS	multiple sclerosis
IUCD	intrauterine contraceptive	MSK	musculoskeletal
	device	MST	morphine sulphate tablets
IV	intravenous	MSU	midstream urine
IVC	inferior vena cava	N&V	nausea and vomiting
IVI	intravenous infusion	Na	sodium
IVU	intravenous urography	NB	*nota bene* (note well)
JAMA	*Journal of the American*	NBM	nil by mouth
	Medical Association	NEJM	*New England Journal of*
JVP	jugular venous pressure		*Medicine*
K$^+$	potassium	NGT	nasogastric tube
KCCT	kaolin-cephalin clotting time	NIDDM	non-insulin dependent
KCl	potassium chloride		diabetes mellitus
kg	kilograms	*nocte*	in the evening
kPa	kilopascals	NR	normal range
L	left	NSAIDs	non-steroidal anti-inflamma-
l	litres		tory drugs
LBBB	left bundle branch block	O&G	obstetrics and gynaecology
LDH	lactate dehydrogenase	obs	observations
LDL	low density lipoprotein	OCP	oral contraceptive pill
LFT	liver function test	OD	overdose
LH	luteinizing hormone	od	once a day
LIF	left iliac fossa	$PaCO_2$	partial pressure of CO_2 in
LMN	lower motor neurone		arterial blood
LMP	last menstrual period	PAN	polyarteritis nodosa
LOC	loss of consciousness	Pap	Papanicolaou
LP	lumbar puncture	PaO_2	partial pressure of O_2 in
LUQ	left upper quadrant		arterial blood
LV	left ventricle	PAYE	pay as you earn
LVF	left ventricular failure	PBC	primary biliary cirrhosis
LVH	left ventricular hypertrophy	pc	*post cibum* (after food)

PCA	patient controlled analgesia	RUQ	right upper quadrant
PCP	*Pneumocystis carinii* pneumonia	RV	right ventricle
		RVF	right ventricular failure
PCR	polymerase chain reaction	RVH	right ventricular hypertrophy
PCV	packed cell volume		
PDA	personal digital assistant	Rx	treat with
PE	pulmonary embolism	SAH	subarachnoid haemorrhage
PEFR	peak expiratory flow rate	SBE	subacute bacterial endocarditis
PID	pelvic inflammatory disease		
PIP	proximal interphalangeal	SC	
PM	*post mortem*	(sub cut)	subcutaneous
PMH	past medical history	SD	standard deviation
PMT	premenstrual tension	SE	side effects
PN	percussion note	SHO	Senior House Officer
PND	paroxysmal nocturnal dyspnoea	SIADH	syndrome of inappropriate ADH secretion
PO	*per orum* (by mouth)	SL	sublingual
PPD	purified protein derivative	SLE	systemic lupus erythematosus
PPF	purified plasma fraction		
PR	*per rectum*	SOA	swelling of ankles
PRN	*pro re nata* (as required)	SOB	shortness of breath
pro tem	as required, on an ongoing basis	SpR	specialist registrar
		SR	slow release
PRV	polycythaemia rubra vera	SRN	state registered nurse
PSA	prostate specific antigen	SSRV	structured small round virus
PTC	percutaneous transhepatic cholangiography	stat	*statim* (immediately)
		STD/STI	sexually transmitted disease/infection
PTH	parathyroid hormone		
PTT	prothrombin time	SVC	superior vena cava
PU	peptic ulcer(ation)	SVT	supraventricular tachycardia
PV	*per vaginum*		
qds	*quarte in die somemdum* (to be taken four times a day)	SXR	skull X-ray
		T	temperature
qid	*quarte in die* (four times a day)	$T_{1/2}$	biological half life
		T3	triiodothyronine
R	right	T4	thyroxine (tetraiodothyronine)
RA	rheumatoid arthritis		
RBBB	right bundle branch block	TB	tuberculosis
RBC	red blood cell	tds	*ter die somemdum* (to be taken three times a day)
RCC	red cell count		
RF	rheumatic fever		
Rh	rhesus	TENS	transcutaneous electrical nerve stimulation
RIF	right iliac fossa		
RS	respiratory system	TG	triglyceride
RTA	renal tubular acidosis/road traffic accident	TIA	transient ischaemic attack
		TIBC	total iron binding capacity

tid	*ter in die* (three times a day)	UMN	upper motor neurone
TLC	tender loving care	URT	upper respiratory tract
TOP	termination of pregnancy	US	ultrasound
tPA	tissue plasminogen activator	UTI	urinary tract infection
TPN	total parenteral nutrition	VDRL	venereal diseases research laboratory
TPR	temperature, pulse and respiratory rate	VF	ventricular fibrillation
TRH	thyrotrophin releasing hormone	VLDL	very low density lipoprotein
TSH	thyroid stimulating hormone	VMA (also HMMA)	vanillyl-mandelic acid
TTA	to take away	VQ scan	ventilation perfusion scan
TTO	to take out	VSD	ventriculo-septal defect
TU	tuberculin units	VT	ventricular tachycardia
TURP	transurethral retrograde prostatectomy	WBC	white blood cell
		WCC	white cell count
TURT	transurethral retrograde tumourectomy	WPW	Wolff–Parkinson–White syndrome
u (U)	units	ZN	Ziehl–Nielsen stain
U&E	urea and electrolytes	Zn	zinc
UC	ulcerative colitis		

Chapter 1
STARTING UP

Day one of your first job is rarely the nightmare you think it will be. Half of it is taken up by firm meetings and introductions to the hospital. During the other half you will be introduced to the wards. It's all over before you know what's happening. You are finally a real doctor. And then it's day two and you have to get on with the job…

Panic?

Never panic. The thing that strikes terror into the hearts of day-one junior doctors is the thought that they, alone, are expected to battle with disease and death when they have never given an IV drug in their life and don't know how to plug in the paddles of the cardiac arrest trolley. That's if they know where to find it. The ward and hospital are often unfamiliar. The whole thing is enough to give you a nasty rash, which many junior doctors do get.

The one thing to remember is: YOU ARE NOT ALONE. You are a modest, essential cog in a vast machine which churns away quite happily whether you know exactly what you're doing or not. You soon will. Nobody expects you to know much on the first day – or even in the first month. And everyone will show you what to do.

People to help you

You are surrounded by people who can help you. All you need to do is to ask them. They include:

1 Nurses who often know more about what you are doing than you do, as they have watched and done it for years.

2 Patients who want to be treated kindly, properly and with as little pain as possible.

3 Other doctors who love to demonstrate their skill at just about everything and are always open to requests for help.

• Problems arise when junior doctors do NOT ask for help. If you feel panic rising in your throat, just ask for help. This is counter-intuitive for self-reliant medics, but it saves lives (yours and the patient's).

• Attend orientation day for junior doctors if the hospital has one. It is useful for finding out what the hospital can do for you. They can be painful and bureaucratic at times but there are often sources of important information.

• If possible contact your predecessors before their last day on the job. They can give you invaluable information about what to expect from your new job (the idea for this book originally came from a request for help from a new junior doctor). In particular, ask them about what your new consultants do and do not like and how to access the computer systems.

• Most people find that they are physically exhausted during their first week of work. Such fatigue passes as you get used to the hospital and new routines.

The Hands-on Guide for Junior Doctors, Fourth Edition. Anna Donald, Michael Stein and Ciaran Scott Hill.
© 2011 Anna Donald, Michael Stein and Ciaran Scott Hill. Published 2011 by Blackwell Publishing Ltd.

Three basic tips

1 Always take the initiative in hospitals. If things are not working, do something about it. Big institutions can become bad places to work in just because no one bothers to address things that are clearly going wrong. Figure out a solution and contact whoever is in charge of the problem, whether it be a doctor, nurse, manager or the porter.

2 Similarly, take initiative in managing patients. Present seniors with a plan for your patients rather than just asking them what to do. Don't be afraid to look beyond what is asked of you. If you feel that a patient has a problem that your team is not interested in then don't just ignore it, take the initiative. Thinking strategically actually makes work more fun and prepares you for more responsibility.

3 Order your work. When tasks are being fired at you from all directions, priority-setting is really important. Try to learn early on which things are super-urgent and which can wait for more peaceful moments. Despite the hype, there is quite a lot of down time in your junior doctor year (unless you are very unlucky or disorganized!).

Other useful start-up information

Dress

It is worth bearing in mind that patients often dress up to the nines to 'visit the doctor'. I once watched an elderly woman with deteriorating eyesight, high-heeled shoes and lopsided make-up hobble over the hospital lawn to visit the diabetes clinic. Having always dressed casually, I dressed my best from then on.

■ Changing from student to doctor mode can put grave dents into your early pay cheques. If nothing else, buy good-quality shoes which will look good and will stay comfortable on your 36th hour.

■ You may get stained with all sorts of unmentionable substances as a junior doctor. *Stain Devils* from supermarkets and household stores can remove most things. Soaking garments in cold water and lots of soap, followed by a normal machine wash removes blood stains.

■ A few hospitals will reimburse you for dry cleaning bills associated with work-related accidents, such as major blood stains on suits. Phone hospital personnel through the switchboard.

■ While wearing theatre scrubs ('blues') on the wards can be all the rage, doing so is an infection risk and frowned on by some hospitals. If you have to wear them outside theatre, remember to change regularly and return them to the hospital laundry to be washed! Wearing them outside hospital grounds is definitely not acceptable.

Equipment

Always carry:

1 Pen (more than one). Black is the only acceptable colour unless you are a pharmacist.

2 Notebook/PDA/piece of paper.

3 Stethoscope.

4 Tourniquet (if you are happy with the hospital's disposable ones this may not be necessary).

5 Torch.

6 Pager/bleep.

7 Cash for food/drink/newspaper.

8 Ophthalmoscope (if not readily accessible on wards) or at least a torch for papillary reactions and looking in mouths.

9 You should also have access to a neurology kit (tendon hammer, orange sticks, neuropins, tuning fork and Snellen's eye chart).

• You may wish to carry everything in a traveller's pouch or a small shoulder bag.

• Things often get misplaced so you should label anything you cannot afford to loose with your name, either by engraving or hospital wrist bands.

• Junior doctors definitely need access to ophthalmoscopes. Ward ophthalmoscopes have an amazing tendency to walk and to run out of batteries. Therefore, buy your own portable ophthalmoscope, and examine people's eyes at every opportunity. It is a great skill to have but takes time to acquire. Pocket veterinary ophthalmoscopes are sometimes the most portable, cheap and reliable, and little known to medics – as they are advertised for vets.

• Ask your ward pharmacist for a couple of aliquots of tropicamide (0.5%) to carry in your top pocket. One to two drops greatly facilitates ophthalmic examination. It takes a few minutes to work. Warn the patient they may have blurred vision and sensitivity to light for a few hours, record the procedure in the notes and tell the nurse. Having failed to do the latter, you are liable to be fast bleeped by a nurse who thinks the patient is coning. It is sensible to dilate both eyes, not only to avoid mistaken neurology but also to allow you to view and compare the fundi. Never use tropicamide in patients with a history of glaucoma or eye surgery. You should also avoid alternatives like cyclopentolate as these can take weeks for the eye to return to normal.

• Consider carrying a ring binder (see Chapter 2) containing important team info, a handful of blood forms; radiology requests; blank drug charts; and history,

discharge summary and TTO sheets. Such a binder allows you to do a lot of the paperwork on ward rounds, before it gets forgotten. It also saves having to dash off to the stationery drawers in the middle, which tends to go down badly with seniors.

First-day paperwork

The first day is mainly paperwork. Here is a checklist of documents to bring:

■ GMC registration certificate
■ Medical indemnity certificate (e.g. Medical Defense Union or Medical Protection Society)
■ Bank details
■ Induction pack and contract from the Trust
■ Occupational health report (and data card if you have one)

Geography

■ Get a map of the hospital from reception to help you learn where everything is.
■ Specifically, find out the location of: blood gas machines, canteen, casualty, wards, radiology department, doctors' mess, drink machines, endoscopy, labs for crucial bloods, nuclear medicine and on-call rooms.

Ward rounds

Think of yourself as the ward round producer (much of it *is* performance). Give yourself at least 15 minutes' preparation time to have everything ready. For each patient, be prepared to supply at the drop of a hat:

1 Patient ID (name, age, date of admission, occupation, presenting complaint).

2 Changes in condition and management since last round (with dates of change).

3 Results (any investigations carried out recently).

4 Assessment (physical, social, psychological).

5 Plan for in-patient management (future investigations, ops, drugs).

6 Plan for discharge (see Discharging patients, below).

It is helpful to print off a list of patients to give to consultants and the senior registrar, which includes 1, 2, 3 and 5 of the above.

■ Unless the patient asks for relatives to remain present, it is generally a good idea to ask them to leave the room while the team examines the patient. Curtains are not sound proof. People will often give more information if their relatives are absent.

■ Ask your registrar which investigations to have available. If your hospital uses an electronic reporting system such as PACS (patient archiving and communications system) then you may wish to access the important scans before the ward round so that your seniors can look at them without too much disruption.

■ Each consultant has up to five pet details that he or she wants to know about each patient. Find out what these are from your predecessor and supply them tirelessly at ward rounds (these could range from occupation to ESR to whether or not the patient has ever travelled to the tropics).

■ Never say that you have done something you haven't, and never make up a result to please seniors. It is bound to backfire. If you realize you have given a piece of information that is wrong, admit it sooner rather than later.

■ Do not argue with colleagues (or anyone else) in front of patients.

■ Get a clear idea of the management plan for each patient. Sometimes instruc-tions may be dealt out in a half-hearted way, only for you to learn later (to your cost) that they were meant in earnest. Do not allow seniors to get away with this. Make definite 'action points' and if your consultant cannot be pressed into being clear, then ask your registrar.

■ If you work with a partner, such as a fellow junior doctor, make sure that jobs arising from the round are clearly allo-cated. Meet up later for a 'paper round' to check important results, prioritize jobs and make sure that everyone is clear about what remain outstanding.

Social rounds

You need to let the social team know how your patient is going to cope (or not) on discharge.

1 Ask yourself: how is this patient going to manage physically, socially and men-tally? Specifically, draw up a list of 'dis-abilities'. These are things that the patient *cannot do*, for whatever reason. From the Barthel Activities Index (Appendix, Barthel score), consider bathing, blad-der, bowels, dressing, feeding, groom-ing, mobility, stairs, toilet, transfer.

2 Have relevant patient details ready (see below). Most are available from the medi-cal notes and the front-page admissions sheet. Otherwise try the nurses, nursing notes, the patient, relatives and the GP.

3 If you are required to give a history, try to include the following points:

● Patient ID.

● Prognosis: short and long term.

● GP and admitting rights to local hospi-tals (usually in the admission sheet at the front of the notes and dependent on home address).

● Type of residence and limitations (e.g. stairs).

- Home support and previous reliance on social services.
- Financial status.
- Special problems which need to be addressed (physical, social, mental, legal).
- Questions you want to ask members of the multidisciplinary team to help you plan for discharge of the patient.

4 Go to the meeting with specific questions you want answered. Make sure you come away with 'action points' – not just vague gestures from various team members about your patient's care (this goes for all ward rounds).

5 Translate medical jargon into normal English for social rounds, as some members of the social team may not be fully fluent in medical acronyms.

6 Familiarize yourself with key people from local rehabilitation services, residential homes, nursing homes and alcohol support services. Effective liaison can prevent or at least curtail hospital admission.

Night rounds

As a junior doctor your experience of night shifts may be limited. However, it is important to do a quick night round before you leave for home. If you are covering overnight this can mean the difference between a relatively happy night and a sleepless nightmare. Even if you are not on overnight you still have a responsibility to leave your patients well tended to for the night shift. This will take the stress of the night cover (which will one day be you) and protect your patients from being neglected while you are away. If you do nothing else, make sure you have checked off the following before going to bed:

1 Analgesia.

2 Fluids.

3 Infusions (on the few occasions where you are required to make them up, leave them in the fridge and tell the nurses where they are).

4 Sedation.

5 Sign for drugs you have verballed during the evening (Chapter 9, Verbals).

6 Ask each team nurse on the night shift if he or she has problems that need sorting out before the morning.

- If possible start your night round *after* the night nurses' start of shift and drug rounds have been completed. This is when they identify problems that you need to deal with before going to bed.
- If you are the covering doctor then tell night staff to bleep you if they are concerned about a patient. Paradoxically, this combined with reassurance and information about worrisome patients cuts down bleeps.
- Inform every team nurse of what to do if a sick patient's condition changes. Sometimes you can set limits for relevant signs (e.g. pulse, CVP, T, BP) beyond which you want a doctor to be called. Write these in the notes. Many hospitals have 'early warning systems' that do this job for you and tell nurses when they should contact a doctor or nurse specialist.
- If bleeped for an apparently trivial matter overnight, try your best not to sound irritated. Be ready to go to the ward, even if only to provide reassurance. Again, paradoxically, this reduces bleeps. If nurses are confident that you will turn up if requested, they will not bleep you ahead of time.
- If the on-call room is a long way from the wards, there may be somewhere that you can sleep on the ward. Ask the sister or charge nurse. Be very careful though as some trust have taken disciplinary action against doctors sleeping in side rooms at night.

Discharging patients

Clearing hospital beds is an invaluable skill that will earn you lots of brownie points from virtually everyone. To clear beds effectively:

1 Make plans for people's discharge on the day they arrive. Ask yourself:

- When will they be likely to leave?
- What will get in the way of this person going home or being transferred?
- What can be followed up in clinic?

2 If possible, write discharge summaries (Chapter 3, Discharge summaries (TTO/ TTA)), sending the TTO (drug prescriptions) to the pharmacists early in the day to avoid delays. Beware of last minute changes to medications if you do this, errors can and do occur.

Work environment

Evidence suggests that upgrading your environment upgrades your work – and you. Old, decrepit NHS hospitals can be depressing. There are ways you can make your particular corner of it a great place to work, even if the rest of the hospital has miles of yellow peeling paint, dripping pipes and corridors of empty wards.

■ There is no crime in asking hospital supplies for better furniture and accessories, like shelving, desk, chairs or bulletin boards. They can always say no.

■ You could take a plant to work.

■ If you have a tiny desk (or no desk), order a better one. Ring hospital supplies and ask if there is a spare one somewhere. Or request a new one. There's nothing like drawers that slide open easily for making paperwork easy. As a doctor with tons of notes to write, you are entitled to a desk of some kind.

■ Consider buying a personal music player. Label it clearly and lock it away. It can do wonders for long winter weekends and nights on call.

■ Put postcards/pictures/photos up in your work area. If you don't have a bulletin board, order one from hospital supplies. Again, some managers frown on this but if it's in an area to which patients do not have access, like the doctor's room, then you should be fine.

■ Most hospitals provide a computer in the doctor's room. Make sure you get as much internet access as local policy allows. Carry a portable USB hard drive. It will allow you to carry your work with you.

■ Bring decent coffee or cocoa supplies to work. A single-cup cafetière, some packs of coffee at the back of the ward fridge and a jar of your favourite spread can upgrade your existence no end.

■ Be nice to your team, bring them biscuits and buy them coffee and they'll do the same for you. Work must be enjoyable and if the people around you are happy then you will be too.

Bibliography

Most junior doctors read little other than fiction during their job. You probably don't need to buy anything you don't already have. A few recommended texts and online resources are:

■ *Pocket Prescriber:* Nicholson T., Gunarathne A., Singer D. (2009) Hodder Arnold, London. A brilliant and truly portable little text, useful for checking those common drugs on a ward round.

■ *Acute Medicine*: Sprigings D., Chambers J. (2007) Wiley Blackwell, Oxford. A comprehensive guide to emergencies.

■ *Pocket Examiner*: Hill C.S. (2009) Wiley Blackwell, London. A pocket-text of clinical examinations.

■ *Oxford Handbook of Clinical Medicine*: Hope R.A. (Editor), Longmore J.M., Wilkinson I., Turmezei T., Cheung C.K. (2007) Oxford University Press, Oxford. A great pocket reference text for medical conditions.

■ *Surgical Talk:* Goldberg A., Stansby G. (2005) Imperial College Press, London. Commonly asked topics for those awkward theatre moments.

■ *The ECG Made Easy* (and sequel, *The ECG in Practice*): Hampton J. (2008) Churchill Livingstone, Edinburgh. An approachable guide to the mysteries of the ECG.

■ *Clinical Medicine:* Kumar P., Clark M. (2009) Saunders, London. Love it or hate it, it probably answers most of the medical questions you could ever ask.

■ *Rapid Medicine*, Sam A.H. et al. (2010) and *Rapid Surgery*, Baker C. et al. (2010) Wiley Blackwell, Oxford. Both are memory joggers for core facts.

■ *Junior Doctors' Handbook*: Published annually by the BMA, free to members. An excellent summary of your rights and useful information for your early years as a doctor.

■ Map of Medicine: A set of 300 flowcharts covering the community and specialist aspects of the 300 'top' conditions. An excellent and interactive quick reference. It is free to NHS professionals in England and Wales; you need an Athens password for the professional version (www.mapofmedicine.com). The read-only version is available through NHS Choices.

Recommended texts for the medical specialties (SHO level texts) include:

■ *Lecture Notes: Respiratory Medicine*: Bourke S. (2007) Wiley Blackwell, Oxford. Beautiful explanations of the pathophysiology and principles of management of respiratory disease. A very good primer for a Chest Unit job.

■ *The Little Black Book of Neurology*: Zaidat O., Lerner A. (2008) Saunders, New York. A concise but very detailed guide to clinical neurology.

■ *Essential Haematology*: Hoffbrand A., Pettit J., Moss P. (updated every reprint; the most recent edition, 2011) Wiley Blackwell, Oxford. A superb book!

■ *Essential Endocrinology and Diabetes*: Holt R., Hanley N. (2006) Wiley Blackwell, Oxford. Another very useful primer for an Endocrine job.

We haven't found any particularly good small books for rheumatology or nephrology so we recommend using the appropriate chapter in any medical textbook such as Kumar and Clark.

For fun and rapid insight into the world you are entering, try the classic: *House of God*, Sham S. (1978).

Chapter 2
GETTING ORGANIZED
OR 'THE FOLDER'

Keeping track of patients and their details can be the bane of your life as a junior doctor. Filling in forms after work is a waste of precious evenings. Fortunately, you can greatly reduce the time you spend chasing paper, patients and results with the core weapon in a junior doctor's arsenal: a folder.

Personal folder and the lists

A well-organized ring-binder folder can save days of time. Unlike a Filofax or PDA, a folder provides a decent writing surface at the bedside and an immediate supply of forms during ward rounds, so that you can do all the paperwork during rounds and don't have to return to the ward later. As well as saving time, a folder means you are less likely to forget things, because you can do many tasks as soon as they are requested. Although they look great and are very powerful, iPads and the like still weigh a lot more than a paper folder and don't synchronize (yet) with hospital electronic medical record systems.

How to make a personal folder

You need one A4 ring-binder folder and brightly coloured dividers. Also consider getting sheets of pre-punched transparent plastic pockets. Fill the folder with all the different forms you use during the day, stacking each type of form behind different dividers. Label the dividers. Stuff blank forms (e.g. blood forms) into the plastic pockets. Useful forms include: blood cards (biochemistry, haematology, bacteriology and cross match), radiology and nuclear medicine request cards, drug charts and fluid charts, spare continuation/history sheets, discharge forms (if these are still paper in your hospital), commonly used telephone numbers, a firm timetable and any foundation assessment forms.

1 You can almost always find a hole-puncher at the ward clerk's desk.

2 Consider sticking common drug regimens to the front of the folder for easy reference. These might include heparin dosing, insulin sliding scales, GTN and morphine infusions, gentamycin dosing and other frequently used antibiotic regimens. Common antibiotic regimens and doses.

3 Hospitals have their own days for doing specialty procedures (such as isotope scans and endoscopy). Colleagues and relevant departments will know what these are. Get a copy of your team's timetable. Find out from your colleagues

The Hands-on Guide for Junior Doctors, Fourth Edition. Anna Donald, Michael Stein and Ciaran Scott Hill.
© 2011 Anna Donald, Michael Stein and Ciaran Scott Hill. Published 2011 by Blackwell Publishing Ltd.

Name	Extension
Accident & Emergency	
Anaesthetist on-call bleep	
Bed manager	
Biochemistry	
Blood transfusion	
Cardiology on-call bleep	
Coronary care unit	
Discharge coordinator	
Doctors' mess	
ECG	
Echocardiogram	
Endoscopy	
Eye clinic	
Food – local takeaway	
Haematology	
Histology	
Intensive therapy unit	
IT department	
Matron	
Medical records	
Medical staffing	

Name	Extension
Microbiology	
Occupational therapy	
Outpatient clinics	
Pain team	
Pharmacy – general	
Pharmacy – drug info	
Physiotherapy	
Porters	
Psychiatry team	
Radiology – CT scanning	
Radiology – general	
Radiology – portable films	
Radiology – secretaries	
Registrar bleeps (your dept.)	
Secretaries (your dept.)	
SHO bleeps (your dept.)	
Surrounding hosp. quickdial	
Theatre list coordinator	
Thrombolysis nurse bleep	
Ward extensions	

Fig. 2.1 Essential telephone numbers.

what you need to bring for team activities such as radiology conferences, academic events and mortality/morbidity meetings.

4 Phone numbers are essential. Making a list early saves a lot of time. You can shrink the list and stick it on the front of your ward folder for easy reference. Another option is to include it in a small font on the bottom of your patient list so it is reprinted each day. Get out-of-hours contact numbers as well. From experience, it is easier to find names if the list is strictly alphabetical. Copy or modify Fig. 2.1 if you like.

In addition to the sundry paperwork above, you will also need to generate three lists daily. These need not be in physical paper form; it can be a digital copy in a PDA or USB memory stick, but a physical one is always handy. Spreadsheets are actually better than word-processors for organizing lists, as they have all kinds of sorting functions. The necessary lists are:

1 The patient list (i.e. the master list)

2 The job list

3 Results sheet

Some doctors combine the three but it is often useful to have a paper copy of each.

Keeping track of patients (List 1)

This is a hassle. People have devised many complex strategies for ensuring that they have up-to-date details for each patient. However you do it, you need information in hand so that you can answer questions on ward rounds; discuss patients over the phone with GPs, nurses and colleagues; write in the notes and do the discharge summary; and request and find results of investigations. The minimum information for this includes:

■ Patient name and hospital number
■ Reason for admission and major details from PMH
■ Main problems now
■ Mainstay of management (e.g. drugs, surgery)
■ Recent results

One way of keeping track of such information is to stick patient labels onto history sheets, leaving a space between each to fill in patient details. Put a line through patients who have been discharged. The labels contain patient IDs. A sheet like this can be made up as patients are admitted in casualty, and stored at the front of a personal folder.

List of things to do (List 2)

The simplest ways to keep track of many tasks are to:

1 Keep a daily list on the back of a card that you can update regularly.

2 Keep a small diary to note down requests for days and weeks ahead (this can be done electronically if you have access to a shared file).

• Write down all requests as soon as you receive them.

X-ray	Give in forms from ward round
	Ask Dr A about Mr B's CT request barium enema for Mr C
Ward 6A	IV line for Mrs D
	Talk to Mr E for colonoscopy
Ward 7B	Vitamin K for Ms F
	Sign verbal for paracetamol

• Try subdividing tasks in terms of *where* they have to be done. This enables you to choreograph your movements around the hospital rather than endlessly dashing from one ward to another. For example:

• Use a checkbox system so you know what things have been done. One system is to tick the box once the task is initiated (i.e. form handed in, referral made, blood test taken) and then convert it into a cross when the result of that is back (an alternative is to colour half a square then complete it).

Results sheet (List 3)

Most hospital systems are able to print off all results from blood or urine tests for the day for a particular consultant, department or ward. Print off one at the beginning (and end) of the day, glance through them to check for any glaring abnormalities and carry it about for the occasion when your registrar asks about the patient's eosinophil count. If the IT fails (as it often will) or you work in a security conscious hospital you may not be able to do this, so just record the results (e.g. from phone calls, lab computers) onto blank labels and you can just peel them off to stick them into patient notes without having to laboriously copy them out. You may still need to record the important results into a table in the notes to chart progress. As a starting point, it is recommended to make sure you note haemoglobin, white count, creatinine, urea, sodium, potassium and c-reactive protein. Certain firms will require different results, for example, a liver job will obviously require transaminases, alkaline phosphatase, bilirubin and clotting on most patients. Those patients on warfarin should always have INR noted. Don't forget to check the date the blood was sent for each of the patients and check the trends. Writing results in notes is important for patients staying longer than a few days or who have stepped down from intensive care

but you don't need to break your back doing it for every single patient.

Data protection and confidentiality

Beware of leaving your folder or any list or USB memory stick lying about. Always carry it in your pocket or in a shoulder satchel. If needing to use your hands to examine a patient or to perform a procedure, make sure you put your folder/list where you won't forget it and where a casual bystander will not be able to just glance at it. Pick up any such lists that your seniors or colleagues are apt to leave about. After you are done with the lists, it is good practice to keep them about for a few weeks before destroying them in a shredder. You may wish to have your teams name and bleep number automatically noted on the top of all lists.

Chapter 3
PAPERWORK AND ELECTRONIC MEDICAL RECORDS

Paperwork or data entry into an electronic medical record (EMR) is not difficult – just boring. As doctors communicate with many people through forms and notes, it is important that they contain clear information. The most important part of paperwork is writing clear, legible patient notes. And the most important part of using an EMR is accurately typing information – the electronic forms are typically the same as the paper ones but may include 'pick' lists. The following refers to paper records but most of it is applicable to EMRs.

Patient notes

Doctors are expected to write in patients' notes at the very least once every 72 hours. However, it is good practice to write something daily and waiting 2 days to fill in notes is unlikely to endear you to the powers that be.

1 Always sign notes and print your surname clearly with your level and bleep number. Some hospitals provide stamps for this purpose.

2 It is useful to ask two things when writing patient notes:

- Do the notes give enough information to treat the patient when I'm not available?
- Will I be legally covered if these notes were ever before a court?

3 For daily notes, there are various standardized ways (so that you don't miss anything) but the most popular is SOAP.

4 Often, the most crucial aspect of any entry in the patient's notes is the Plan. It has to be clear whether something written in the notes has been arranged. With shift systems in place and plenty of handovers, it is often difficult for someone reading the notes to tell what is already in motion and it can be exasperating to discover 5 days down the line that the echocardiogram had never been requested. For decisions which may have to be made in your absence, it is essential to document clearly a decision tree, for example, 'If systolic BP drops below 100 mmHg, stop GTN infusion'.

5 If you're not sure about how to document a patient's condition, flick back through previous notes and see how others approached it.

6 It is helpful for subsequent readers if you include the time, date and place (e.g. casualty) in the margin of notes. Also, if you are documenting a ward round, it is useful to note the surname and designation of the person leading the round.

The Hands-on Guide for Junior Doctors, Fourth Edition. Anna Donald, Michael Stein and Ciaran Scott Hill.
© 2011 Anna Donald, Michael Stein and Ciaran Scott Hill. Published 2011 by Blackwell Publishing Ltd.

SOAP

Subjective data (e.g. history and examination)
Objective data (e.g. blood results, imaging)
Assessment (e.g. active and inactive problems)
Plan for future

7 If you are called to see a patient, briefly document (even if the call was trivial):

- That you saw the patient.
- The time and date.

8 It is foolhardy to write anything in the notes that you would not want the patient or relatives to read; they have legal access to the notes.

9 It is perfectly admissible to write 'no change' or words to that effect if nothing much has happened to the patient but be careful that there hasn't been an important change you have missed. Writing 'Patient well, continue' doesn't look good if they've actually been spiking temperatures or have deteriorating renal function!

10 Don't forget to document the social or psychological aspects (e.g. whether the patient is cheerful, sad or fed up).

Accident forms

When called to see a patient who has had an accident (e.g. fell out of bed):

1 See the patient as soon as possible. Nurses are legally liable unless they make sure you see the patient. Never be short with a nurse who is making a reasonable request even if you are very busy. It is their job and if they push you to see their patient they are probably doing it well.

2 Ask the patient what happened and which part hurts the most. After a quick 'ABC' emergency assessment check the following:

- Temp, BP, pulse and respiratory rate.
- Consciousness level (see Appendix, Glasgow Coma Scale (GCS)).
- Skin for bruising, bleeding, cuts and fractures.
- Bone tenderness and shape for fractures. Frail patients can sustain fractures with remarkably little fuss. Especially look for hip, wrist and scaphoid fractures. Examine the skull carefully if the patient hits his or her head. Consult with your senior if there is sign of serious injury or drowsiness – the patient may well need a CT head scan (see Chapter 14, Skull X-rays; CT head – some emergency indications).

3 Sign an accident form (the nurses will give you one). Filling it in is self-explanatory.

4 Also write in patient's notes. Include:

- Time and date
- Brief history of accident
- Brief examination findings
- A plan including a note that you be contacted if the patients vital signs deteriorate or there is concern
- That you signed an accident form

5 Ask the nurses to continue observations at regular intervals.

6 Think about how the accident occurred. If possible, make a plan with the nurses to prevent future accidents. There may be a falls assessment sheet that needs to be filled in. Consider referral to other teams as necessary, for example, a hospital falls team.

7 Consider carrying a couple of accident forms in a personal folder (see Chapter 2, Personal folder and the lists); it saves time in the middle of the night.

Table 3.1 Conditions for which it may be possible to fill out serial forms.

MI:	
On admission	
Days 1–3	Lipids (only worth doing within 12 hours of infarct; unreliable post-MI for 3 months)
	Serial cardiac enzymes
	Serial ECGs
Warfarin initiation	Check the INR at least:
	Every day for 1 week
	Every week for 3 weeks
	Every month for 3 months
	Every 8 weeks after that
Renal failure:	
Daily	Urea, creatinine and electrolytes
TPN:	
Daily	Creatinine and electrolytes
Mon, Wed, Fri	LFT, calcium, phosphate, alkaline phosphatase
Weekly	Magnesium, zinc, FBC, urea
IV fluids	Daily urea, creatinine and electrolytes
Post-op bloods:	
Next day	Urea, creatinine, electrolytes and FBC

Blood forms and requesting bloods

■ Ask haematologists and biochemists which details on blood cards are essential. Often there are spaces on the card for information that isn't needed.

■ Write your bleep and ward number clearly on blood cards so the labs can contact you if necessary.

■ Two good times to fill in forms are during the daily ward round and when writing in patients' notes. Having forms ready saves time.

■ Where possible, anticipate patients' blood needs and write forms in bulk. For example, if someone has had a suspected MI, you can write out a stack of cardiac enzyme forms on admission, or on the ward round the next day, for 3 days. Conditions for which it is sometimes possible to fill in serial forms include those shown in Table 3.1.

■ Try having a separate plastic bag or a hook or paper clamp for each day of the week in the doctors' office. You can write serial forms at the start of the week and see at a glance who needs what. Alternatively you can stack forms chronologically on a clipboard.

■ One way of keeping track of patients' tests is to write 'FBC' and date under the patient's label in your patient list (Patient notes, above).

■ If you don't have a phlebotomist, don't despair. Taking bloods in the morning enables you to sort out patients' problems before the ward round and enables you to say good morning to patients on a one-on-one basis. Make sure you take round a trolley like the phlebotomists do. This has remarkable effects on one's efficacy.

Consent

(see Chapter 15, Consent)

Death and cremation certificates

(see Chapter 8, Death certificates; Cremation forms and fees)

Discharge summaries (TTO/TTA)

(also see Chapter 1, Discharging patients and Chapter 5, Information about patient discharge)

The discharge summary or 'TTO' or 'TTA' (To Take Out or Away) is a sheet that junior doctors write for patients to take to their GPs. It enables GPs to continue with outpatient care until the more detailed discharge letter arrives (if indeed one is sent from your unit, this was traditionally the job of the consultant or a senior doctor but sometimes these are not sent). The TTO is also the prescription form that the nurses use to order drugs for patients to take home with them (although some hospitals provide a separate form for this function). Many units now have electronic TTAs that incorporate the medications with space for a freehand discharge letter.

1 Get the GP's name and address from the patient or the front page of the notes.

2 Complete the TTO before the patient leaves! Occasionally you may arrive on a Monday morning to find uncompleted TTAs waiting for you, but avoid this as far as possible. Include:

• Patient details
• Name of consultant
• Name of ward
• Diagnosis
• Important results (positive and negative)
• Treatment given
• Treatment on discharge
• Follow-up arrangements
• What the patient has been told
• Your name and bleep number

3 Patients are often delayed in hospital because TTOs have not been written. Write them as soon as possible so that drugs can be fetched from the pharmacy. Patients and nurses will love you for this. You can prepare TTAs in advance but DO NOT sign them off until the day the patient is actually leaving. It goes without saying that prepared TTAs will need a final check for any recent changes.

4 If you have a paper system you can carry a bunch of TTOs on ward rounds so that you can write them on the spot when the decision is made to send someone home. This means that you can check any discharge details with the team, and the form can be sent to the pharmacy straight away. If you are on an electronic system and a decision is made to send a patient home on the ward round do a quick mental check to make sure there are no outstanding issues you are unsure about like follow-up time or anticoagulant plans.

5 Phone the GP on discharge if the patient:

• Self-discharges
• Is in an unstable condition
• Has complex home circumstances

- Dies
- Needs an early visit

6 Consider phoning the GP if you are discharging a patient with particularly complex or sensitive care needs, such as elderly people living alone or terminally ill patients. They will appreciate it and your patient will receive better care.

Drug charts

(see Chapter 9, Drug charts)

Drug prescriptions

(see Chapter 9, Writing prescriptions)

Handovers

Before you go home, to bed or away for the weekend you will need to 'hand over' your patients to the doctor who replaces you. It need not be a formal handover, but it is recommended that it be more detailed than just 'There's a Mrs Smith on Ward 4 to be seen. See you in the morning'. Obviously how much detail you tell your successor depends on whether or not they are familiar with the patients – bear in mind that they may not know them at all. In these changing times of the European Working Time Directive, handover is becoming ever more frequent and important. You need to make sure your successors know:

1 Who your patients are, which ward they are on and why they are in hospital.

2 A brief summary of the management of each patient (e.g. awaiting surgery tomorrow, NBM, needs continuous morphine infusion for pain relief but stable). Also, list out the jobs which have been done and those which haven't.

3 Likely complications or difficulties and how you have been dealing with these to date.

4 Anyone (doctor/nurse/relatives) who may be contacted if problems arise.

5 If you are handing over to a locum who is new to the hospital, you will help him or her enormously by spending a few minutes sharing key information about the layout of the hospital and how to perform routine tasks (see Chapter 17, Locums).

Referral letters

If you need to refer a patient to another team, you can phone the registrar of that team and leave relevant details in the patient's notes (if they are not available then consultants are often surprisingly helpful so long as the request is reasonable). Alternatively you can write the consultant a letter. If you write a letter, include the following:

1 Address the letter to the consultant of the other team.

2 Name of your consultant, yourself and your bleep number.

3 Name of patient, age, sex, DOB, hospital ID and current location (e.g. ward/home).

4 Name of patient's GP.

5 Specific question(s) your team needs answered.

6 Relevant clinical history and examination findings.

7 Recent investigations (including negatives).

8 When you need his or her advice by (write this in a humble way!).

Try to anticipate which investigations the other team might need, and have them ready. For example, surgeons almost always need a recent FBC, clotting, group and save, and maybe an ECG and CXR if they are considering theatre. Gastro-enterologists, or any specialist doing a biopsy, will want an INR if investigating liver complaints. See Chapter 11, Specialist referrals and investigating the medical case for a list of investigations that different specialists are likely to need.

Self-discharge

However it may feel, hospitals are not prisons. Unless patients seem likely to incur life-threatening harm to themselves, you cannot restrain them from leaving hospital (even when it is patently idiotic for them to do so). If your patient decides to leave against your advice, try the following:

■ Explain to them why they should stay and the risks they are taking by leaving.
■ Inform your senior.
■ Have the patient sign a self-discharge note. This is usually available from the ward clerk. If necessary, you can write one yourself. It is a good idea to have a second witness to sign the note:

> I, (*Jo Bloggs*) hereby state that I am leaving (*Name of Hospital*) against medical advice on (*today's date*). Witnessed by Dr (*Your surname*, *today's date*) and (*Colleague's name*, *today's date*)
> (Jo Bloggs' signature)
> (Your name and signature)
> (Second witness name and signature)

■ Rarely, you may consider using the Mental Health Act to section a patient and restrain them from leaving. Always seek senior advice before doing this unless you are very familiar with this (Appendix, Mental Health Act).

■ Make a brief note of what happened in the patient's notes.
■ Inform the patient's GP that the patient has self-discharged.

Sick notes

You may be asked to write a sick note for patients to verify that they have been unable to work. There are two types of sick notes you can write:

1 If the patient is *not* trying to claim state benefit, they may request a handwritten note on hospital-headed paper. The easiest way to address it is 'To Whom It May Concern' along the top, followed by something like: 'Mrs A has been an inpatient at the X Hospital from 24–30 April and will be unable to return to work until 7 May.' Sign and date it, block print your name and position under your signature as well as the name of the patient's consultant. In this kind of letter, you should *not* disclose the diagnosis. If in doubt, ask your senior. Such forms are often supplied free from hospital juniors or at a substantial price by GPs!

2 If the patient *is* trying to claim state benefit after leaving hospital they can self-certify for the first 7 days of absence from work due to ill health. They can obtain the *SC2* form from their employer. Similarly, for the self or unemployed an *SC1* form can be obtained from the department of work and pensions. This means that you shouldn't have to write one for a patient unless they will clearly need an extended period of absence in which case you can normally find forms on the ward that require a signature. I would always check that the patient is happy for you to write any medical details on such a form before issuing it. Again, ask your senior if you have any doubts about it.

Chapter 4
ACCIDENT AND EMERGENCY

Working shifts in A&E can be a lot of fun, or it can result in the weekend from hell, working 'til you drop'. As usual, being organized and armed with a few hints makes a big difference to coping well.

General

During both medical and surgical takes you see the same handful of conditions most of the time (see below). Whatever your baseline knowledge, you soon become adept at treating them.

■ Do not be afraid to ask nurses for advice. They have generally seen it all before and they know the regulars.

■ You can spend a lot of time looking for equipment in casualty. Try preparing batches of forms and bottles when things are quiet. Suggested forms include (per patient): two history sheets, drug chart, fluid chart, X-ray form, blood cards, consent form.

■ Try equipping yourself with a metal trolley at the beginning of the shift. It helps to keep your equipment in one place and gives you a surface to work on.

■ Stick a yellow plastic bag to the edge of the trolley for rubbish; it saves trips to the garbage with packaging. A small yellow sharps bin is ideal if you can find one.

■ Tape two or three sheets of paper to your 'take' desk. Use these to note down accepted patients (a patient identification sticker is ideal), so as not to lose track of expected (and received) patients. These sheets can also be used to document tentative and confirmed diagnoses, the results of initial tests, and the ward to which the

patient is sent from casualty. You can then use the sheets to give a good handover or lead the post-take round.

■ Dehydration is a real problem if you work without a break in casualty (or anywhere else for that matter). Suggest to the medical or surgical hospital manager that a drinking water dispenser be installed in casualty. Drink as much fluid as you can!

■ Take meal breaks ruthlessly. Hold the fort for your colleagues and have them do the same for you. No one works efficiently with hypoglycaemia.

Admitting and allocating patients

1 Ask medical and nursing colleagues about the local routine for admitting and allocating patients during take.

2 When a GP telephones you to admit a patient:
● Be polite.
● Have paper and pen ready.
● Listen first.
● Take down the name, age, problem, hospital number, GP name and number and when to expect the patient's arrival.
● Phone casualty or the ward with the patient's details.
● Let your senior know that the patient is coming in and their main complaint.

The Hands-on Guide for Junior Doctors, Fourth Edition. Anna Donald, Michael Stein and Ciaran Scott Hill.
© 2011 Anna Donald, Michael Stein and Ciaran Scott Hill. Published 2011 by Blackwell Publishing Ltd.

3 If you accept a patient from a GP, then you are obliged to clerk them, even if it is obvious that they need to be transferred to another specialty. Try, therefore, to transfer the call to the right specialist *before* the patient arrives, or you will end up seeing the patient, however inappropriately.

4 You may bear the brunt of poor bed allocation. Consider negotiating with admissions, the managing sister or charge nurse ('bed manager') and clinical managers to work out a better system. It helps to know the wards' bed status when working in A&E, so you can send patients where you want them. In many hospitals nearly all patients will be shipped to an 'Acute or Medical Assessment Unit' from where they will be either discharged home or, if their stay is likely to be more than a few days, to a team elsewhere in the hospital.

Keeping track of patients

■ Try keeping a sheet of paper with patient stickers down one side with results of baseline tests and a thumbnail sketch of the patient next to each sticker. This is invaluable for post-take ward rounds.

■ If you are missing results, be conscientious in checking them before retiring. It is better to find out an unwelcome result late and when you are looking forward to going home rather than when you return the next day and something tragic has happened. Being uncompromising about this requires will power!

■ If you urgently need a result after midnight, you can usually get recent results by phoning the laboratory technician on call. Likewise, there is usually a duty biochemist or haematologist on call.

■ Whatever you do, get results for patients before you go to bed and make

sure you have them ready for the post-take ward round.

■ If results are not back before you go to bed, inform the next person taking over to just have a glance at the results when they are received. You should really document in the notes who is going to check the results when they arrive, or at the least that this job has been 'handed over'.

Medicine

On admission, complete for each medical patient:

1 A focused history and examination (finding the middle ground between an inadequately brief history and an extended essay takes experience).

2 Baseline tests:

● Bloods: FBC, U&E, glucose, ESR, CRP (consider clotting screen and LFT)
● Urine: MSU and dipstick
● ECG
● Radiology: CXR (consider erect CXR if suspected perforation)

3 IV access.

4 Fluid chart for 24 hours.

5 Drug chart.

The most common medical emergencies

1 Haematemesis (peptic ulcer or gastritis)

2 Acute coronary syndrome (including myocardial infarction and unstable angina)

3 Stroke (infarct or haemorrhagic)

4 DVT and PE

5 'Off legs' or collapse

6 Overdose

Overdose

Junior doctors in medicine see many patients who have overdosed. A&E get the slashed wrists and other forms of bodily mutilation, but you have to deal with people's gastric contents. Do not panic with overdose patients. There is usually more time than you realize to sort them out and the vast majority have not taken devastating overdoses. You can (and should) get senior medical and nursing assistance if the patient *is* in a critical condition. They may need transfer to ITU. Never wash out an uncooperative or unconscious patient without the supervision of an anaesthetist.

In general

■ If in **any** doubt about how to treat someone, phone the 24-hour National Poisons Information Service/Toxbase hotline (switchboard and A&E staff will have these numbers). Their staff will tell you exactly what to do, according to your patient's symptoms and history.

> **National Poisons Information Service**
>
> 0844 892 0111 (www.toxbase.org)

■ The *BNF* has an excellent section on treatments for different substance overdoses at the beginning of the book (look under 'Poison' in the index). We have not tried to replicate the *BNF* information here, as it is more detailed and up to date in the *BNF* itself.

Treating the patient

First, quickly assess the patient

1 If the patient is unconscious, perform basic airway management and seek senior help urgently. Make sure you have control of the airway and if the GCS is falling or <8, or the respiratory rate is low then consider early intubation. Check the airway for obstruction, dentures or vomit in any unresponsive patient.

2 If the patient is drowsy or unconscious, alert an anaesthetist to intubate the patient for a washout. Get senior advice. The patient may need to be transferred to ITU.

3 Quickly check for and treat hypoxia, hypotension and hypovolaemia (from vomiting), hypoglycaemia, hypothermia and arrhythmias. Ask the nurses to do a capillary blood glucose, ECG, BP and pulse oximeter reading, particularly if the patient is semi-conscious. Consider doing a blood gas and, if necessary, a rectal temperature.

4 Secure IV access. Consider immediate, rapid IV fluid if the patient is in shock.

5 Take the following samples from the patient:

- Biochemistry sample
- FBC (at least one)

Consider requesting storage – in case there is need to do further tests.

- Clotting screen and INR

Acute liver failure will cause a rising prothrombin time.

- Sample of vomitus (to biochemistry)

Label with time, date and suspected substance.

- Arterial blood gas

Changes usually occur only after several hours or days, but a baseline is useful.

It is standard practice to check drug levels (principally salicylate and paracetamol) for all overdose patients. Patients may conceal or simply not realize how many tablets they have taken, or whether they contain these substances. Paracetamol levels should be taken not less than 4 hours after ingestion, aspirin

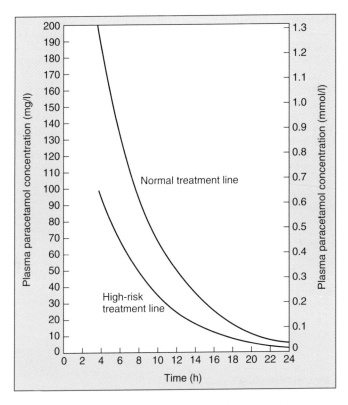

Fig. 4.1 Chart to decide who should receive Parvolex. (Reproduced with kind permission from the Department of Analytical Toxicology, University of Wales College of Medicine.) People at or above the treatment lines should receive treatment in accordance with guidelines published in the British National Formulary, *providing they have no contraindications.*

not less than 6 hours, longer may be necessary if the tablets have enteric coating.

■ Always collect at least one sample of blood from the patient, regardless of what they claim to have taken.

■ Lethal paracetamol overdoses may not become apparent for several days, when the person starts to go yellow. **Always assume that the person has taken paracetamol, and more than they say they have.** The

Parvolex treatment chart found in A&E (see Fig. 4.1) is used to assess whether or not the patient needs treatment with a Parvolex infusion (N-acetylcysteine – see the *BNF* for dosage) to counteract a paracetamol overdose. Take blood levels at least 4 hours (but less than 8) after the patient has ingested the tablets.

■ If the level is *on or above* the line, the patient needs urgent treatment or risks fatal liver damage. Be prepared for potentially serious side effects, including bronchospasm, hypoglycaemia, shock and vomiting. Glucose should be checked hourly. Patients may not be sure when they took the overdose. Newer guidelines suggest erring on the side of treatment if uncertain. However, if you feel unsure about whether to treat or not, get senior advice quickly.

■ Levels *below* the line do not usually require treatment unless the patient has existing liver damage or is taking enzyme-inducing drugs such as carbamazepine. Consult with your senior. Levels need to be rechecked to make sure that they are not rising.

■ Aspirin overdose causes a wide anion-gap metabolic acidosis and may be associated with a respiratory alkalosis (due to direct stimulation of the respiratory centres), so consider serial ABGs. Features include tachypnoea, tachycardia and tinnitus.

Second, decide if the patient needs to be washed out

Washouts (gastric lavage)

■ Once a common procedure this has fallen out of vogue but may still have a role in some overdoses.

■ NEVER wash out an unconscious patient without first intubating the patient with an anaesthetist's assistance. Consider washing patients out within:

■ 4 hours for anything except corrosive agents and petrol.

■ 6 hours for opiates and anticholinergics.

■ 12 hours for salicylates, aminophylline, tricyclic antidepressants.

■ Ask someone to show you how to do your first few washouts.

■ Gum boots and a plastic apron save your clothes during washouts.

■ Be sure to use *warm* water to wash the patient out. Cold water is painful and may induce vasospasm and angina.

■ Monitor oxygen saturations and have suction equipment ready.

■ Coat the hosepipe with lubricant jelly before insertion; it makes it much easier to swallow.

■ Do not forget to follow the water washout with a bottle of charcoal solution (e.g. 50 g in 200 ml of water) to prevent further absorption.

■ Save a specimen jar of vomitus for biochemical analysis.

Patients refusing treatment

You *can* section someone who refuses to be treated (see Appendix, Mental Health Act) if you think they have taken something that may be lethal. Obviously use this as a last resort. Sectioning someone is a complex process and may have serious consequences for them. Get senior advice. Sometimes when faced with the prospect of being sectioned, patients change their mind about being washed out.

Third, do a more thorough history and examination

I If possible, get a thorough history from the patient *as well as* from whoever is accompanying them. If possible, try to ascertain:

A What precipitated the attempt?

● Intention at time of overdose (did they mean to kill themselves?)

● Previous intentions (have they felt like this often?)

● Was the attempt impulsive or premeditated?

● Did they try to avoid being found?

● Did they leave a note?

- Did the patient take illicit drugs or alcohol?
- Did the patient have specific problems that caused them to consider suicide?

B How likely are they to try to kill themselves again?

- How do they feel about being alive?
- Do they still want to die?
- Psychiatric disorder, especially depressive disorders with insomnia, anorexia and weight loss.
- Chronic/serious physical disorder.
- Alcohol dependence.
- Social isolation.
- Unemployment.
- Male.
- <50 years old.

2 Examine the patient thoroughly.

3 Perform a mini-mental test score (see Appendix, Mini-mental test score).

Fourth, discuss the patient with your senior regarding continuing supportive care and more definitive treatments. Additionally you will probably need to refer the patient to the psychiatrists.

Surgery

On admission, you should complete:

1 History and examination.

2 Baseline tests:
- Blood: FBC, U&E, clotting screen, glucose, amylase, G&S or cross-match
  Urine: MSU and dipstick, consider pregnancy test
- ECG
- Radiology: AXR, consider erect CXR

3 IV access (some centres prefer this to be done by the anaesthetic team in theatres unless the patient is for extended fasting, check your local policy).

4 Fluid chart for 24 hours.

5 Consent – this should only be taken by someone capable of doing the procedure in question.

6 Drug chart.

- It is cruel to leave patients in acute pain. Ambulance staff and nurses may not give pain relief until a doctor has seen them. If someone has renal colic, for example, you may be able to diagnose this quickly and prescribe analgesia accordingly. You must remain aware of pitfalls (like the vasculopathic renal colic patient who actually has an aortic aneurysm that is dissecting to the renal vessels).
- Diclofenac sodium (Voltarol) provides effective pain relief for renal colic. It can be given IM or by suppository.
- Very occasionally, patients who are seeking opiates *or* a stay in hospital may fake surgical conditions. Look for needle marks, small pupils and odd histories. If you suspect a patient is faking pain, ask for senior advice. It is extremely dangerous (and unethical!) to 'punish' addict patients (or anyone else) with inadequate pain relief. If your patient is an opiate addict *and* has a real surgical condition, then they will need extra relief for severe pain.

Most common conditions for surgical emergency admissions

1 Acute abdomen (appendicitis and other RIF pain, UTI, obstruction, IBD, IBS)

- Always be aware of the possibility of pregnancy or gynaecological conditions in young women with abdominal pain. It must be routine to request pregnancy tests on urine specimens.

2 Renal colic

3 Changing catheters

• Urological conditions, such as changing catheters, renal colic and haematuria, can sometimes be referred to the urologists.

Medical and surgical assessment units (MAUs and SAUs)

Over the past 10 years these units have become the norm, chiefly to take the stress off A&E and meet the 4-hour target, but also to begin the initial assessment and management of patients within the first 24 hours of admission. If your hospital has these units, it is likely you will see many of your medical or surgical patients in the unit rather than in A&E. All the same principles in A&E apply to these units with the added benefit of having the entire team (from junior doctor to consultant) and the majority of the patients in one place.

Fast-track patients

Some patients (usually with time-critical conditions although many others are beginning to fall under this banner) will be triaged directly into pathways for rapid assessment, investigation and treatment. Common pathways include: myocardial infarction, acute stroke, GI haemorrhage and head injury.

■ Be familiar with the local policy as these pathways are designed to lighten bureaucracy, reduce errors and generally make things easier for you.

■ There may be a designated person in charge of all such admissions, who should be more than happy to help out with any problems.

■ These pathways will be audited so be aware of the critical factors in these pathways (e.g. thrombolysis times, grading of severity).

■ Also, remember that these pathways also apply to inpatients, not just to new patients coming in.

Chapter 5
BECOMING A BETTER DOCTOR

Postgraduate medical education used to be fairly limited, to the detriment of doctors' morale and brain cells. Although the reforms have been controversial, certain aspects of medical education are rapidly improving. There are many things you can do to keep your work interesting and to prevent the whisky bottle from becoming too attractive!

Foundation programmes (for UK readers)

Foundation programmes are compulsory for all UK graduating doctors. Even though schemes have been in place since 2005, most programmes are continuing to mature. The scheme is intended to streamline the training of junior doctors so as to ensure that all junior doctors develop a set of core generic skills and to reduce the bottleneck when entering the registrar grade. Foundation programmes are divided into 2 years (FY1 and FY2) that are now usually paired.

FY1 trainees are comparable to the pre-registration house officers in the older system and are frequently still called that. Placements are of variable length between 3 and 6 months, but most programmes have six placements of 4 months each across a 2-year programme. Typically, a minimum of 3 months in each year represents surgery and medicine. The third placement in each year is often in primary care or gynaecology (A & E can come under the umbrella of medicine or sur-

gery). During the first year, if not already dictated during your job selection, you will have an opportunity to put forward your preferences for placements in FY2. Discuss your choices with your educational supervisor and friends, but ultimately you should choose your placements based on your interests as well as any gaps you may have in your experience. It will be useful when applying for specialist training posts if you can demonstrate a clear path from your initial foundation jobs to the specialty you wish to pursue, for example, a GP trainee may want initial experience in general medicine and surgery before undertaking specialized rotations in paediatrics and obstetrics/gynaecology. The official line is that the foundation jobs you undertake will not influence selection to specialist training; this is largely true but subtler aspects of selection like audit experience, procedural skills and perceived commitment to specialty may indirectly influence candidate ranking.

In addition to the usual foundation rotations there are also currently a number of academic rotations (called ACFs, or academic clinical fellowships, at specialist trainee level). These were designed to encourage more clinicians into academia and improve the output of translational research. They are (generally) fairly competitive and give protected time, either each week or as a block, to academic work – be that research or teaching. The perceived sacrifice is that many academic jobs are in Cinderella specialities. Regardless of whether you choose an academic or regular foundation job, you will still need to complete the same core foundation competencies. Once these are complete you will be competing for the same jobs, with the same application forms, regardless of what you did during foundation training. This means that what you do with your time is much more important that what job you are allocated.

It may be worth noting that a core commitment of the NHS is to try to accommodate flexible training. This extends to, and includes, the foundation years. Some doctors are now choosing to take a 'year out' of their Foundation programme (a TOFP 'time out of Foundation programme'). This is generally granted so long as you have a very clear aim that will benefit the health service/foundation school you are at in the long run. It currently requires approval from the head of your foundation school. Although it will no doubt change in the future, it is also possible to complete one of the two foundation years in another country. The same competencies will still need to be completed and you will need to have a clinical consultant contact abroad who is willing to support you and sign the necessary paperwork. However, many young doctors are now taking this option (usually, and unsurprisingly, to travel to Australasia) with the support of their foundation schools.

Assessments

Your meetings with your educational supervisor should be focused on the progress of your training. This will largely be based on your assessments. Although a rapidly changing area, the assessment tools currently in use include:

1 Mini-PAT (peer assessment tool) and TAB (team assessment behaviour)
You pick a range of assessors from among your peers, your seniors and other non-medical staff, and they complete questionnaires about your clinical skills and conduct on the wards. You fill one in as well, and the results are collected, made anonymous and presented to you in your meetings with the educational supervisor. This exercise is aimed at finding out your strengths and weaknesses. It can be very demoralizing to discover your weaknesses (or what other people *think* are your weaknesses) but you should not shy away from selecting more critical assessors. Although compulsory for progression, these assessments are not currently used in any competitive sense so you should choose assessors who are likely to give you an honest appraisal – in the long run they will help you become a better doctor.

The alternative that is being increasingly used in many foundation schools is the 'TAB'. This is another type of multisource feedback questionnaire that allows a number of co-workers (typically 10) to comment on your performance and, in particular, your attitudes and behaviour.

2 Mini-CEX (clinical evaluation exercise)
You will have to find several clinical scenarios to be assessed on. These are extremely varied and can be found in the curriculum of your foundation school. The assessor is usually a senior registrar, consultant or GP. It can be difficult to arrange an occasion where a real clinical scenario, assessor and you coincide. The best way is to find the

assessors first and then tag along on their daily routine so that when a scenario pops up, he or, she can just assess you doing it immediately. Alternatively reminding an assessor about an interesting patient you saw that they know is usually adequate to prompt them into completing the assessment.

3 DOPS (direct observation of procedural skills)

You will have to find a variety of clinical opportunities to demonstrate your prowess. The procedural skills do not need to be complex, they can be fairly routine and straightforward (e.g. venepuncture, taking an ECG) and will happen at least once a day on every ward. As such, there will be no shortage of occasions to be assessed. That said, if you have a mind to go into a particular specialty (e.g. anaesthetics) an interview panel will probably be more impressed if you pull out examples of several central line insertions you have done than if you can only prove your ability to take blood. The trick again is to find the assessor first and then offer to perform the task that the assessor was going to do.

4 CBD (case-based discussion)

This is the more traditional format where you pick actual cases you have seen to discuss with your consultant or other senior medical team member. History-taking, examination, differential diagnosis, investigation, management, record-keeping and ethical aspects are areas you will have to cover. If you see surgical pre-admissions or patients on an acute-take, then these are easy opportunities to complete the task. If you rotate through accident and emergency, this also offers many opportunities for near complete clinical encounters.

There are minimum numbers of assessments you will need to do, but do not be limited by them. The more

assessments you have, the more you will learn and the more you will have in your logbook as evidence of adequate training. At foundation level, a surgical logbook is not required but again is recommended for those with a surgical bent (you will need one soon regardless and may regret not documenting all those early exposures).

In addition to these 'minimum' prescribed assessments, you are expected to be a lifelong learner and a 'reflective practitioner'. The latter means taking time to think about events that you have been involved in (both positive and negative) and searching for the underlying lessons they can teach you. Most doctors do this in a fairly heuristic way of their own accord but formalizing the process will allow you to consciously guide your own development. Written records of such events, in addition to being a good way to strengthen your learning and portfolio, will also give you a bank of memorable clinical episodes that will be manna when it comes to interviews.

Moving on from the Foundation programme

Selection into specialist training is fairly complex and can differ markedly depending on your specialty choice. In addition, it is liable to change rapidly over the coming years. However, as we currently stand in 2010–2011 there are two main groups of specialties – those that have a period of core training (general surgical/core medical/psychiatry/acute medical and anaesthetics) followed by further competitive selection into subspecialties; and those that are 'run-through' and do not have a stage of further selection. The latter includes specialties such as general practice, pathology, neurosurgery, ophthalmology, microbiology, paediatrics, obstetrics & gynaecology and public health. Orthopaedics is currently run through only in certain deaneries. For more information on the selection process see www.mmc.nhs.uk.

Skills you acquire in the Foundation programmes may form part of the selection process but previous experience in the specialty is not mandatory so do not despair if you didn't get the placement you wanted in FY2. The best way to insulate your career from changes in policy is to keep comprehensive records of *all* aspects of your clinical development as you go along. This should ideally include all courses, exams and a logbook of procedures, particularly covering all the skills relevant to your specialty.

In terms of postgraduate exams, it is currently possible to enter for the first part of the MRCS (surgical membership) exam as soon as you are granted a medical certificate; the final part can then be completed whenever the candidate is ready. For MRCP (medical membership) you need at least 12 months experience (i.e. complete FY1) to enter the first part. Once this is completed you can again sit for the final two parts whenever you are ready. The Foundation programme as a whole does *not* support trainees to complete these exams as foundation doctors, so don't expect any help with study leave or funding. However, this is not the stance taken by many other bodies and with both general medicine and surgery requiring full membership by mid-ST level, it may be prudent to keep an awareness of these from an early stage. For the other specialties (anaesthetics, pathology, psychiatry, emergency medicine, etc.), it is not usually possible to sit for any exams until on a training programme, and it is certainly not allowed to complete

them. There are lots of diplomas that can be completed if you are itching to work on your postgraduate CV; the *BMJ* careers section has good articles on most of them.

Information technology

It is becoming impossible to practice medicine without some rudimentary literacy of things digital. Most people will be familiar with using computers for word-processing, email and web-surfing, but there is a lot more out there.

■ Junior doctors move around a lot and with the plummeting cost of computers, laptops are so much more practical. Decent laptops or an iPad cost from about £500 and it will mean that during on-call lulls, you can spruce up your CV, write up that case report, or whatever. Be sure to get permission if connecting your computer to hospital equipment (e.g. printers, network points). There are numerous smaller alternative devices now available and many of the more business-orientated mobile phones have word-processing capability.

■ PDAs (personal digital assistants) are becoming ever more popular and come in several flavours, like iPhone, Palm™ and PocketPC™. Each type has a lot of medical software including formularies, patient list software, medical calculators and textbooks, but are usually not inter-compatible. Most medical software (especially formularies) are designed for North American doctors so they may not always be relevant. The ubiquitous Apple iPhone™ is now the choice of many doctors and has a range of handy medical applications for calculating medical formulae. A range of medical texts and learning tools are also available for download. This is likely to enter a fierce battle with Google's™ imminent 'android' phone that utilizes a Linux-based system.

■ All UK hospitals now have networked computer systems for accessing patient details, blood results, ordering tests and such. Learn how to use most of their functions early, and it will make being a junior doctor a lot easier.

■ Mobile phones in hospitals is a controversial area. The best advice is to follow local hospital policy (and not the behaviour of your consultant!). At the very least it will make it less likely for patients and relatives to follow suit and start answering calls during ward rounds!

■ Digital photos or video are best taken formally. No furtive clicks of the X-ray box! The written consent of the patient should be explicit about what the images can be used for and a copy of it should be filed with the patient's notes. Remember that you are responsible for the images. The medical photography department can help for more difficult photos (e.g. fundi) or get better pictures of clinical signs for case reports and the like.

■ Carrying a portable USB key makes carrying electronic documents around a lot easier and allows you to work on whatever hospital computers you find. Just make sure that you don't carry confidential information, should you lose the USB key. Some hospitals now only allow encrypted USBs from their IT department to be used. Breaches of these rules are taken extremely seriously.

The internet

Using the internet in the NHS is fraught with precautions and limitations. All hospitals will have local policy about the level of internet access and what is allowed. Be very aware of this. A few pointers:

■ Be very careful with confidential or potentially sensitive information in emails, particularly if you try to forward emails from work to home email addresses (the opposite way round is generally much easier).

■ Keep discussions of clinical cases anonymous even in closed teaching sessions like grand rounds.

■ The hospital intranet will often have archives of local policy, the local formulary and contact details of various people.

■ Keep hospital email and personal email distinct. Most hospitals are giving doctors' their own email account. You can get a universal NHS one at www.nhs.net; this is highly recommended as it is likely you will be working within the NHS for a long time. In addition, many people like www.doctors.net.uk.

Online medical databases

NHS Evidence is a good starting point for clinical information. This includes useful resources like clinical pathways represented in the Map of Medicine (NHS approved clinical flowcharts) and Prodigy (a summary of evidence-based information for primary care). Take a little time to familiarize yourself with this NHS service – it is improving all the time!

Other web sites rich in online content are:

■ The *British National Formulary* at www.bnf.org can save you time if you cannot find the ward's *BNF*. Your hospital should have a subscription to it.

■ PubMed at www.ncbi.nlm.nih.gov/PubMed

■ The General Medical Council at www.gmc-uk.org

■ *British Medical Journal* at www.bmj.com

■ *Journal of the American Medical Association* at www.jama.ama-assn.org

■ The British Thoracic Society at www.brit-thoracic.org.uk has very detailed guidelines on the diagnosis, investigation and management of respiratory disease.

■ EMedicine at www.emedicine.com is a useful quick reference on common and rare diseases. It is directed towards US doctors, though. A comparable UK service is offered by www.gpnotebook.co.uk

■ A portal for doctors at www.doctors.net.uk offers free email, forums and other useful content.

■ www.whonamedit.com provides the ward round trivia about all those eponymous conditions.

■ NHS Choices at www.nhs.uk includes an encyclopaedia for patients; it is a useful resource where patients can educate themselves about their condition. It is well designed and includes professional resources like the Map of Medicine.

Keeping up with the literature

The information and technology explosion is real. How on earth can you keep up with the literature? Actually, you can. There are several ways to keep up to date with stacks of international journals with minimal fuss (we wish we had known about them when we were students):

■ Adopt a 'problem-based' approach to reading. This means reading whatever you need to answer real questions rather than blindly scanning journals with minimal retention and maximum boredom (see Evidence-based medicine, below). You will remember much more of what you read if your patient depends upon it and you'll probably also find it more interesting. The age-old advice of reading up on clinical conditions

you see still holds true, and review articles, while not only more up to date than chapters in books, are often of a much higher quality.

■ Read review articles before you read other kinds of studies. Good-quality systematic reviews, especially those using meta-analysis, are the most efficient studies to read[1] because they combine the results of many individual studies, adding statistical power and giving you an efficient overview of the topic. Much of the write-up in these studies flows around methodology and may become tiresome unless you are specifically appraising the literature. However, if you can convince yourself relatively quickly that this is adequate, then the conclusions are often very useful and clinically relevant.

■ Learn to critically appraise what you read so that you can evaluate studies yourself rather than relying on the authors' conclusions. It is true that most published studies, even in leading medical journals, do not have reliable results because the study methodology was not rigorous enough. Critical appraisal is a simple process that enables you to be much more discriminating in what you read (see Evidence-based medicine, below).

Evidence-based medicine

Evidence-based medicine is a central tenet of being a good doctor. Basically, evidence-based medicine involves using research findings to give clinicians much more statistical power in interpreting everyday clinical data rather than relying on anecdotal evidence. Not only do people who practice evidence-based medicine find that they become more aware – and critical – of research findings, but they quickly become adept at solving difficult problems and find that they can engage better in medical debates. Evidence-based medicine can be practiced by teams or by individuals.

Evidence-based medicine involves carrying out three key steps:

1 Ask a clear question about the problem you are trying to solve (e.g. Should I anticoagulate an elderly woman with asymptomatic atrial fibrillation?).

2 Search the literature for good-quality evidence using a structured, hierarchical search that gives you the most statistically powerful research first. Search first for systematic reviews, second for randomized controlled trials and lastly for other types of studies.

3 Critically appraise (or evaluate) the evidence you have found to see whether or not its findings are reliable and relevant to your situation. To do this you need a list of questions, which help you to assess the methodology of the research. There are various books and courses to boost these skills.

In practical terms, it means you should always approach whatever you do with an inquisitive mind and a level of scepticism (i.e. 'Why am I doing this?', 'Is there any evidence that doing things this way is better than doing it some other way?') And if in doubt, look it up (see Online medical databases, above).

Clinical governance and paraclinical work

In addition to all the work directly involving patients, you should strongly consider getting involved in the other aspects of medicine. Not only is it a worthwhile learning experience, it is good on your CV and occasionally enjoyable! The amount of paperwork and the organizational obstacles can be very daunting but your seniors (registrars and consultants) should be very supportive.

Clinical governance is increasingly important for all junior (and senior) doctors. As a minimum, you should know what it means and how to go about the process of audit.

Clinical governance is defined by the system through which NHS organizations are accountable for continuously improving the quality of their services and safeguarding high standards of care, by creating an environment in which clinical excellence will flourish. It is traditionally classified in terms of the seven pillars

1 Clinical effectiveness and research

2 Audit

3 Risk management

4 Education and training

5 Patient and public involvement

6 Using information and information technology

7 Staffing and staff management

Clinical audit

Clinical audit is simply the measurement of clinical practice and its effectiveness with the aim of improving it. It is useful to get involved in clinical audit as you will learn a lot about correct management, the common pitfalls and the difficulties in implementing change in a large organization. You can easily get involved in an existing audit by speaking to the relevant consultant or your hospital audit department. Alternatively, you can start a new one. Retrospective audits are generally easier to conduct than prospective ones unless your daily work overlaps with audit. You can start by looking at local or national guidelines. Then figure how to measure whether they are being followed. Here are some `tips:

■ Design a form with all the data parameters you want to collect.

■ Pop into the clinical coding department. Here you can get a list of clinical codes that fit the scope of your audit. From there, you can get hold of a list of patients.

■ Don't try to track down all the notes yourself. Your clinical audit department is far more efficient at getting them. Sometimes, if you give them your blank forms, they will collect the information from the notes for you!

■ Spreadsheet programs are very good at sorting out the data once you have collected it.

■ Find an occasion to present it. Invite everyone involved.

■ Do not forget to think up solutions to any deficits you discover.

■ If you are working in the same hospital for more than a few months, consider repeating your audit once your recommended changes have been implemented. An audit cycle is not truly complete until it has been repeated at least once.

The audit cycle:

Step 1: Identify an issue or problem.

Step 2: Set criteria and establish a 'gold standard'.

Step 3: Observe practice and collect data.

Step 4: Compare performance with criteria and standards (data interpretation).

Step 5: Implement change.

Step 6: Re-audit to establish effectiveness of change and 'close' the loop. If the process is repeated again it becomes an audit 'spiral'.

Case reports

There is an element of luck in writing a case report, since you need an interesting case to write about. However, a good case need not be a rare one; common cases can be just as good, especially if there were pitfalls in the diagnosis or management of the patient.

■ You will likely need pictures or videos of any diagnostic imaging so make sure you get consent from the patient and involve the photographic unit.

■ The *BMJ* or the *Journal of the Royal Society of Medicine* has good formats to follow.

■ Good case reports are short and succinct. Journals are rarely interested in any superfluous details.

■ Your case report does not need to follow strictly the chronology of events in the patient. By holding back on the result of an investigation till the end of the case report, you create necessary drama!

Courses

Education is more than just working on the wards, attending grand rounds and reading books. There is a wide array of courses one can take on; these are regularly advertised in the *BMJ* careers classified sections and fall into several broad groups:

■ Examination courses are aimed at doctors sitting for postgraduate exams and try to condense 5 years of medical school into about a week. Often overbooked so consider it early. Despite what you may hear, it is not necessary to attend these courses to pass an exam. They are largely based around boosting confidence.

■ Skills training courses are extremely varied from the more clinical ones like the Resuscitation Council's ALS courses to less clinical ones like courses teaching interview technique. Resuscitation Council courses are invaluable, and should be top on the list of courses to do. It is now a requirement that ALS is completed by the end of FY2 in many foundation schools. Check which courses are compulsory or organized by the deanery before using up your own time and money.

■ Lecture courses are generally more suited for more senior doctors but may be interesting, particularly if in a field that you like.

All these courses are usually expensive. Your postgraduate centre is likely to have funds for junior doctors for this express purpose but they will be limited. Alternatively, speak to your educational supervisor about funding them.

Professionalism

No one teaches you how to be a professional. Don't worry if the transition from student to doctor is full of bumps and jolts – it certainly was for us. There isn't much mystery to being 'professional'; it's mostly about communicating well, building relationships and being responsible for what you say and do. However, this is no small thing to accomplish.

Communication

For an enjoyable job, good communication is essential. As a junior doctor, you will make about 30 phone calls for every patient you admit. You may interview up to 5000 people during the year. You will write volumes of notes that others will rely on and that might one day be used as evidence in court. You will physically touch thousands of people.

Although most medical schools do teach communication or relationship skills, you are still supposed to largely pick them up from your seniors. As you have probably already observed, many seniors are singularly lacking in personal and communication skills. It pays to develop your own skills; they will save you bleeps, headaches, time and lawsuits. Over 90% of UK medical defence cases result from poor communication rather than from negligence per se. Most so-called ward 'personality clashes' can be solved by effective and imaginative communication.

1 It is really important and difficult to write legibly at 3 a.m. Write for others as you would have things written for you. A fountain pen can force you to write legibly (or it can make things even worse!).

2 Write your name and bleep number on ward boards. This is very helpful for the nursing staff if you are on call (e.g. 14 May cover: Jo Bloggs' bleep 1413). Never deliberately omit your bleep from the notes, the doctors who do this are unprofessional and potentially compromise their patients' care. It doesn't take many episodes of trying to get hold of a member of a visiting team who did not leave their contact details to understand the importance of this.

3 Let people know if you are very distressed about something. Try not to transform grief or fatigue into defensive behaviour, such as silence or arrogance. People are usually pretty good at helping you out if they know what's up, you don't have to tell everyone but having a confidant such as your educational supervisor or a sympathetic senior can be invaluable.

4 ESP (extra-sensory perception) is not a reliable form of communication; short notes and phone calls work much better.

5 We have all been yelled at unreasonably by colleagues at some time. Try not to take it to heart or to say something you will later regret. There are some disillusioned and depressed folk out there, just bristling for a fight. If they do have a legitimate point underlying their intemperance, learn the lesson and move on. That said, if you experience sustained and unprofessional bullying from another member of staff (which does happen in hospitals), you should seek to stop it, either by standing up to the person concerned (easier said than done) or by taking the problem to a trusted senior or manager. The BMA helpline can assist with such things too, for example, by helping to identify whom to take the case to next. Do not ignore it.

6 Most junior doctors lose their heads from time to time. Don't be afraid to say you're sorry. People usually respect apologies.

7 If conflicts arise, some useful tips include:

- Ask yourself, are you sure you're right?
- Does it matter?
- Try turning difficult questions back to the patient. For example, you can ask them: 'What makes you ask that question?'
- Try to appear calm, despite what you may feel inside.

8 There are many resources to help people understand choices about treatments more thoroughly, such as videos, pamphlets and online information. Contact a lecturer nurse, librarian or district health authority to find out if any are readily available.

9 Use an interpreter if necessary. Interpreters can usually be contacted through the switchboard or the casualty nursing staff.

Consultants and senior registrars

■ Each consultant will have about five things that they want to know about each patient (sometimes for no apparent reason). Find these out early and supply them tirelessly, no matter what they are. Your predecessor is usually a good source of this kind of information.

■ NEVER say you've done something when you haven't.

■ Impress your seniors by being straightforward and by knowing your patients well. This matters much more in your job than having read the latest *NEJM*.

GPs

You will talk and write to many GPs; some you will get to know quite well. The following are some recommendations from a number of GPs, including Joe Rosenthal, a GP who also teaches at the Royal Free Hospital in London:

1 Phone requests for admission:

- Have paper and pen ready.
- Be polite.
- Listen first.
- Take down: name, age, problem, hospital number, GP name and number, expected time of admission.
- Ask for a list of the patient's medications, particularly if the patient may be confused.
- Inform casualty.

2 Phone the GP on discharge if the patient:

- Self-discharges.
- Is in an unstable condition.
- Has poor home circumstances.
- Dies.
- Needs an early visit.

Don't rely on the post!

3 Discharge letter. Complete *before* the patient leaves. Many are now electronic but ensure that it includes:

- Patient details.
- Name of consultant.
- Name of ward.
- Diagnosis and important negative findings.
- Treatment given.
- Treatment on discharge.
- Follow-up arrangements.
- What the patient has been told.
- Your name and bleep number.

4 Think about the resources the GP has in his or her surgery. Try to avoid things like 'repeat CXR in 1 month' on the discharge form. The GP is not an outpatient service and it may be much more difficult for them to arrange certain tests than it is for you. If there are loose ends requiring tests in future, set up a clinic appointment.

Nurses

It is crucial to get on with nurses, who are fantastic allies. They know most of what you need to know as a junior doctor and are usually keen and willing to teach you. Nurses are trained in a range of things that doctors aren't and vice versa, so the teams are complementary – remember this and use it to your advantage! Here are some hints for starters:

■ Always introduce yourself to nurses and other staff when you're new on a ward.

■ Always tidy up after yourself. Especially tidy up your own sharps. Most needlestick injuries arise from sharps someone else left hidden.

■ Tidy up your trolley after any procedure. Find out in the first couple of weeks how to make up your own trolley and how to pack it away.

■ Don't expect nurses to do things they are not qualified to do. Nurses may have extended roles (such as IV drug administration) but they may not. Nurses can be struck off much more easily than doctors.

■ Do unto nurses as they do to you. Make them cups of tea or coffee or offer to do an IV round if you're on the ward without much to do. This helps to create an easy, generous atmosphere on the ward, which makes coming to work much more fun.

■ To avoid heaps of bleeps, ask nurses to write down tasks and have one nurse bleep you with the list every couple of hours or so. Tell them you will return to do a round at a specific time (or at a particular hour – say between 4 and 5 p.m.).

■ If you foresee problems with a patient overnight, discuss these with the nurses. Arrange 'bleep thresholds' for foreseeable problems. Instructions such as 'call me if his systolic falls below 100' may seem superfluous, but they suggest that you are on top of the problem and indicate your willingness to respond promptly. This reduces the frequency of those 'just thought you might like to know…' bleeps.

■ If multiple bleeps are a real problem, consider arranging a meeting with the medical or surgical manager and nursing staff to work out a better system. This is the sort of thing hospital managers are employed for. Talk to your senior if he or she is supportive. Try not to jump into this though if you are new to a job; often with a little time you will find that a system that seems strange or untenable actually works quite well.

■ If you have a plan in your head for a patient, or can foresee a problem a patient might have (e.g. a delayed discharge date), let the nursing, social work and occupational therapy staff know so they can help you with it rather than having to nag you for information.

■ Write instructions to nurses in the medical notes, but also tell them.

■ Save time: get to know how team nursing works on your ward. Basically, team nursing means that nurses work in independent, often colour-coded teams, each of which looks after a certain number of patients. Do not try to elicit information about a 'red' patient from a 'green' nurse (see Team nursing, below). Also don't be surprised if nurses assume that doctors work in a similar fashion – more junior staff may assume that only a certain number of the patients are 'yours'.

■ Nurses often work in three 8-hour shifts or sets of 12.5-hour shifts. Their rota is usually kept in the nurses' office. It may be helpful to know when a particular nurse will be available.

■ Try not to interrupt nurses when they are meeting for the shift 'report', on handover or on their breaks. Remember that breaks are sacred to nurses; if there is something urgent then another nurse will always be covering their patients.

Helpful things to know about nurses

■ Nursing grades (varies between hospitals):

Student nurse: attends university for 3–4 years (shorter for graduate programmes).
Staff nurse: graded D–F (A–C are auxiliary nurses also known as health-care assistants or HCAs).
Sisters: graded F–H (usually).
Nurse managers: graded H–J.
Lecturer practitioner: senior specialist nurse who teaches and advises more inexperienced staff.

Nurse practitioners: gradually increasing in number but are still relatively thin on the ground in the UK. They are very experienced and are able to do a lot of what junior doctors do.

■ Nursing jargon:

Bank nurse is a nurse hired temporarily from a 'bank' agency, comparable to locums.
Charge nurse is a male version of ward sister.
Team nursing means that nurses work in colour-coded teams, each of which independently cares for different groups of patients. It means that nurses get to know their patients better. It also means that nurses may not know much about patients who aren't assigned to their team. If you want to know about a 'blue' patient, ask a 'blue-team' nurse.
To 'special' is to provide intensive nursing for a seriously ill patient.
Ward sister is the female version of charge nurse who may have overall responsibility for the patients.
Modern matron, reintroduced by the government over the last few years in an attempt to return to traditional standards of cleanliness and care, is a senior nurse who oversees a department and is largely occupied with managerial and administrative duties.
Back/Late shift is the shift from approximately 2 p.m. to 9 p.m.
Early shift is the shift from approximately 7 a.m. to 2 p.m.

■ Things nurses hate most:

> Doctors treating them like
> second-class citizens.
> Doctors not answering bleeps
> reasonably quickly (so they have
> to wait by the phone for ages).
> Doctors leaving sharps (and other
> rubbish) around.
> Doctors not explaining things well
> to patients and not informing the
> nurse what they found out from
> the patient.

Patients

(see also Chapter 8, Breaking bad news)

Listen to patients, even if you think their worries are trivial. Remember that you don't have to solve all their problems. Just listening can be a huge help.

■ If you do not have time to listen to a patient properly, either organize for someone else to listen (such as their nurse) or tell the patient that you will sit down with them later. Preferably give the patient a time and stick to it.

■ If you cannot make it back to talk to a patient, phone their nurse to tell the patient so they are not left waiting.

■ Avoid medical jargon when talking to patients. Even words you might assume are common parlance like abdomen are foreign to many patients; just try asking non-medics what a prostate is!

■ Give people information in bite-size chunks that they can manage. This is especially important for people who are anxious or when you are relaying frightening information.

■ Use conceptually clear diagrams wherever possible to explain yourself. Remember that anatomically correct diagrams may be more confusing than conceptually clear ones.

■ Be straightforward with patients. Answer questions honestly, even if it means saying that you don't know.

■ Do not be pushed into committing yourself to a diagnosis or prognosis if you do not have good evidence for it.

Patients' families

Patients' families suffer terribly from lack of information from hospital staff. You can greatly alleviate this with minimal effort and you will be showered with gratitude. If possible, take the patient's nurse with you to ensure continuity of care. There are two main problems you can easily help with: patient discharge and informing families about their relative.

Information about patient discharge

Making arrangements for home care can be a major ordeal, particularly for families where everyone works. You should start thinking about the logistics from the moment the patient is admitted. You can make a big difference if you or the nurse can let the family know as soon as possible:

1 When (and if) the patient can go home; if possible, morning or afternoon. It may be possible for your patient to leave at a time that is convenient for family routines.

2 Special instructions that the patient will need to follow at home and when they should go and see their GP.

3 Drugs that will be needed and when in the near future.

4 Who they can contact if something goes wrong.

Hints

■ Find out the discharge procedure from nurses.

- Be aware of hospital visiting hours so that you can tell families when patients are admitted.
- Liaise with nurses, social workers and occupational therapists, as they often have important information for patients and their families on discharge.
- Remember that many people will not challenge a doctor and may endure a lot of hassle to do what you say, even when it makes no difference to the ward. If families are looking bothered, ask them what's wrong. You may be able to help with little effort.
- Imagine the patient was your relative and you had to look after them – what would you need to know?
- Ask family members if they have any questions.

Information about what's wrong with the patient

(see Chapter 8, Breaking bad news)

Your main duty is to care for the patient, not their family; you should get the patient's permission before divulging information to any family member. Taking time in a non-stressful environment to explain things to family members can be invaluable. Families remember how doctors explained things to them. Key features that we find make a difference include:

- Take the family to a private room. This enables people to remember information and ask questions.
- Try to get rid of your bleep. Hand it to a colleague.
- Have all investigations and findings to hand. Be ready to answer lots of questions and be ready to admit uncertainty.
- Write in the notes what you have told the family and tell the nursing staff; this is very important in cases with a poor prognosis.

- Have tissues and cups of tea handy if possible.
- If possible, collect all family members for one chat. Have the family nominate one family member to be the spokesperson. This is helpful in big scattered families as it helps you avoid getting caught in the middle of family disputes and repeating yourself everytime a family member turns up.
- If news is very bad or unexpected, it may be courteous to ask your senior to see the family first.

Confidentiality

Breaches of confidentiality may be both unlawful and amount to professional misconduct, and you may be called upon to justify any such breach. Keeping confidentiality is not always as easy as it sounds – you may need to discuss patient histories with many people, both within the hospital and the community. The following guidelines should help you to keep legal confidentiality:

- Refer to patients by name as little as possible.
- Do not discuss confidential information with people over the phone unless you are certain of their identity and that they are authorized to receive the information.
- Never discuss patients in public places, such as lifts and hospital canteens.
- Never discuss anything with the press if approached. Refer immediately to your consultant or the hospital manager.
- Refer police officers to your senior; do not feel pressured into discussing patients if you are unhappy.
- Take care when discussing patients over the phone. Transfer ward calls to the doctors' office wherever possible.

It is easy to find yourself shouting above the noise of a ward only to find that the entire ward can hear you.

■ Remember that curtains are not sound-proof. If you have confidential or delicate information to convey or obtain, consider taking the patient to a side room.

■ Do not talk about patients so that they may be identified outside of imme-diately relevant hospital settings. For example, don't tell your dinner guests stories about patients that they may rec-ognize, even if you don't name them. It is better to avoid this kind of thing alto-gether, however entertaining it may be.

■ The MDU and MPS both have 24-hour advice lines if you are a member.

Exceptions to keeping confidentiality
(see Chapter 17, Whistle-blowing)

There are common-sense exceptions to confidentiality, such as when you have good reason to believe that the patient is likely to cause death or serious harm to him- or herself or others. Sometimes it may not be clear cut as to whether you should or shouldn't respect confidential-ity. For example, if a patient admits a crime to you, should you tell anyone about it? Whichever is the case:

■ Always ask your consultant for advice.

■ Document your decision and other relevant information in the notes to cover yourself in the event of a court case, or complaint. Your medical defence insurer can advise you if you are in any doubt.

Consent

(see Chapter 16, Public health and health promotion)

References

1 Milne R., Chambers L. (1993) Assessing the scientific quality of review articles. *Journal of Epidemiology and Community Health* **47**, 169–170.

2 Breaking Bad News: Regional Guidelines from The National Council for Hospice and Palliative Care Services (2003). (Available at www.dhsspsni.gov.uk/ breaking_bad_news.pdf)

Chapter 6
CARDIAC ARRESTS AND CRASH CALLS

You will almost certainly be a junior member of the hospital crash team. If you are first on the scene, the absolute priority is to ensure adequate ventilation and perfusion – basic life support. It is one of the few occasions when a well-learnt plan of action is essential.

Cardiac arrest calls

You do not have time to 'make a diagnosis'. Stay calm and then:

1 Check if the patient is unresponsive; if this is the case then:
- Shout for help.
- Turn the patient onto their back.
- Open the airway using head tilt/chin lift and make sure it is clear. Finger sweeps are out of vogue but look in the mouth.
- Assess for signs of life for 10 seconds (look/listen/feel for breathing, and feel carotid pulse).

2 Once you have confirmed cardiac arrest get help (preferably in the form of the resuscitation team). All UK hospitals should now use the standard 'crash call' number: 2222.

3 Ensure the airway is secure (using adjuncts if necessary) and that someone (preferably two people working in rotations) commences adequate CPR (30 chest compressions followed by 2 breaths). Help if necessary. Maintaining a cardiac output is key in prolonging life, compressions *must* be effective. In-hospital basic life support guidelines are available at http://www.resus.org.uk/pages/inhresus.pdf

4 Attach a defibrillator, ideally with a cardiac monitor. If no cardiac trolley is readily available, a portable automated external defibrillator (AED) may be available. These AEDs provide voice prompts and are portable.

5 Use the advanced life support algorithm in Fig 6.1; based on the new Advanced Life Support (ALS) guidelines (version 5) by the Resuscitation Council (UK). We strongly recommend you read the guidelines in full (available from the Resuscitation Council (UK) web site or the resuscitation officer in your hospital).

Hints

1 Find out how the defibrillator works and learn the layout of your hospital's arrest trolley. Ensure you enrol on an Intermediate life support or Advanced Life Support (ILS, ALS) course as soon as possible (these are usually organized by your foundation school during your FY1 and FY2). If you do not know how to attach the defibrillators used in your hospital you must learn how to do so as soon as possible.

2 Always wear gloves. Ideally you should also use 'universal precautions', these include a mask, eye shield and

The Hands-on Guide for Junior Doctors, Fourth Edition. Anna Donald, Michael Stein and Ciaran Scott Hill.
© 2011 Anna Donald, Michael Stein and Ciaran Scott Hill. Published 2011 by Blackwell Publishing Ltd.

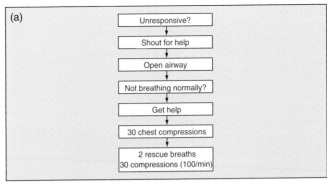

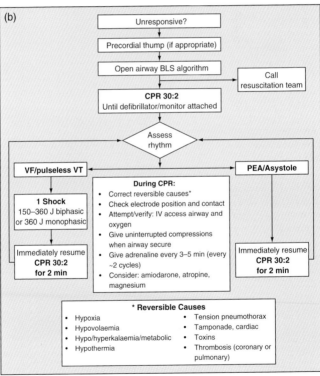

Fig. 6.1 Protocol for (a) basic life support and (b) advanced life support (adults). Reproduced with permission from Advanced Life Support, 5th edition. The Resuscitation Council (UK).

protective clothing. Be aware of sharps that may not have been disposed of properly, particularly those thrown on the floor or stuck in a mattress.

3 Note the time of the crash call so you can keep track of how long the resuscitation has been in progress. If there are an adequate number of people nominate a scribe to note time and events.

4 The crash team will usually consist of a medical registrar (the team leader), an anaesthetist, specialist trainees, and FY trainees, as well as nursing staff. It may feel chaotic but it is important that everyone has an allocated role (usually delineated by the team leader) to ensure the call is run smoothly. As a junior, this may be in the form of performing compressions, scribing/keeping time, gaining access/bloods/ABGs, giving drugs or tracking down the medical background. If you are unsure of your role, ask!

5 It is useful to know the patient's medical background although this is not a priority. Look for risk factors:

• Bleeding (e.g. oesophageal varices, recent surgery, bleeding disorder).

• Pneumothorax (e.g. recent central line placement, chest drain, surgical procedures).

• Pericardial tamponade (e.g. recent chest trauma, recent MI).

• Pulmonary embolus (e.g. recent DVT, major pelvic surgery).

• MI (e.g. history of IHD).

• Electrolyte imbalance, especially K^+ (e.g. anuric patient after major surgery, patient with severe renal impairment) and glucose levels (always make sure a BM has been done).

• Drug overdose (e.g. dilated/constricted pupils, IVDU (intravenous drug user) track marks, smell of alcohol).

The commonest unexpected cardiac arrest calls in inpatients are due to pulmonary embolus and electrolyte imbalances.

6 Cardiac arrest is traumatic for other patients on the ward. Use professional language and stay calm.

7 After an unsuccessful call, be sensitive to the fact that nurses and other doctors may have a close relationship with the patient.

8 Always check that he patient is not 'not for resus in the event of cardiac arrest'. This should be written clearly in the notes (see 'DNR orders' below). When in doubt, your duty is to attempt to save the patient's life.

9 If you are with a very unwell patient who you suspect might arrest in a few minutes, get help fast (e.g. getting your seniors or putting the call out).

'Do not resuscitate' (DNR) orders

This is a complex area and a frequent cause of complaint and litigation. It is one of the most common reasons for the GMC to take doctors to task. Make sure you read the joint statement from the BMA and the Resuscitation Council (available at http://www.resus.org.uk/pages/dnar.pdf or from the BMA medical ethics department – tel. 020-7383-6286, email ethics@bma.org.uk). The key points are as follows:

1 The decision not to resuscitate should only be considered when the likelihood of success is very small.

2 Your consultant is responsible for resuscitation status. Do not change a patient's resuscitation status (in either direction) without discussing the case with your senior. Always document that you have done so in the notes and state the rationale for the decision. Document the decision clearly – don't use codes like 'not for 2222'.

3 Good communication is essential. All decisions should be discussed with the entire medical team, the nursing staff, the patient (providing he or she is mentally competent) and the family.

4 The decision should take into account the views of the patient, family, close friends and staff. Note that if a competent patient chooses to decline CPR, this decision must be upheld. However, patients may not demand CPR against the opinion of the senior clinician; they are nevertheless entitled to a second opinion. If the patient lacks mental capacity or defers to the medical team, the consultant is responsible for the decision.

5 If the patient has given an advance directive ('living will') while mentally competent, this must be followed, even if the patient is now mentally incompetent.

6 'Not for resus' does not preclude any measures short of cardiopulmonary resuscitation (this may have to be explained to the family). This is in contrast to patients on a palliative pathway like the 'Liverpool Care Pathway' – used for patients who are terminally ill or unlikely to survive and are believed to die over the next few days; these are designed to ensure that patients are pain free and comfortable at their time of death. Medical treatments aside from those providing symptomatic relief are withdrawn and crash calls should not be put out for these patients.

7 Resuscitation status should be continually reviewed in the light of changes to clinical condition.

8 In the event of an arrest where the status is unclear, resuscitation should be attempted.

9 If in doubt about these guidelines, ring your defence union (they have a helpline for just such difficulties).

Chapter 7
COMMON CALLS

This section provides help with problems you are likely to get bleeped for. In particular, it helps you to exclude serious conditions and to initiate mainstay management.

How to use this section

Like a recipe book, this section lists basic protocols for common calls. We recommend the following:

■ When first using the chapter, read the short blurb immediately beneath each call, which lists the most likely causes of each problem and things to watch out for. Differential diagnoses are listed in the way that makes them easiest to remember. Most of the time, this is in order of likelihood in the hospital setting.

■ Feel free to scribble in the margins and make modifications to each 'recipe' in light of the clinical context and seniors' preferences. You probably will not need to carry out each step for every patient.

The Hands-on Guide for Junior Doctors, Fourth Edition. Anna Donald, Michael Stein and Ciaran Scott Hill.
© 2011 Anna Donald, Michael Stein and Ciaran Scott Hill. Published 2011 by Blackwell Publishing Ltd.

■ Remember that unusual presentations of a common condition are more common than common presentations of rare conditions.

■ To make this section easy to use in the middle of the night, we have kept abbreviations to a minimum. If in doubt, please refer to the abbreviations list (see Prelims, Abbreviations). Drug abbreviations are as follows:

od	once in 24 hours
bd	twice in 24 hours
tds	three times in 24 hours
qds	four times in 24 hours
PO	orally
SC	subcutaneously
IM	intramuscularly
IV	intravenously
nocte	at night
mane	in the morning
stat	straight away
T	one tablet
TT	two tablets

Considerations for all ward calls

■ Never hesitate to call your seniors. It is their job to back you up. However, like everyone else, seniors do not like to feel dumped on. Unless it is a dire emergency, make sure you have assessed the problem thoroughly and if possible make a provisional differential diagnosis and management plan. Resist the temptation to call them as soon as you find a problem, unless it is immediately life-threatening. You may find that after you have assessed the patient, you do not feel the need to contact them immediately.

■ If you need help, always refer problems upwards (to seniors) not sideways (to other new doctors). Be sure not to mistake the illusion of competence that some of your peers display with real competence. No one will support you if things go wrong and your only source of advice was someone at the same level as you.

■ Always examine patients in a good light even if it means switching on the main light.

■ Even in dire emergencies, act steadily and reassure the patient. If you need urgent senior help, stay with the patient and ask someone else to get hold of your senior.

■ The key to managing simultaneous bleeps is to prioritize tasks according to urgency and location in the hospital.

■ Keep emergency routines fresh in your mind throughout the year. Patients can deteriorate when you least expect it, such as on convalescent wards.

■ Before going to bed, check that you know where to find: ophthalmoscope/otoscope, stethoscope, patella hammer, blood-taking equipment, catheter sets, blood gas machines, ECG machine and blood fridges (this is particularly important – if in doubt they are usually near the theatres or the ITU).

■ While on call, if you are going to sleep then wear theatre scrubs.

■ If you are tired or woken from a deep sleep, try washing your face in cold water and mentally preparing yourself for the problem you are about to deal with. Consider differential diagnoses as you walk to the ward.

■ After seeing patients, sit down with their notes and review their history to make sure you have not missed something, and document your findings.

■ Whatever you are called for, don't forget to check the drug and fluid charts. A common error of junior doctors is not realizing that a patients urine output is falling.

■ When tired, try not to argue with nursing or medical colleagues. If you feel you are being bleeped unnecessarily, take the matter up when you are well rested.

■ Do not be too hard on yourself if everything seems daunting. It is! Experience is the only way to develop good clinical judgement and familiarity with practical procedures. You will learn to cope; sometimes it just takes a little time.

Abdominal pain

Your priority is to exclude peritonism and obstruction. Common causes of non-acute abdominal pain, such as UTI, constipation and post-op pain, are not life-threatening but may require treatment.

When answering your bleep, ask for:
■ BP, pulse and temp.
■ A dipstick of the urine to look for protein and blood.
■ Keep the patient NBM.

Differential diagnoses

Intestinal obstruction
■ Constipation
■ Adhesions
■ Hernia, volvulus, tumour
Peritonism
■ Inflammation/infection of any intra-abdominal organ (e.g. pancreatitis)
■ Perforated viscus

■ Complications of pregnancy
■ Ruptured ectopic pregnancy (a life-threatening emergency)
■ Other gynaecological causes (ovarian torsion, etc.)
■ Leaking abdominal aortic aneurysm (a life-threatening emergency)
■ Intestinal infarction
Peptic ulceration/gastritis
Extra-peritoneal causes
■ Urinary retention
■ UTI
■ Wound abscess
■ Basal pneumonia
■ Inferior MI (often with associated N&V and bradycardia)
■ Retroperitoneal bleed or abscess
■ DKA

On the ward

1 See the patient immediately. *If flat*, call for senior help and commence basic life support. See The moribund patient, below.
2 If the patient is stable, take a more thorough history and examine the patient. Don't forget to consider:

• Medical history: alcohol, diabetes, IBD, IHD, recent procedures, previous surgery, and shingles.

• Pain – localization and radiation, onset, character, relieving or aggravating factors, associated symptoms.
• LMP and gynae history (previous peritonitis, pelvic surgery, pelvic inflammatory disease, and previous ectopic pregnancy; intrauterine devices predispose to tubal pregnancy).
• PR and faecal occult blood.
• Extra-abdominal causes.
• *Exclude peritonism* and differentiate between localized or generalized peritonitis: fever, guarding, rebound tenderness, absent bowel sounds.
• *Exclude obstruction*: no flatus, no bowel motion, vomiting, cramping abdominal pain and abdominal distension. Check hernial orifices – this is vitally important and cannot be done reliably through clothing.

3 Investigations to consider:

• FBC, clotting and G&S.
• U&E, Ca^{2+}, amylase and glucose.
• ABGs if acutely unwell, or if you suspect pancreatitis or intestinal ischaemia (both cause a metabolic acidosis and the lactate will be raised).
• Radiology: erect CXR (free air under diaphragm, pneumonia), supine/erect AXR (check for air–fluid levels, intestinal distension, calcifications, air in biliary tree).
• ECG and cardiac enzymes to rule out MI.
• MSU for UTI (a common cause of abdominal pain in hospital) and urinary dipstick for blood or protein.

Hints

■ Do not delay analgesia. Opiates do not mask the rigidity and rebound tenderness of peritonism.
■ Involve the surgical team early if necessary.
■ Gastritis and non-perforating peptic ulcers can cause severe epigastric pain but not true peritonism. The pain is usually relieved within minutes by antacids.
■ Consider bowel infarction in patients who are acutely unwell with abdominal pain in the absence of peritonism.
■ Free air under the diaphragm may persist for more than a week after abdominal surgery or laparoscopy, and in such a situation it becomes an unreliable sign.

Anaemia

You will usually be called by the lab for gross anaemia. In this case, your immediate concerns are to exclude bleeding and heart failure. Chronic anaemia should always be investigated before transfusion unless the patient is acutely compromised, since donor blood may mask the cause (see Table 7.1). By far, the commonest cause of anaemia in the UK (other than menorrhagia) is occult GI blood loss.

Table 7.1 Differential diagnoses of anaemia.

Low MCV (<96 fl)	Normal MCV (76–96 fl)	High MCV (>96 fl)
Iron deficiency	Acute blood loss	B_{12} or folate deficiency
Chronic bleeding (e.g. GI)	Haemolysis	Liver disease
Nutritional	Chronic infection	Alcoholism
Thalassaemia	Chronic inflammation	Marrow infiltration
Sideroblastic anaemia	Malignancy	Hypothyroidism
	Pregnancy	Reticulocytosis
	Chronic renal failure	Acquired sideroblastic anaemia

On the ward

1 See the patient and assess the need for transfusion. Try to avoid transfusion until the diagnosis is clear, unless:

- Hb is dangerously low (<6 g/dl), although it is still usually possible to take samples for investigation prior to transfusion.
- The patient has symptoms (feeling faint, SOB at rest, tachycardia, angina, postural hypotension or has had serious acute blood loss).

Where possible, avoid transfusions in patients with:

- Haemoglobinopathies, especially thalassaemia. They can usually cope with low Hbs. Consult with your senior and a haematologist.
- B_{12} deficiency, as it may precipitate heart failure.

2 Take a history and examine the patient. Do not forget to consider:

- Occult GI bleeding – dyspepsia, weight loss, change in bowel habit.
- Menorrhagia.
- Medication (NSAIDs, drugs causing haemolysis, marrow suppression).
- Recent procedures or operations.
- Jaundice, skin rashes, lymph nodes.
- Abdomen: splenomegaly, ascites.
- PR and FOB (used for screening in the UK but not in hospital practice as it is non-specific).
- CVS – signs of infective endocarditis, prosthetic valves (can cause haemolytic anaemias).
- CNS – signs of peripheral neuropathy or dementia (B_{12} deficiency).

3 Investigations to consider:

- Repeat FBC and reticulocyte count.
- G&S or crossmatch.

- Iron studies (iron, ferritin, total iron binding capacity, transferrin saturation), B_{12}, folate and blood film.
- U&E, liver function tests.
- LDH, reticulocyte count and haptoglobin level are useful markers of haemolysis.
- Other tests (e.g. bone marrow biopsy), according to the differential diagnoses.

Hints

■ Patients with chronic anaemia are particularly susceptible to heart failure following transfusion. Check for existing heart conditions; discuss with your seniors first and transfuse them as slowly as possible. In those with heart failure or at risk of fluid overload, it may be necessary to give furosemide with each unit.

■ Iron-deficiency anaemia is not an end diagnosis – you need to investigate its cause. The commonest are occult GI blood loss due to peptic ulcer disease or colonic tumours, menorrhagia, poor diet and pregnancy.

■ Be alert to mild anaemia when checking routine blood results. Slight Hb deficits are easy to miss and can be an early sign of serious disease.

■ Leukoerythroblastic anaemia means there are primitive red and white cells in the peripheral circulation. The patient may need a bone marrow biopsy and investigation for occult malignancy.

■ Consider intra- or retroperitoneal bleeding in acute anaemia and no external evidence of haemorrhage. Look for bruising in the flanks or around the umbilicus.

Arrhythmia

While abnormalities in the heart rate and rhythm are relatively common and seldom life-threatening, never be afraid to call the crash team *before* the patient arrests! You are not expected to diagnose and manage arrhythmias without senior advice.

When answering your bleep
Ask nursing staff for pulse, BP and temp. Give O_2 if the patient is unwell.

On the ward (initial management for all arrhythmias)

1 See the patient. Check ABC. *If flat*, have someone call the crash team and commence CPR. Give 100% O_2; get nurses to attach a cardiac monitor.

2 If the patient is well and stable, take a brief history and examination. Do not to forget to consider:

- Cardiac symptoms (chest pain, palpitations, breathlessness, nausea, syncope, swollen ankles) and heart conditions (IHD, MI, valvular heart disease, rheumatic fever).
- Pulse rate and rhythm.
- Circulatory status. Is the patient in shock? (Low BP, cold peripheries, sweaty.)
- Signs of cardiac failure (raised JVP, peripheral oedema, basal inspiratory crackles, gallop rhythm – third and/or fourth heart sounds).

3 Do an ECG, and compare with previous ones.

4 Scan the patient's notes for details of current condition and treatment.

5 Document your findings and notify your senior.

ARRHYTHMIAS WHEN THE PULSE IS IRREGULAR WITH A NORMAL RATE

Atrial fibrillation (normal rate)   Ventricular ectopics
Wandering atrial pacemaker   Variable AV block

On the ward

1 Severe symptoms are unusual. First do an ECG and then examine the patient. Atrial fibrillation and ectopics are common. Check the notes and find the most recent ECG for comparison. Is this a new problem?

2 In most cases, the arrhythmia is not significant. However, if the ECG reveals atrial fibrillation or multiple, frequent ectopics:

- Examine the patient for heart failure (raised JVP, basal crackles, swollen ankles) and mitral valve disease (murmurs, added sounds).
- Consider thyroid disease.

3 Investigations to consider:

- U&E, FBC, ESR, serial cardiac enzymes, Troponin.
- Serial ECGs (AF is common post-MI).
- Consider T_4, TSH, digoxin levels and an echocardiogram.

4 Discuss further management with your senior.

5 If atrial fibrillation is compromising the patient, it may require immediate treatment with electrical or chemical cardioversion. The key decision is rate versus rhythm control.

Hints

■ Measure and document both peripheral pulse rate and apex rate.

■ AF is associated with MI, IHD, mitral valve disease, thyroid disease, hypertension, pericarditis and other causes of a dilated atrium. Rarely, it is associated with atrial myxoma, infiltration, endocarditis and rheumatic fever. It is common following cardiac surgery, when it is usually temporary but may require short-term treatment with an antiarrythmic like amiodarone.

New onset AF should usually be treated with anticoagulation. This may not be suitable in long-standing AF or in those with a high risk of falls but it should always be considered, particularly in-hospital where treatment dose Low Molecular Weight Heparin (LMWH) (e.g. 1.5 mg/kg of enoxaparin) can easily be administered.

BRADYARRHYTHMIAS (ARRHYTHMIAS WITH A SLOW RATE)

Sinus bradycardia

Sudden stress, severe pain, post-systemic infection

Inferior MI

AV heart block

Second-degree heart block: intermittent block with or without an elongated PR interval

Third-degree heart block: complete heart block

Drugs: amiodarone, beta blockers, calcium channel blockers, digoxin

Faulty sinus node: sick sinus syndrome, infiltration

Hypothyroidism and hypothermia

Raised ICP

Jaundice

On the ward

1 See the patient and assess ABC. Bradycardic arrhythmias can be serious. *If flat*, call the crash team and start CPR if necessary. Give 100% O_2.
2 If the patient is stable but symptomatic, inform your senior and:

- Consider urgent ECG and U&E.
- Review all 'suspect' drugs (see above).
- If symptomatic with sinus bradycardia or AV block, give atropine 0.5 mg IV (up to 3 mg in 24 hours). If bradycardia continues, get help. Consider starting an adrenaline infusion 2–10 μg/minute or transcutaneous pacing as a bridging measure while the patient waits for longer-term pacing.
- Consider urgent digoxin levels.

3 If the patient is asymptomatic, do an ECG and discuss with your senior.

Hints

■ A fourth heart sound with bradycardia is common following inferior MI.

■ A history of recent collapse requires urgent assessment even if the patient is currently asymptomatic.

TACHYARRHYTHMIAS (ARRHYTHMIAS WITH A FAST RATE)

Sinus tachycardia (regular rhythm, normal waveform)

■ Hypermetabolic states, for example, fever, anxiety, hyperthyroidism

■ Drugs, for example, digoxin, nitrates, nicotine, sympathomimetics, theophylline

■ Shock, sepsis or hypovolaemia of any cause

■ Heart failure

Supraventricular tachycardia

■ Atrial fibrillation with fast ventricular response (fast AF) (rhythm will be irregular)

■ Atrial flutter (has regular rhythm; often 300 atrial beats per minute, with a ventricular response at 150 bpm, that is, 1:2 conduction)

■ Atrial tachycardia (has regular rhythm)

■ WPW syndrome (rhythm is regular unless AF supervenes)

■ Nodal (junctional) (rhythm is regular)

Ventricular tachycardia

On the ward

1 See the patient. Assess ABC. *If flat*, call the crash team, request an urgent ECG and start CPR if necessary. Give 100% O_2.

2 If the patient is stable, do an urgent ECG and consider a cardiac monitor. On the basis of the ECG, decide if the patient has sinus tachycardia or an arrhythmia.

• If the ECG reveals a sinus tachycardia, treat the underlying condition.

• If the ECG reveals an arrhythmia, you need to differentiate between SVT and VT, which can be difficult (see Hints, below). Seek senior advice if you are unsure.

3 For the specific management of SVT or VTs, see Table 7.2a and b.

Hints

■ Broad rule of thumb in discriminating between SVT and VT:

– SVTs have narrow complexes (<140 ms) and are not necessarily associated with serious underlying heart disease.

– VTs have broad complexes (>140 ms) and indicate serious underlying heart disease.

■ Carotid sinus massage can cause sinus arrest, especially in the elderly, or if the patient has had a recent MI or is digitalized. Use only if urgent action is required.

■ Atrial tachycardia with heart block is commonly associated with digoxin toxicity.

■ Discriminating VT from SVT with bundle branch block is not easy, and you should seek senior help. If the patient is compromised, treat as VT.

■ Whether the patient has a VT or SVT, you need to identify and treat the underlying cause, in addition to treating the arrhythmia.

Table 7.2a Managing supra-ventricular tachycardias.
If the patient has SVT and hypotension, get help fast. The patient may require
50–100 J of synchronized Dilation and Curettage (DC) cardioversion

Atrial fibrillation	Non-AF SVT
■ Irregularly irregular pulse and no p waves on ECG.	■ If the patient has SVT that is not AF, they may need immediate treatment, but discuss with your senior first.
■ Commonest type of SVT. Common causes of fast AF in the hospital setting include MI, PE and pneumonia.	■ Most SVTs respond to IV adenosine. Ensure that the patient is on a cardiac monitor and that a resus trolley is close to hand. Inject 3 mg adenosine with a flush rapidly into a large peripheral or central vein. If there is no response after 1–2 minutes, give 6 mg, and then a further 12 mg if necessary. Expect facial flushing, nausea and transient breathlessness. Warn the patient of transient chest pain when you inject the adenosine.
■ First-line treatments of acute fast AF are rate control (with digoxin) or rhythm control (with amiodarone or synchronized cardioversion).	
■ Digoxin controls the ventricular rate, but does not resolve the fibrillation. Amiodarone can restore the rhythm but requires large vessel IV access. Both these agents need a loading dose (see Chapter 9, Drugs).	

Table 7.2b Management of ventricular tachycardias.

■ Treat pulseless VT in the same way that you would VF (see Advanced life support guideline, p. 40).

■ Sustained VT usually precipitates shock unless treated with DC cardioversion (100–200 J), so seek urgent senior help. Note that a broad complex tachycardia may be SVT with bundle branch block but should be treated as VT until proved otherwise.

■ Investigations to consider:

U&E, Ca, Mg, Troponin, FBC if acutely unwell. Consider T_4 and TSH.

Drug levels as appropriate: digoxin, theophylline and anti-arrhythmics.

ABGs and CXR if acutely unwell.

Calcium

Most labs report total serum Ca^{2+}, of which about half is bound to albumin. If the albumin levels are low, the lab result will underestimate total Ca^{2+}. To correct roughly for hypoalbuminaemia, add 0.02 mmol/l $\times$ the albumin deficit to the laboratory result, or ask for an ionized Ca level which need not be adjusted for albumin (a special tube is required). Albumin deficit is defined as 40 minus measured albumin level.

Hypercalcaemia

On the wards, this is often spurious and often an incidental finding. However, true hypercalcaemia may need to be corrected. Rarely, it requires urgent treatment.

Differential diagnoses

■ Spurious: tourniquet left on too long or blood taken from the drip arm
■ Hyperparathyroidism (primary and tertiary)
■ Malignancy – bony metastases, myeloma, paraneoplastic syndrome
■ Drugs – thiazide diuretics, excessive ingestion of Ca^{2+}-containing antacids, excessive vitamin D intake
■ Rarer causes: granulomatous diseases (e.g. sarcoid, TB), endocrinopathies

---

On the ward

1 See the patient. Check that the result reflects true hypercalcaemia. In hospital, hypercalcaemia is usually an incidental finding and is frequently 'spurious', due to dehydration, venous stasis, taking blood from an infusion arm or abnormal albumin (see Differential diagnoses, above). However, a corrected Ca^{2+} of above 3.5 mmol/l usually requires treatment.

2 Exclude acute symptoms that require urgent treatment (anorexia, vomiting, abdominal pain, impaired mental state, dehydration). If acutely symptomatic:

● Seek senior advice.
● Consider: saline diuresis: 3–6 l normal saline/24 hours IV and furosemide 40–120 mg 2–4-hourly according to response. A CVP and urinary catheter is useful to monitor fluid balance (a catheter is also kinder if the patient has difficulty getting to the loo).
● Avoid phosphates until Ca^{2+} levels are normal or risk deposition of Ca^{2+} phosphate ('metastatic Ca/Pi deposition').
● Consider hydrocortisone (especially useful in malignancy, sarcoid and vitamin D intoxication), calcitonin or mithramycin therapy.

3 If the patient has true hypercalcaemia but is not acutely unwell:

- If dehydrated, request that the patient drink enough fluid to maintain a urine output of about 2–3 l/day. If very dehydrated or unable to drink, consider IV fluids.
■ Investigate the cause of hypercalcaemia, exclude renal impairment and correct abnormal K and Mg levels (see investigations below).

4 Investigations to consider:

- U&E, ESR, phosphate, alk phos, Mg^{2+}.
- ECG. Review CXR.
- Consider plasma Igs, serum and urine electrophoresis, urinary Bence-Jones protein, skeletal survey, bone marrow biopsy (myeloma investigations) and PTH levels.

Hypocalcaemia

Like hypercalcaemia, hypocalcaemia can be spurious and may be caused by acute hyperventilation. Hypocalcaemia is rarely an emergency, unless Ca^{2+} is < 1.5 mmol/l (risking laryngospasm).

Differential diagnoses
■ Spurious (low albumin as in malnutrition or chronic malabsorption, blood taken from drip arm)

■ Acute hyperventilation
■ Major systemic illness, especially pancreatitis
■ Hypoparathyroidism – thyroid surgery or neck irradiation
■ On TPN without adequate Ca^{2+}
■ Vitamin D deficiency – malabsorption, renal disease, phenytoin or phenobarbitone
■ Excessive ingestion of phosphate

On the ward

1 Assess the severity of the patient's condition. Check that the result is not spurious. Look for peripheral or oral paraesthesia, carpopedal spasm, Chvostek's sign (tapping over the facial nerve induces facial twitch), confusion and tetany.

2 If hypocalcaemia is symptomatic or Ca^{2+} < 1.5 mmol/l, seek immediate senior advice and institute treatment to prevent laryngospasm. Give 10% Calcium gluconate 10–20 ml in 50–100 ml 5% dextrose over 5 minutes (not faster), followed by 1–2 mg/kg/hour IV for 6–12 hours according to response. Correct the Mg^{2+} deficiency and measure the phosphate level. If the phosphate is high, discuss with senior. The patient may need phosphate binders and slow correction of Ca^{2+}, as too rapid correction can result in metastatic deposition of Calcium phosphate.

3 Asymptomatic hypocalcaemia (Ca > 1.75 mmol/l) does not require immediate treatment. Give oral supplements (2–4 g daily in divided doses) that contain cholecalciferol (most do – see the *BNF*).

4 Investigations to consider:

- U&E, Mg^{2+}, phosphate.
- Amylase, parathyroid hormone or others according to the differential diagnosis.

Hints

To avoid undetected hypocalcaemia in patients on TPN, check Mg^{2+} and Ca^{2+} measurements at least weekly, and more frequently if acutely unwell.

Chest pain

Chest pain always requires urgent attention. While angina, oesophagitis and oesophageal spasm are the commonest causes of chest pain, never forget pulmonary embolus in the hospital setting.

When answering your bleep
Ask the ward staff to:

- Find an ECG machine.
- Repeat the vital signs.
- If the patient has a history of IHD, prescribe sublingual GTN 5 mg over the phone and start 40% O_2.

Differential diagnoses
(*do not miss these!*)

- Heart
- Angina (IHD, LVH/HOCM)
- *Acute MI**
- Pericarditis or myocarditis, including post-MI Dressler's syndrome
Lung/pleura

- *Pulmonary embolus**
- *Pneumothorax**
- Pleurisy/pneumonia
Aorta
- *Dissection**
- Aneurysm
GIT
- Oesophageal spasm
- Oesophagitis/gastritis
- Pancreatitis, cholecystitis, peptic ulcer
Other
- Shingles
- Costochondritis
- Rib or vertebral collapse
Sudden onset of central chest pain
- Exacerbation of IHD
- MI
- Oesophageal spasm
- PE or dissecting aneurysm
- Pneumothorax
- Rib fracture

On the ward

1 Assess the patient. *If flat*, get help (e.g. crash team) and institute emergency treatment:

- 100% O_2 via an on-rebreathing mask.
- IV access.
- Urgent U&E, FBC, cardiac enzymes, ABGs.
- ECG (stat) and ECG monitor.
- Urgent mobile CXR.

2 If the patient is stable, take a thorough history and examination. Do not forget:

- T, BP, pulse and circulation (well-perfused or cold and clammy)?
- The key to the diagnosis is the history. Specifically:

(a) Ask a lot about the pain itself. Have they had this pain before? Do they have known IHD or oesophagitis/oesophageal spasm? Does the pain feel anginal? Is it relieved by GTN? Relieving or precipitating factors (exercise, posture, food)? Pain lasting less than 30 seconds, stabbing or sharp in quality and highly localized is unlikely to be due to ischaemia.

(b) Any N&V (common with MI)? Recent falls or trauma?

- Listen for pleural and pericardial rubs (often missed).
- If there are odd chest noises, think of pneumothorax.

3 Investigations to consider:

- ECG ± CXR.
- IV access if you suspect an MI.
- Repeat ECG in 1–2 hours (there may be no ECG changes in an early MI).
- U&E, troponin and cardiac enzymes. Consider blood gases, FBC, clotting and G&S if embolus, anticoagulation or surgery is likely.
- D-dimers are sensitive but not specific for emboli. That means that if the d-dimer level is low, the chance of an embolism is very low (reassuring). However, if the level is high, it could be an embolus or just as easily a different diagnosis. Very high levels can suggest disseminated intravascular coagulation (DIC).

4 Discuss with your senior.

Hints

■ Pain radiating to either arm, neck or jaw suggests a cardiac cause.

■ Sublingual GTN will often provide immediate relief of angina and is a useful diagnostic aid. It also relieves oesophageal spasm, but over a few minutes.

■ Oesophageal spasm or severe anxiety sometimes causes ischaemia-like changes on the ECG. Seek advice if unsure.

■ A tachycardic patient may also show rate-related ischaemic changes but these do not normally occur with a simple sinus tachycardia.

Confusion

Beware of unexpected confusion in patients. In particular, hypoxia is common, but easily missed in the elderly. Never assume disorientation or dementia without first excluding serious medical causes and ascertaining the patient's usual mental state.

When answering your bleep

■ Ask for a ward capillary blood glucose test ('BM stick' – this stands for *Boehringer Mannheim* the old name for *Roche Diagnostics*).

■ Temp, BP, pulse and urine dipstick.

■ Pulse oximetry if available (see Pulse oximetry, below).

Differential diagnoses

'DIM TOP' (Mike's South African acronym!)

■ **D**rugs (especially sedatives and analgesics)

■ **I**nfection (anywhere; commonly UTI and pneumonia)

■ **M**etabolic – hypoglycaemia, Na., K., Ca, liver or renal failure

■ **T**rauma (concussion, subdural haematoma)

■ **T**oxins (alcohol withdrawal, drugs, others)

■ **O**xygen deficit (hypoxia) – pneumonia, pulmonary oedema, PE, respiratory depression (opiates), anaemia

■ **P**ain and discomfort (any cause, including urinary/faecal retention)

■ **P**sychiatric/dementia

■ **P**erfusion abnormalities (stroke, TIA)

■ **P**ost-op confusion (hypoxia, urinary retention, infection, drugs, abnormal electrolytes, pain, blood loss, disorientation, alcohol withdrawal)

On the ward

1 Assess the patient's general condition and vital signs. If the patient is very agitated or violent, get help from nurses and porters. Consider sedation but be careful; it is a form of chemical constraint and is difficult to defend in many situations in the UK. Please check with a senior if you are considering sedation. If you do sedate a confused patient with any history of trauma, you are obliged to CT them – try and agree this with radiology before the sedation!

2 If the patient is stable, take a history and examination. Don't forget to:

• Specifically exclude cardiac and respiratory distress. Consider pulse oximeter readings, ABGs and CXR. Hypoxia is a surprisingly common cause of confusion that is easily missed.

• Perform a mini-mental test score. Is the patient truly confused or just disorientated, in pain or angry?

• Ask about recent falls, funny turns or previous strokes/TIAs. Is the patient in atrial fibrillation or do they have a patent foramen ovale or carotid artery disease?

• Check possible infection sites (IV lines, UTI, chest, surgical wounds) and palpate for a full bladder or packed colon (urinary retention is a common cause of confusion).

• Look at the fundi for papilloedema – a hard sign of raised ICP (e.g. in subdural haematoma) and assess the CNS for localizing signs (inc. pupil reactions). Pupils are often naturally asymmetrical (anisocoria or Adie's pupil), but in the context of confusion or neurology this cannot be assumed.

• Check drug and fluid charts and review the medical background.

3 Ask the nursing staff or a relative about the patient's usual mental state. Is this a new occurrence?

4 Investigations to consider:

- U&E, glucose, FBC and ESR, ABGs.
- Blood cultures.
- Liver function tests (including clotting).
- Plasma Ca^{2+} in patients with malignancy.
- MSU.
- ECG.
- CXR, CT head.

Hints

■ Nurse the patient in a moderately lit room and minimize noise. Give repeated reassurance to the patient. A well-loved family member or a familiar nurse is invaluable.

■ Consider nursing the patient on a mattress on the floor. Some hospitals have special 'soft-walled' beds. Bed rails and 'hand ties' are regarded by most nursing staff as unnecessary and potentially dangerous. Physical restraint is rarely used in the UK.

■ Secure NG tubes and IV lines with bandages. It is occasionally necessary to put mittens on the patient's hands.

■ If you have excluded serious causes, consider short-term sedation with a benzodiazepine (diazepam 5–10 mg IV slowly, repeated after 4 hours if necessary). For shorter effect, use lorazepam 1–2 mg (25–30 µg/kg) IV slowly, repeated after 6 hours if necessary. Use with caution in the elderly.

Alternatives include:

– Haloperidol 5–10 mg IM or PO.

– Chlorpromazine 50–100 mg IM or PO (caution in cardiac patients). (Both haloperidol and chlorpromazine are especially useful in the more acute setting. Have a resus trolley to hand. You may need to wait 10–20 minutes for the drug to take effect.)

– In alcoholic patients, consider clomethiazole instead (see Chapter 10, Alcohol withdrawal).

■ You may not find any cause for the patient's confusion. Patients may simply be disorientated from a change in environment; but make sure you exclude serious medical causes before making this diagnosis. Clear, repeated explanation about where the patient is and why can be helpful, as is a small map showing where the toilets are and how to call for nursing assistance.

Constipation

Constipation is common in hospital due to hospital food, immobility, drugs and having to use a bedpan. Remember that it is a symptom and not a diagnosis. It is better for the patient to treat the cause than to blindly prescribe laxatives. Always be alert to obstruction and its causes (particularly tumours). Post-op ileus is common, usually resolves by itself and should never be treated with laxatives!

Differential diagnoses

Poor (low roughage) diet
Immobility
Drugs
• Ca^{2+}-based drugs (e.g. antacids) • Ferrous sulphate • Opiates • Tricyclic antidepressants • Anticholinergics
Embarrassment at using a bedpan (or unavailability/unwillingness of staff to assist)
GI tract

• Pain (anal fissures, haemorrhoids, recent surgery) • IBS • Obstruction (acute and subacute) from any cause, especially tumours • Ileus (pseudo-obstruction)
Metabolic
• Dehydration • Endocrine – hypothyroidism • Hypercalcaemia, hypokalaemia
Neurological
• Spinal cord compression/lesions

On the ward

I See the patient. Exclude:

• Intestinal obstruction (vomiting, abdominal pain or distension, high pitched or absent bowel sounds). If present, you must exclude a tumour and other sinister causes like strangulated hernias (see Abdominal pain, above).
• IBD (this can cause constipation; never prescribe laxatives in these patients without first consulting your senior).
• Pain/embarrassment which inhibits straining. Have they had recent surgery? In certain surgeries (like cardiothoracic), it is important that patients do not strain for prolonged periods.

2 Take a brief history and examination. Don't forget:

• To ask the patient how often they usually open their bowels.
• PR (faecal impaction, anal fissure). It is essential that you perform a PR – much serious pathology can be missed if this is omitted. 'If you don't put your finger in it, you'll put your foot in it'.
• Drug and fluid charts.

3 Investigations are seldom necessary but consider:

• K$^+$, Ca^{2+}, FBC.
• T$_4$ and TSH only if you suspect hypothyroidism.
• Sigmoidoscopy or colonoscopy if malignancy is suspected. While faecal occult blood is a good community-screening test, it has little role in inpatient management.

4 Management. For simple constipation:

• Ensure adequate hydration and mobilize if possible.
• Bulk-forming agents: Bran cereals or ispaghul husk (Fybogel or Metamucil).
• Stool softeners: Docusate sodium 200 mg PO bd (cheap) or lactulose 15 ml PO bd (expensive).

- Stimulants: Senna or bisacodyl. Glycerine suppositories if NBM. Co-danthrusate (danthron docusate) is effective but reserved for very elderly or terminally ill patients due to risk of danthron-induced tumours.
- Enemas, for example, phosphate enema 100ml PR.

5 Consider prophylaxis for patients at risk of constipation (bedridden, e.g. post-op, stroke or patients on regular opiates):

- Stool softeners (docusate sodium 100mg/day, or lactulose 10ml/bd) and/or stimulants (senna 1–2 tablets daily) or enemas. Adjust dose to symptoms.

Diarrhoea

By far the commonest cause in hospitals is drugs (antibiotics and laxatives), but infection should always be considered. Less common but important to consider is obstruction with overflow. In all cases, the patient may need to be rehydrated.

Differential diagnoses

- Anxiety and pain
- Drugs: laxatives, broad-spectrum antibiotics leading to *Clostridium difficile* infection, antacids containing Mg sulphate. Also cimetidine, colchicine, cytotoxic agents, digoxin or thiazide diuretics
- Intestinal obstruction with overflow (neoplasm)
- Faecal impaction with overflow, especially in elderly patients
- Infection
- IBD, other causes of intra-abdominal inflammation, ischaemia, etc.
- Non-specific in association with other diseases

On the ward

1 Exclude dehydration (BP lying and sitting, JVP, mucous membranes). Also check renal function.

2 Directed history and examination:

- Risk for intra-abdominal sepsis (recent surgery, diverticular disease), IBD, immunocompromise (including HIV).
- N&V, blood or mucus PR.
- Peritonism or impaction.
- Drug chart for new drugs, laxatives, antibiotics.

3 If the patient is otherwise well and an infective cause is unlikely with no evidence of colitis or intra-abdominal mischief, send a stool sample for MC&S and consider an antidiarrhoeal agent like loperamide.

4 If the patient has systemic signs or is taking antibiotics:

- Take a fresh stool specimen for MC&S and *Clostridium difficile* toxin.

- Bloody diarrhoea (dysentry) can be caused by polyps, ischaemic or pseu-domembranous colitis, cancer, IBD or infection with shigella, campylobacter, salmonella or haemorrhagic forms of *Escherichia coli*.
- Consider sigmoidoscopy and biopsy if the patient has bloody diarrhoea or the stool culture is negative.

5 Further investigations to consider:

- U&E; FBC to check WCC. Amylase (pancreatitis) and coeliac serology/jejunal biopsy if signs of malabsorption. Thyroid Function Tests (TFTs) if thyrotoxicosis suspected.
- Electron microscopy (EM) of stool specimen for viral infection (SSRVs).
- Inflammatory markers (CRP and ESR) especially if known IBD.
- Special cultures/stains in immunocompromised patients for cryptosporidia, mycobacteria, etc.
- Plain abdominal X-ray (to look for colonic distension and obstruction) if pain or known IBD.

6 Irrespective of the cause you must ensure adequate hydration.

- Oral rehydration regime (see *BNF* – oral rehydration).
- IV fluids if severe or the patient cannot drink (see Intravenous fluids, below).

Hints

■ Barrier nursing is advisable until infection is ruled out.
■ Wash your hands between patients.
■ Be wary of diarrhoea in patients on steroids. Their abdomens may be 'silent' despite serious intra-abdominal mischief.

■ If no cause is found, then consider referral to a specialist. There are numerous rarer causes of diarrhoea including carcinoid syndrome, VIPoma, amyloidosis, Addison's disease, laxative abuse, lactose intolerance and tropical sprue that may need to be excluded.

Electrocardiograms

Do not get too worried about interpreting ECGs during your first job. While the range of potential anomalies is bewildering at first, practice really does make perfect and junior doctors are only expected to diagnose a handful of important conditions (see Common ECG diagnoses, below). For a more complete guide consult Hampton's *ECG Made Easy* and *ECG in Practice* (see Chapter 1, Bibliography). Whatever the ECG diag-nosis, remember to treat the patient, not the ECG!

Common ECG diagnoses

■ Atrial fibrillation (no P waves, rate can be fast or normal)
■ Recent or past MI (see below)
■ Third-degree heart block (no relationship between P waves and QRS complexes)
■ Ventricular tachycardia

Basic ECG parameters to consider

- Rate: 60–90 bpm (lower in athletes).
- Rhythm: irregular or regular.
- Axis: normal: from $-30°$ (aVL) to $+120°$ (III) (some use from 0° to 90°)
- P waves: present/absent before each QRS complex?
- PR interval (start of P wave to start of QRS): constant? Normal interval: 120–200 ms (3–5 small squares).
- QRS interval: up to 120 ms (3 small complexes: squares) is 'narrow' and

represents normal conduction system. If greater than this or 'wide', then the origin of the rhythm is likely to be ventricular unless there is bundle branch block. Check height of the R waves. Are Q waves present?

- ST segment: isoelectric (i.e. on segment: baseline – this is the line between the T wave and the P wave)?
- T waves: upright or inverted (flipped)?

If the ECG is abnormal, consider each parameter systematically:

Abnormal rate and rhythm

Atrial tachycardia
- QRS rate >100/minute.
- Narrow QRS (<120 ms) (except in SVT with BBB or WPW syndrome).
- P wave abnormal (shape, size, upside down, swallowed by QRS, or with short PR interval).

Sinus arrhythmia
- Normal P waves, QRS complexes and rate.
- Regularly irregular. Rate varies with breathing (variation in cardiac output related to venous return as a result of altered intrathoracic pressures).

Atrial fibrillation
- No P waves.
- Irregularly irregular timed narrow QRS complexes.

Atrial flutter
- Saw-tooth baseline of atrial depolarization.
- Regular QRS complexes. Often the 'saw' to QRS is regular and constant at 2:1, 3:1 or 4:1.

AV nodal rhythm
- Narrow QRS complex.
- P waves hidden within the QRS complex or just preceding it (very short PR interval). P waves may be inverted.

Ventricular tachycardia
- Wide QRS (>120 ms), rate >150/minute.
- Abnormal T waves.
- P waves often absent or may have no relationship to QRS complexes. Regular rate.

Note: If there is a rapid QRS rate without P waves, a wide QRS (>120 ms) indicates VT (unless there is pre-existing BBB) whereas a narrow QRS (<120 ms) indicates AV nodal tachycardia.

Calculating the axis

1 If the QRS is predominantly positive in I and II, the axis is normal.

2 If the QRS in lead I is negative and III is positive, the axis is to the right 'arRiving together'.

3 If the QRS in lead I is positive and II and III are negative, the axis is to the left 'Leaving each other'.

4 Alternatively find a lead in which the QRS complexes have equal positive and negative deflections. The axis lies 90° to that lead.

5 To determine the actual axis, see Fig. 7.1. The precise axis can be determined from an ECG with trigonometry but is not clinically necessary.

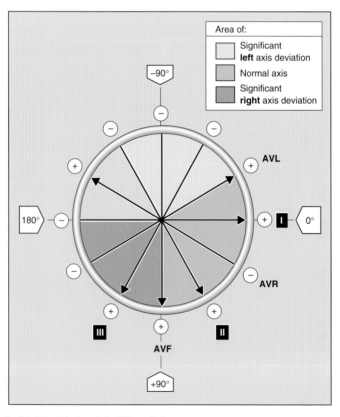

Fig. 7.1 Determining the axis for ECG examination.

P waves

1 Indicate atrial depolarization and are best seen in leads II and V_1.

2 Large left atrium (p. mitral): bifid and wide (>110 ms), P wave in II, biphasic in V_1.

3 Large right atrium (p. pulmonale): peaked P waves (>2.5 mm). Look at lead II.

4 No P waves: atrial fibrillation.

5 Negative P wave in I is either dextrocardia if QRS complexes become smaller from V_{1-6} OR 'technical' (due to lead misplacement) if there is normal R wave progression from V_{1-6}.

PR interval

Delay indicates abnormal AV conduction, that is, heart block.

1 First-degree HB: prolonged PR interval in each cycle but all P waves conducted, that is, followed by a QRS complex.

2 Second-degree HB:

• Type I: Progressive lengthening of the PR interval then followed by a non-conducted P wave is called the Wenckebach phenomenon (type I).

• Type II: some P waves are not followed by a QRS complex. May find 2 (or 3) P waves before a QRS complex, that is, 2:1 (or 3:1) block. P wave rate is normal.

3 Third-degree HB: no relationship between P waves and QRS complexes. Ventricular escape rhythm <50/minute. QRS usually wide.

4 A consistently short PR interval indicates conduction down accessory pathways (e.g. WPW). May be associated with 'slurred' upstroke of the QRS.

QRS complexes

Wide complexes (>120 ms) indicate abnormal ventricular depolarization, occurring in VT, ventricular extra-systoles, complete heart block or bundle branch block.

1 Ventricular extra-systoles: no P wave, *early* QRS and abnormally shaped QRS complex, abnormal T wave. Next P wave is 'on time'. Isolated extra-systoles are a common normal finding (particularly in young, fit people). They should, however, become less frequent as a person exercises. A *late* QRS is not an extrasystole but instead a 'rescue beat'. They are not normally a concern unless there is structural heart disease or post infarction when they are associated with increased risk of death.

2 LBBB: RSR 'W' pattern in V_1, 'M' pattern in V_6. Inverted T waves in I, aVL, V_{5-6} (remember the mnemonic 'WiLLiaM'). The presence of LBBB may mask underlying infarction. Once you have identified a LBBB, further comment is generally unreliable. It is associated with acute MI, aortic valve disease, cardiomyopathy and may be seen after cardiac surgery.

3 RBBB: RSR 'M' pattern in V_1, 'W' pattern in V_6. Inverted T waves in V_{1-3}, deep and wide S wave in V_6 (remember the mnemonic 'MaRroW'). Often a normal variant but can be associated with IHD, acute massive PE, congenital disease or cardiomyopathy.

4 Ventricular strain/hypertrophy: inverted T waves and depressed ST segments in the appropriate chest leads (V_{1-3} for RV and V_{4-6} for LV).

5 RVH: R wave larger than S wave in V_1 and no RBBB, deep S in V_6. Sometimes right axis deviation and 'p. pulmonale'. NB: a dominant R in V_1 is seen in posterior infarction with RBBB.

6 LVH: the Framingham voltage criteria is R wave in V_6 >25 mm in height OR combined voltage of R wave in V_6 and S wave in V_1 >35 mm in height. If these criteria are strictly adhered to, then there would be an overdiagnosis of LVH in the young and healthy. There is occasionally an associated left axis deviation. Causes of LVH include heart failure and outflow disorders including Aortic Stenosis (AS) and HOCM.

ST segment and T waves

1 Depressed ST segments: ischaemia, digoxin toxicity ('inverted tick' ST depression and inverted T waves in V_{5-6}), posterior myocardial infarction.

2 Elevated ST segments (always serious): infarction, coronary artery spasm (variant angina), pericarditis/myocarditis (saddle-shaped ST segments in all leads), ventricular aneurysm, posterior ischaemia.

3 ST changes in MI:

- Inferior MI: Leads II, III and aVF.
- Anterior MI: Leads V_{2-5}.
- Lateral MI: Leads I and aVL ('high'), and V_{5-6}.
- Septal MI: Leads V_{1-4}.
- Posterior MI: ST depression in V_{1-2} and prominent R wave with upright T waves in V_{1-3} (poor R-wave progression).

4 T wave inversion is often non-specific but in the context of chest pain points to critical ischaemia. Widespread T wave inversion is interestingly seen in massive cerebral events like subarachnoid haemorrhage. A similar picture may be seen in neuromuscular disease, for example, Freidreich's ataxia associated with cardiomyopathy.

Table 7.3 Diagnosing infarction sites by ECG changes.

Site of infarction	Changes seen in leads
Anterior	V_1–V_2
Septal	V_3–V_4
Lateral	I, II, aVL, V_5–V_6
Inferior	II, III and aVF
True posterior	Dominant R in V_1 (exclude RV strain and RBBB)

Important ECG abnormalities to recognize

Myocardial infarction

Sequence of changes (see Table 7.3):

1 At first the ECG may be normal.

2 Within 6 hours, tall T waves and raised ST segments are evident.

3 Within 24 hours, T waves invert and ST segments normalize.

4 After 24 hours, Q waves are evident and ST segments are normal.

NB: T wave inversion may or may not persist. Q waves persist.

Pulmonary embolism

There are often no ECG changes:

1 Sinus tachycardia.

2 Evidence of RV strain/hypertrophy (see above).

3 Right axis deviation.

4 RBBB.

5 Deep S in I, Q wave in V_3, inverted T in V_3 ('SI, Q3, T3'). An unreliable sign.

Hyperkalaemia

1 Tented 'tall' T waves ('Pot makes T').

2 Small or absent P waves.

3 Widened QRS complexes (this is with severe hyperkalaemia and eventually 'stretches out' into Torsades de Pointe VT or VF).

4 No ST segment.

5 Note that if there is *hypo*kalaemia, there will be an absent T wave, prominent U waves, prolonged PR interval and ST depression.

Finally, before making any diagnosis on the basis of an ECG remember to first check the patient (and that the ECG is from the correct patient!). Second, check the ECG leads and attachments. Third, check the calibration (is the trace running at the correct rate and voltage?).

Eye complaints

Except for the simplest problems, junior doctors are not generally expected to diagnose or treat eye diseases. Do not be afraid to seek an ophthalmological opinion. Ophthalmologists are usually keen for referrals and can teach you a lot.

The acute red eye

Differential diagnoses: conjunctivitis, foreign body, corneal ulceration or herpes keratitis, acute glaucoma, acute iritis.

On the ward

1 Take a brief history and examination. Don't forget:

- Clinical background, especially diabetes and other systemic diseases.
- Visual acuity, discharge, corneal lustre.
- Pupils: shape, direct and consensual responses.
- Ophthalmoscopy to assess red reflex (normal in conjunctivitis and simple foreign body) and fundus.

2 Unless the cause is obvious, notify your senior and seek ophthalmological opinion.

- If the problem is unilateral, ask about previous history of shingles (look for periocular vesicles) or iritis (which often recurs in the fellow eye). Conjunctivitis or ulceration can also be unilateral.
- Exclude conjunctivitis: the eye usually feels itchy, gritty and tears. Vision, corneal lustre, pupillary responses and red reflex are all normal. Purulent discharge suggests bacterial conjunctivitis. Look at the pattern of redness/injection. Intensity of injection around the periphery suggests conjunctival inflammation; whereas injection around the cornea suggests corneal or intra-ocular inflammation.
- Exclude acute glaucoma: the eye is red and painful, the pupil is hazy and fixed and the patient sees halos around lights. Seek urgent ophthalmological assistance.

3 Exclude a foreign body: the eye usually tears. Foreign bodies are sometimes hidden under the inside of the upper lid. Invert the upper lid over a small spatula (cotton bud or orange stick). Bear in mind that the sensation of having a foreign body in the eye can also be caused by corneal ulcers and acute keratitis.

Sudden loss of vision in one or both eyes

This is always an emergency. Seek immediate ophthalmological advice. Differential diagnoses are: acute glaucoma, central artery or vein occlusion, amaurosis fugax, optic neuritis, retinal detachment, severe hyperglycaemia, temporal arteritis.

Floaters

Floaters are usually condensations of vitreous, but can be blood, bits of retina or inflammatory cells. They are normal with age, but if they have appeared recently or suddenly, seek an ophthalmological opinion.

Falls

While most falls in hospital are trivial, they are a common cause of fracture in the elderly. You need to sign an accident form when called to investigate a 'fall' (see Chapter 3, Accident forms).

When answering your bleep

Consider asking for a ward glucose test and blood-pressure measurements.

Differential diagnoses

■ Simple accident (slippery floor, disorientation, frailty, generalized weakness)
■ Poor vision (no glasses, cataracts)
■ Drowsiness from drugs, especially sedatives and recent anaesthesia
Occasionally:
■ Loss of consciousness: TIA, fit, vasovagal, postural hypotension, vasodilator and other drugs, cough/micturition syncope, arrhythmias/MI, PE, mitral/aortic stenosis, hypoglycaemia, anaemia
■ Poor motor function/balance: generalized weakness from illness, Parkinson's disease, cerebellar disease, peripheral neuropathy, multiple sclerosis

---

On the ward

1 See the patient. Nurses are legally liable until the patient is seen by a doctor.

2 Ask the patient what happened and which part hurts the most. Don't forget:

• Temp, pulse and BP, including postural drop.
• Consciousness level (see Appendix, Glasgow Coma Scale (GCS)) and mini-mental test score if appropriate.
• Skin for bruising, bleeding, cuts and fractures.
• Bone tenderness for fractures. Frail patients can sustain fractures with remarkably little fuss. Especially look for hip, wrist and scaphoid fractures. Examine the skull carefully if the patient has hit their head. If there are signs of head injury or drowsiness, consider a CT head (see Chapter 14, CT head – some emergency indications).
• Drug and fluid charts (sedatives, hypoglycaemic agents, vasodilators – especially ACE inhibitors, anti-arrhythmics).

3 Investigations to consider:

• U&E, FBC (looking particularly for raised WCC) and glucose.
• MSU.
• ECG.
• The patient may need cardiac investigations later (e.g. ECHO, 24-hour ECG).

4 Sign an accident form (ask the nurses for one). If the patient appears well, 'No apparent injuries on examination' is sufficient.

5 Write in the patient's notes. Include:

• Time and date.
• Brief history of accident.
• Brief examination findings.
• That you signed an accident form.

6 Ask the nurses to continue to do regular observations and to contact you if the patient's condition deteriorates. If the patient has hit their head, consider requesting neurological observations.

7 Think about causes to the fall. Plan with the nurses how to prevent future accidents.

Hints

■ Many falls are caused by patients being in an alien environment, particularly in elderly patients with poor righting reflexes. To prevent future falls, show patients the call button and remind them that they need to call the nurse for toilet assistance after anaesthetics or sedatives. If the bed needs to remain raised high off the floor, caution patients about the drop before stepping down onto a slippery floor.

■ Fractures or simple bruising in the elderly can lead to substantial blood loss. Never forget to check limbs for occult fractures.

■ Sudden loss of consciousness is most commonly caused by fainting, postural hypotension and arrhythmia. MIs and TIAs rarely present with syncope alone.

Fever

In hospital, fever is most commonly due to infection, blood transfusions and drugs. When called at night, the major concern is to exclude bacterial infection.

Differential diagnosis

Think 5 Ws: wind (i.e. respiratory), wound (including lines), water, walking (DVT) and wonder drugs

■ Infection, especially UTI, phlebitis, pneumonia. More common in diabetics

■ Drug-induced, for example, antibiotics, allopurinol, ibuprofen

■ Common during blood transfusions

■ Thrombosis and secondary infarction: DVT, PE, MI, ischaemic bowel

■ Tumours

■ Alcohol withdrawal

■ Hyperthyroidism

■ Inflammatory and vasculitides, especially IBD, rheumatoid arthritis

■ Post-surgery

On the ward

I See the patient. Check T, pulse and BP and check the charts. Fever above 40°C requires urgent action. If there is any chance of shock (tachycardia, hypotension with warm peripheries), ensure large bore IV access and commence IV fluid resuscitation. Take blood cultures (at least two sets). Discuss IV broad-spectrum antibiotic cover with your senior.

2 Exclude immunosuppression and diabetes. Check the patient's history, latest WCC and glucose. In either case, look vigorously for infection site (see The immunocompromised patient with fever, below p. 72).

3 Try to localize the source of infection. Don't forget to consider:

• Asking about abdominal pain, cough, chest pain, diarrhoea, dysuria/frequency, prosthesis/heart valves, rashes, rigors/chills.
• Recent surgery or invasive procedure.
• Recent sexual contacts, travel abroad (TB, malaria, amoebiasis).
• Drugs.
Common sites for infection:
• Chest, wound/line sites, bladder.
• Skin, leg ulcers.
• ENT (remember ears). Check for meningism.
• IV lines, catheters, drains – how long have these been in place?
• Do not forget to examine the genitalia, do a PR (ischiorectal/prostatic abscess), and consider PV (PID). Check joints for tenderness and swelling.

4 Consider other diagnostic possibilities (see Table 7.4). Check the legs for DVTs.

5 Investigations to consider:

• Urine dipstick and MSU.
• FBC (for white cell differential). U&E, CRP, ESR. Blood gases or pulse oximetry if you suspect a PE or pneumonia.
• Blood cultures.
Consider further investigations:
• Other cultures (sputum, stool, CSF, wound swabs, catheter tips).
• Radiology (CXR, AXR, sinus X-ray, US, CT scan, ECHO).
• Serology.

6 Management. Take cultures and decide whether to start antibiotics straight away:

• You should start antibiotics if the patient is immunocompromised or diabetic as these patients can deteriorate rapidly (see On the ward, below).
• If the patient is otherwise well, has a temp of <38.5°C and is not immuno-compromised or diabetic, you can usually prescribe an antipyretic and withhold antibiotics until you have test results (e.g. WCC). Have the nurses call you if the temp rises and discuss with your senior if in doubt. Conservative management is usually appropriate for patients in the following circumstances, if their temp is <38.5°C:
• Up to 24 hours post-op or following invasive procedures.
• Following blood transfusion (see Blood transfusions, below).
• If antibiotics started in the past 24 hours.
• Paracetamol (1 g 4–6-hourly) is a good antipyretic. For fevers above 40°C, prescribe tepid sponging and fanning.

- If SBE is a possibility, you need to take three sets of blood cultures from different sites and at different times (3–6 hours apart). Do not start antibiotics before consulting with your senior, as starting antibiotics before a diagnosis is confirmed may prevent isolation of an organism which makes effective treatment much more difficult.
- Remember to make best use of your microbiology department. They are usually eager to help you.

Table 7.4 Common post-operative causes of fever.

Days 1–2	Days 2–4	Days 5–10
Atelectasis ± infection	DVT	As for days 1–4
Aspiration pneumonia	Pulmonary embolism	Deep abscess formation
UTI	Wound infection	

The immunocompromised patient with fever

A patient is defined as immunocompromised if they have WCC $<2 \times 10^9/l$, an absolute neutrophil count $<1 \times 10^9/l$ (neutropenia), are HIV-positive with a low CD4 count and are on high-dose steroids or other immunosuppressants.

On the ward

1 Take a quick history and examination (see On the ward, above) remembering:

- The patient can have weird organisms in weird places, including the CNS.
- Check *all* orifices.
- They can deteriorate rapidly (within hours). Seek senior advice early.

2 Investigations:

- Culture everything!
- If there is a central line, take peripheral and central blood cultures (include a culture from each lumen of triple lumen cannulae).

Be careful when drawing blood from peripheral veins, which may be few, and in particular from immunocompromised patients, such as cancer patients. Consider using small-gauge needles and butterflies.

- Take stool, urine, sputum, MSU and wound swabs, including from around the entry site of indwelling IV lines. Get advice from a microbiologist for special stains and cultures of sputum and stools for AFBs, PCP, *Cryptosporidium*, etc., if HIV-positive.

- Consider removing lines and culturing the tips (cut using sterile technique – sterile scissors, gloves – and send to microbiology in a sterile container). Discuss with senior before removing any line you cannot easily replace!
- Recheck FBC for neutrophil count, platelets and Hb.
- U&E and glucose. Consider amylase, G&S, clotting, ESR, CRP.
- CXR (mobile).
- Specimen for serology if patient is new.

3 Start broad-spectrum antibiotics once cultures are taken. Antibiotic policy changes rapidly, so check the latest protocol with a microbiologist or pharmacist. Oncology and haematology units usually have a written management protocol available. An aminoglycoside plus a beta-lactam, with or without extra anaerobic cover (metronidazole), is usual. Add flucloxacillin if a staphylococcal wound or line infection is likely.

Fits

Your aim is to prevent the patient from harming themselves and to end the fit as soon as possible. Most fits last less than 5 minutes and do not require active treatment, but prolonged fits require urgent treatment to prevent hypoxia and brain damage. The 'kindling' theory has not been proven irrefutably in humans but can be summarized as 'fits beget fits' by lowering subsequent seizure thresholds. In the case of paediatric seizures status epilepticus 'continuous or recurrent seizures without recover that persist for 30 minutes or greater' can lead to mesial (medial) temporal sclerosis – a form of epilepsy that may require partial unilateral hippocampal resection to resolve the epilepsy. Similarly, the longer a seizure persists the harder it usually is to terminate.

When answering your bleep
■ Ask for a ward glucose to be done.
■ Note the time you were called and proceed immediately to the ward.

Differential diagnoses

■ Epilepsy (this diagnosis requires a 'tendency to seize', that is, at least two fits; this can be triggered by omitted antiepileptic doses)
■ Drug or alcohol withdrawal
■ Hypoxia (fever in children)
■ Stroke, particularly subarachnoid haemorrhage
■ Infection or inflammation of the brain and meninges
■ Metabolic causes: hypoglycaemia or hyperglycaemia, deranged Ca^{2+}, Mg^{2+}, Na^+, thyroxine, urea, bilirubin (liver/ renal failure)
■ Post-traumatic (subdural haematoma)
■ Drug overdose – tricyclics, phenothiazines, amphetamines
■ Non-epileptic seizures (pseudo-seizures)
■ About half the cases are idiopathic

On the ward

1 Place the patient in the recovery position. Protect the patient's head with a pillow.

2 Do not forcibly restrain the patient, if possible, as it tends to prolong the fit.

- Give 100% O_2 by face-mask and insert an oral airway if possible, but never force one. The risk of choking on the tongue is less than that of choking on a tooth!
- Establish IV access. Get help if you are struggling.
- For adults give 2–4 mg lorazepam (IV bolus) or rectal diazepam (5–10 mg) if IV access is impossible. If the fit does not terminate within 5 minutes of IV therapy, repeat IV diazepam 5 mg/minute up to 20 mg or until significant respiratory depression occurs.
- If not already done, check blood glucose with blood glucose stick. If the patient is hypoglycaemic (glucose < 2.5), give 50 ml of 50% dextrose IV immediately. Flush the line with saline as concentrated dextrose is highly irritant. Alternatively give glucagon (1–2 mg IM or SC).

3 If the patient is still fitting, call your senior. Meanwhile, if the patient is not already dosed with it, give phenytoin 1000–1500 mg (15–18 mg/kg) IV slowly (not exceeding 50 mg/minute). Watch for hypotension. If the patient has been taking phenytoin, the next step is phenobarbitone (15 mg/kg IV or IM slowly up to 100 mg/minute) – but get senior advice first. The patient may need ventilation. The final step in termination is general anaesthesia, commonly with thiopentone.

4 Once the fit has terminated:

- Examine the patient for localizing CNS signs, evidence of raised ICP (check fundi, BP and pulse).
- The patient will probably sleep deeply for some time.
- Consider consequences for the patient's driving licence (see Appendix, Fitness to drive).

5 Investigations to consider:

- FBC, U&E, blood glucose, liver biochemistry, Ca^{2+}, Mg^{2+}.
- ABGs.
- Blood cultures if febrile.
- CXR.
- CT scan if the cause is unclear and there are localizing neurological signs, papilloedema or head injury.
- LP if suspected bacterial meningitis (exclude a space-occupying lesion first, preferably with CT. If unsure, ask your senior. LP in the presence of an obstructed CSF flow can cause coning).
- Toxicology screen if indicated by the history.
- Blood for anticonvulsant levels (some hospitals can do these within an hour).

Hints

■ If you arrive after the patient has stopped fitting but it sounds like a typical grand mal seizure, discuss prophylaxis with your seniors. If known epileptic, consider why they fitted now: Does it fit with their usual pattern of seizures? Intercurrent infection. Alcohol abuse. Poor adherence to treatment.

■ A useful alternative to phenytoin (especially for alcoholics) is a ready-mixed 0.8% clomethiazole solution for IV infusion, run in 40–100 ml over 5–10 minutes.

■ If you suspect malnourishment or chronic alcohol abuse, give thiamine 100 mg IV.

■ If you arrive and the patient is still fitting, spend a few moments observing the seizure to confirm that it is a generalized seizure and still continuing. Do not rush to terminate the seizure with drugs if it is witnessed and known to be <5 minutes. Most generalized seizures self-terminate within minutes.

Intravenous fluids

If you have never done it before, prescribing IV fluids can look horribly complicated. It isn't, providing you keep an eye out for the cardinal sins of IV hydration:

1 Over hydration, risking heart failure.

2 Electrolyte imbalance, especially Na^+ and K^+.

3 Phlebitis.

4 Unnecessary and expensive if the patient can drink!

How to prescribe IV fluids

1 Decide on the daily volume of fluid required:

● Look at the fluid chart each day to make sure that you are keeping up with (and not grossly exceeding) daily losses. Remember that in addition to recorded losses (urine, faeces, vomit), people lose 500 ml/24 hours in insensible losses.

● The average person needs 3 l/24 hours (each litre given 8-hourly).

2 Decide on which fluid(s) to use:

● Most patients can be given a daily total of 2–3 l of fluid in ratio of 2 l of 5% dextrose water to 1 l of normal (0.9%) saline. These should contain a total of 40 mmol of K^+ and 60–120 mmol Na^+ in 24 hours. This is typically written up as shown in Table 7.5.

3 Exceptions:

● Replace saline with dextrose water in patients with liver failure or ascites (the overactive renin-aldosterone system in these patients tends to retain salt).

● Avoid dextrose water in patients recovering from DKA or with hyponatraemia.

● Potassium imbalance is easy to achieve with IV fluids – and easy to correct. Measure electrolytes daily and adjust the K^+ accordingly. If the K^+ is suddenly very high, repeat the sample. Spurious hyperkalaemia can occur if you take blood from the drip arm, leave the tourniquet on too long or haemolyse the cells.

• Hyponatraemia is a common and potentially lethal complication of IV hydration. If the patent's Na^+ begins to creep below 135 mmol/l, the first step is to reduce the total IV fluid load and substitute dextrose with normal saline (see Hyponatraemia, below).

Table 7.5 Example of typical fluid chart.

Date	Fluid	Added drugs	Rate	Volume	Signature
01/05/10	Normal saline	+20 mmol KCl	125 ml/hr	1000 ml	J. Bloggs
01/05/10	5% dextrose		125 ml/hr	1000 ml	J. Bloggs
01/05/10	5% dextrose	+20 mmol KCl	125 ml/hr	1000 ml	J. Bloggs

Table 7.6 A rough guide to the electrolyte content and daily production of body fluids.

Fluid	Na^+ (mmol)	Cl^- (mmol)	K^+ (mmol)	HCO_3^- (mmol)	Daily volume (ml)
Sweat	50	40	5	~	Variable
Gastric	60–100	100	10	~	1500–2000
Bile	140	100	15–30	15–30	200–800
Pancreatic	140	75	5	70–120	200–800
Ileal	140	100	5	15–30	2000–3000
Diarrhoea	50	40	35	45	Variable

Hints

■ Patients with fever require about 10% more fluid for every degree Celsius >37°C.

■ At least daily, examine elderly patients for signs of fluid overload and reduce fluids if necessary. Check the fluid charts and request daily weighing.

■ See Table 7.6 for a rough guide to body fluid content.

Upper gastrointestinal bleeds

Always attend to GI bleed calls urgently: these patients can deteriorate rapidly, and small bleeds can herald major bleeds. Most reported bleeds, however, are minor and do not require urgent action.

While answering your bleep
Ask for BP and pulse to be taken as you head for the ward. If your nurses can get large bore IV access, then ask them to do so and draw bloods.

On the ward
The basic approach for all upper GI bleeds is the same:

1 See the patient. Wear universal precautions and then assess the severity of the bleed.

2 If the patient is hypovolaemic or at high risk for a major bleed (see High-risk and hypovolaemic patients, below), then they will require urgent treatment. To assess for severe hypovolaemia, check the BP, pulse and JVP (pulse >100/minute, sweaty and pale, cold peripheries, postural drop >20 mmHg and JVP imperceptible when lying at 30° or less).

3 As usual, treat on the basis of clinical findings. Remember that a small initial fall in Hb could be associated with a massive life-threatening bleed. Acute bleeds do no immediately alter Hb.

4 High-risk patients:

• Age >60 years • Melaena (which may be a substantial upper GI bleed) • Severe bleed • Re-bleed in same admission • Patients on anticoagulant therapy • Coexistent cardiac, respiratory or renal failure • Known or suspected oesophageal varices or cirrhosis.

High-risk and hypovolaemic patients
If the patient is hypovolaemic or a high-risk patient

1 Notify your senior immediately.

2 Remove false teeth. If hypotensive, give 100% O_2 and lower the patient's head.

3 Insert two cannulae (one in either arm), as big-bored as you can manage, even if the patient's bleeding seems to have stopped.

4 If pulse >100 bpm or there are other signs of a major bleed, give 500 ml of colloid or crystalloid as fast as possible and repeat if necessary while waiting for blood.

5 Urgently crossmatch 4–6 units of blood. Use O-negative blood if the patient is still unstable after 3 units of colloid and a crossmatch is not available.

6 Do FBC and clotting studies. Transfuse until haemodynamically stable (pulse down, BP rising and steady, warm peripheries, good urine output); 80% of bleeds stop spontaneously but 20% re-bleed.

7 Insert urinary catheter. Monitor urine output.

8 Consider inserting a CVP line, especially if the patient has a cardiac history or difficult venous access (consult your senior). Keep CVP in the mid to normal range (there is a risk of a re-bleed if the pressure is kept too high).

9 If the patient is anticoagulated at the time of the bleed, anticoagulation will need to be reversed. Discuss with your senior as to the best drug and dose to use.

Further investigations and ongoing medical management (discuss with your senior)

1 U&E. Bear in mind that urea is often raised due to blood in the gut, so look at the creatinine to assess renal status.

2 ECG and CXR in high-risk patients.

3 Give IV ranitidine (50 mg tds) or IV omeprazole (80 mg over 1 hour) followed by a continuous infusion of 8 mg/hour for 72 hours. Administration is only evidence based if given for recurrent bleeding ulcers post-endoscopy.

4 Monitor: pulse, BP, urine output ± CVP hourly until stable. Slow the rate of a blood transfusion once the pulse is less than 90 bpm and BP systolic is greater than 100 mmHg. Ask to be called if there are signs of:

• Re-bleed • Further haematemesis or melaena • Pulse rate rises (by more than 10 bpm) • Systolic BP drops by more than 10 mmHg • Urine output is less than 0.5 ml/kg/hour • The patient becomes confused.

5 Repeat clotting studies if patient has had more than 4 units transfused. You may need to give FFP.

6 Repeat FBC daily. Transfuse if Hb less than 8 g/dl or if symptomatic so that Hb > 10 g/dl.

7 Daily FBC, U&E. Repeat G&S if necessary (if previous sample used up).

8 Ensure 2 units of packed red cells are available for 48 hours after haemostasis.

9 Keep the patient NBM for 12 hours (longer if surgery is likely), and for at least 8 hours before endoscopy.

10 Ensure that the patient is on the next endoscopy list (usually the following morning) and that the endoscopist is informed. Obtain the patient's consent.

11 Discuss high-risk patients with the surgical team, so that surgery can be arranged more smoothly if the patient deteriorates.

Low-risk patients
If after initial assessment the patient is well and at low risk of bleeding (e.g. only coffee-ground vomitus, no melaena, normal pulse, BP and JVP, warm peripheries):

• Take a history and examination to exclude the risk of a big bleed • Insert a large cannula (just in case) and consider repeating a FBC and G&S • Inform your senior • Ask the nurses to monitor vital signs • Most patients will require no further action.

Hints

■ Confirm with the patient that they have had true haematemesis, not haemoptysis or an occult nose bleed.
■ Vomitus can look like coffee grounds and contain small amounts of blood if the patient has not eaten for several days.

■ In acute bleeds, the reported Hb lags approximately 12 hours behind the actual red cell loss. The *minimum* amount for transfusion is 1 U/g of Hb deficit; be guided by the clinical signs.

Lower gastrointestinal bleeds

Major lower GI bleeds, usually heralded by fresh or altered blood PR, are much less common in the hospital setting than upper GI bleeds, but can be just as serious. If called for a lower GI bleed, first exclude local causes such as piles and fissures and remember that major upper GI bleeds can present with altered blood PR. Follow the protocol for upper GI bleeds, with the possible addition of an urgent sigmoidoscopy. Discuss with your senior.

Glucose

You may be called for abnormal ward glucose readings. While *hyper*glycaemia is rarely an emergency, patients can die or suffer brain damage from *hypo*glycaemia so need urgent attention.

On the ward

Hypoglycaemia is usually caused by oral hypoglycaemic agents, poor insulin control and faulty ward glucose readings:

1 See the patient. If they are alert and well, repeat the blood glucose stick and take a sample for an urgent glucose test from the laboratory. Give them a concentrated sugar drink, such as sweet tea, or a hypostop drink and some biscuits.
2 If the patient cannot drink or is unconscious, administer 50 ml of 50% dextrose IV immediately. Flush the vein with 50 ml of saline, as concentrated dextrose is highly irritant. Also, it is acceptable to give 1 mg glucagon SC or IM.

3 Check the drug chart and recent insulin or oral hypoglycaemic doses. Adjust as necessary. Consider other, much rarer, causes of hypoglycaemia in the hospital setting, including liver failure and acute alcohol consumption.

4 Ask the nurse to repeat ward glucose readings. If the patient was semi-conscious or unconscious, repeat at least hourly until stable. Ask to be called if ward glucose readings are lower than 5 or more than 11 mmol/l.

5 If patient overdosed on long-acting insulin or oral hypoglycaemic agent, set up a 10% dextrose drip and adjust rate according to blood glucose readings (4–6-hourly once fully conscious and readings normal). Keep drip running for at least 48 hours.

Hyperglycaemia is commonly caused in diabetics by acute illness, corticosteroid treatment and test error. Hyperglycaemia in non-diabetics may be caused by blood being taken 'upstream' from a glucose-containing drip, from latent carbohydrate intolerance which may be unmasked by sepsis, acute stress (e.g. MI) and steroids, and from laboratory error. Be guided by the clinical state of the patient. Do not overreact to mildly elevated blood glucose (e.g. 11 mmol/l) on a single occasion. This can be investigated once the patient is over their acute illness. Hyperosmolar complications take days to develop, while DKA and Hyper Osmolar Hyperglycaemic Non-Ketotic Coma/State (HONK) have a dramatic clinical presentation.

1 See the patient. Repeat blood glucose stick and also send blood for urgent bio-chemistry glucose analysis. Make sure the sample is not taken from a 'drip' arm.

2 Check urinary ketones. If these are positive, do an ABGs and manage as for early DKA. If negative and the lab glucose result is greater than 22 mmol/l, the diagnosis is more likely to be HONK – give an immediate dose of insulin (5–10 U Actrapid SC) and discuss with your senior.

3 If the patient is diabetic with consistently elevated blood glucose, consider changing their drug management.

Hints

■ Laboratory venous blood glucose results are often around 10% higher and more accurate than finger-prick assays.

■ Type II diabetes may require insulin for control during acute illness (see Chapter 15, Diabetes). Do not be afraid to give if indicated.

Haematuria

In the hospital setting, haematuria is commonly caused by UTI or catheterization. However, haematuria may be the first sign of serious renal tract disease, such as tumour or renal parenchymal disease (see Table 7.7).

On the ward

1 Exclude vaginal or anorectal bleeding (common sources of false-positives).

2 Test for UTI: send an MSU and repeat the dipstick (look for protein, leukocytes and nitrites – the later are relatively non-specific). If symptomatic (dysuria, frequency ± low grade fever), treat for UTI once the MSU is sent (see Chapter 11, Renal medicine).

3 If a UTI is unlikely or the patient is unwell, discuss with your senior. Consider other causes (see above) and further investigations in light of the clinical context:

- Urine cytology.
- FBC, ESR, CRP, U&E.
- AXR for calculi; urogram.
- Repeat urinary dipstick daily until diagnosis is clear.

Table 7.7 Differential diagnoses of haematuria (consider the anatomy of the renal tract).

Renal parenchyma	Renal tract	Extra-renal (systemic)
■ Glomerulonephritis	■ UTI	■ Bleeding diathesis
■ Cystic disease	■ Trauma (e.g. catheters)	■ Vasculitis (e.g. SLE)
■ Tumours	■ Calculi	■ Malignant hypertension
■ Analgesic nephropathy	■ Prostatic disease	■ Emboli
■ Tuberculosis	■ Tumours	■ Sickle cell disease
	■ Bladder inflammation (e.g. infection)	

Hints

■ Urinary catheters can cause slight haematuria and usually do not require active treatment unless infection or non-trivial trauma is present.

■ If the urinary dipstick reveals significant proteinuria (2+ or more), renal parenchymal disease becomes more likely than a UTI. A very fresh sample of urine must be examined urgently for casts, etc. Commence a 24-hour urine collection to measure protein and creatinine clearance.

■ If no red cells are seen on microscopy despite significant dipstick positive haematuria, consider haemolysis or myoglobinuria (rare).

■ Anticoagulation within the therapeutic range rarely causes haematuria, but may unmask renal tract pathology. Repeat the clotting studies and discuss with your senior.

Headaches

Tension headaches are common in hospital. However, a severe headache with additional symptoms can be serious. The key to the diagnosis is the history.

Differential diagnoses and key symptoms

■ Tension headache: no associated symptoms. Pain can be severe, usually symmetrical and band-like.

■ Migraine: usually history of previous episodes. Severe, throbbing pain which may be unilateral or asymmetric. May have prodromal symptoms (visual symptoms such as flashing lights, tunnel vision, cranial nerve deficit rarely lasting more than 1 hour, N&V, photophobia). Classic history makes the diagnosis, but exclude other causes if drowsy, neurological deficit or visual symptoms. A variant is cluster headaches: unilateral pain becomes severe around one eye which becomes red, swollen and watery. Episodes last up to 1 hour, and can occur several times a day.

■ Sinusitis: dull, unilateral or central frontal headache. Local tenderness.

■ Drug-induced: especially nitrates, digoxin, tricyclic antidepressants, benzodiazepines (the morning after).

■ Meningitis, encephalitis: photophobia, stiff neck, ± fever and rash. Requires urgent LP (if no signs of raised ICP or focal neurology) and antibiotics.

■ Subarachnoid haemorrhage: sudden onset of severe headache (like an explosion in the head) and meningism. Occasional atypical history (small leaks) mimicking meningitis. CT scan ± LP (showing red cells uniformly spread throughout the CSF).

■ Raised ICP: present on waking, often associated vomiting. May have blurred vision, raised BP, slow pulse.

■ Brain abscess: non-specific pain. Diagnosis requires index of suspicion and CT. A raised CRP in this context should not be ignored.

■ Hypertensive encephalopathy: always markedly elevated BP (diastolic >130 mmHg) and other signs of malignant hypertension (see Hypertension, below).

■ Subdural haematoma: elderly, alcoholic, anticoagulants, head trauma.

■ Acute glaucoma: usually presents with a dull pain behind the eyes which the patient may describe as a headache. Early: mildly injected conjunctiva. Later: overtly red eyes. There may be an arcuate scotoma. Urgent ophthalmology referral required.

■ Temporal arteritis: patient >50 years old. Subacute onset of frontal headache. Commonly associated with fever, malaise, myalgia, weight loss, unilateral blindness or other visual disturbance (indicating imminent occlusion of the ophthalmic artery). A typical history, tender temporal arteries and a markedly raised ESR establish the diagnosis. Temporal artery biopsy should be undertaken but may be negative.

On the ward

1 See the patient. Briefly exclude emergencies (meningitis, encephalitis, subdural haematoma, subarachnoid haemorrhage, acute glaucoma, temporal arteritis) with symptoms and signs (see Differential diagnoses and key symptoms, above).

2 Perform a history and examination. Ask the patient if he or she has had similar headaches before (consider tension headaches, migraine and sinusitis). If history is typical for tension headache or migraine and if there is no evidence of fever, stiff neck, raised ICP or temporal artery tenderness, then prescribe analgesia (see below). If, however, the headache is persistent, you should examine:

- Pupils and fundi (raised ICP).
- ENT (otitis media, sinusitis).
- CNS (especially cranial nerves).
- Gait (if history suggestive of space-occupying lesion).
- Palpate temporal arteries for tenderness.

3 Investigations to consider: If the history is typical for a tension headache or migraine, and there are no sinister signs, then no investigations are necessary. Otherwise consider (depending on clinical context):

- ESR, CRP.
- LP and CT scan, sinus X-ray.
- Temporal artery biopsy, but a negative result does not exclude skip lesions.

4 Treatment: Once the rare but serious causes are excluded, mild-moderate cases can be managed with 1 g of paracetamol 4–6-hourly PRN. 10 mg metoclopramide IV is also shown to be very effective in acute migraine as it counteracts the effects of acute gastric stasis. If the patient is already on paracetamol, try ibuprofen (400–600 mg qds) unless NSAIDs are contraindicated. The next line of therapy is triptans – these are usually started in specialist clinics. Narcotic analgesia is not recommended except in occasional, severe headache. Other preparations used in migraine include ergotamine and prednisone. Be aware that chronic analgesic headaches (due to overmedication) are not uncommon. Migraine prophylaxis includes propranolol titrated up from 20 mg.

Hints

■ Always consider meningitis in patients with fever and headache, although any febrile illness may have an associated throbbing headache.

■ The scalp may be tender with tension headaches, migraine, temporal arteritis or shingles.

■ Be alert to depression in patients with recurrent tension headaches or migraines.

Hypertension

Hypertension is common but rarely requires treatment in the middle of the night unless there is evidence of heart failure, malignant hypertension or severe renal disease.

On the ward

1 Recheck BP and pulse. Note previous readings. Make sure you use a big enough manometer cuff if the patient has large arms. Exclude:

- Heart failure: raised JVP, basal crackles, swollen ankles, enlarged liver.
- Malignant hypertension: headache; confusion or depressed level of consciousness; deteriorating vision. Perform fundoscopy to check for fresh retinal haemorrhages, and dipstick urine for haematuria/proteinuria.
- Renal failure: check urine output and recent creatinine result.

2 If heart failure, malignant hypertension or renal failure, start to treat the cause and call the medical registrar for further management.

3 Otherwise, an elevated BP alone is seldom an indication for treatment. However, if the diastolic BP is greater than 130mmHg, put the patient to bed and prescribe an oral beta-blocker (if no contraindication – be very careful in patients with existing cardiac disease) or a calcium channel blocker and aim to reduce the blood pressure slowly over 2–3 days. Slow release of nifedipine can cause a dramatic fall in BP, so do not use without consulting your firm's policy. Call your senior if there is no response within 1 hour.

4 If the patient is in pain or anxious (common causes of elevated systolic pressure), provide analgesia and reassurance as appropriate.

Peri-operative hypertension

(see also Chapter 15, Surgery)

Pre-op hypertension: Most anaesthetists will not anaesthetize a patient with a diastolic BP >100mmHg. Discuss prescribing 10mg of nifedipine PO or further sedation with the anaesthetist or your senior. Five milligrams SL nifedipine will reduce the blood pressure within 5 minutes and may be repeated. Ensure the anaesthetist is aware of the problem. They may prefer to manage the patient with IV labetalol. Note: many analgesic drugs vasodilate and cause a drop in blood pressure after induction. *Post-op hypertension* is often related to pain and will settle with adequate analgesia. If persistent, discuss with your senior.

Hints

■ Do not treat hypertension for at least 48 hours following a stroke. Dropping the BP under these circumstances can cause brain damage due to infarction and loss of the ischaemic penumbra.

■ Raised ICP can cause hypertension and bradycardia (Cushing's reflex).

Hypotension

Hypotension is a common call, particularly post-op. Hypotension is seldom an emergency, but while on the phone ask how far the BP has fallen. A fall in systolic BP of >20mmHg is significant and >40mmHg (or systolic BP

<80 mmHg) is an emergency (see The moribund patient, below). Trends are more important than absolute values.

Differential diagnoses

■ Low blood volume (bleeding, dehydration)

■ Low peripheral resistance (post-general anaesthetic, infection, vasovagal, anaphylaxis, drugs: ACE inhibitors, nitrates, antihypertensives)

■ Poor cardiac function (arrhythmia, CCF, PE, tamponade, acute MI, valve failure, myocarditis, cardiomyopathy)

On the ward

1 See the patient and repeat the BP. If well but feeling faint, vasovagal or drug causes (including general anaesthesia) are likely. Drop the patient's head and raise the legs. Check the drug chart and do an ECG. Observe.

2 If unwell, feel their peripheries.

• If the patient has cold, clammy peripheries, consider:
– Hypovolaemia (bleeding or dehydrated: JVP down).
– Cardiac causes (MI, arrhythmia: raised JVP. Check for irregular pulse, basal crepitations, history of IHD, chest pain).
– PE (raised JVP, short of breath. Check for DVT, often no signs).
– Anaphylaxis (wheezy, short of breath, new drug started).
• If the patient has warm peripheries, consider sepsis (JVP variable, fever). Check for source of infection (chest, abdomen, urine, skin, cannulae, surgical wounds). Exclude immunocompromise (see The immunocompromised patient with fever, above). Note that in some patients, severe sepsis may cause circulatory shutdown (cold peripheries) without going through a stage of vasodilatation.

3 Treat according to the cause.

• If hypovolaemic:
– Place the patient's head down.
– Insert large bore IV cannulae. Give rapid IV fluid – colloids are usually first line.
– Face-mask O_2 100% (at least in the short term).
– Catheterize and monitor urine output.
– Consult your senior.
• If cardiac causes are most likely:
– The patient may go into shock. Get senior help and do an ECG stat.
– Give face-mask O_2 100% (at least in the short term).
– Sit the patient up if it is more comfortable for them.
– Arrange for a mobile erect CXR.
If septic:
– Large bore IV access, rapid IV fluids.
– Face-mask O_2 100%.
– Blood cultures (two times) are mandatory, FBC, U&E.
– Consult your senior urgently before giving broad-spectrum antibiotics.
• Less common causes:

– PE. Do urgent ECG, CXR and ABGs. Discuss anticoagulation with your senior.

– Anaphylaxis. Give 100% O_2; adrenaline 0.5 ml of a 1:1000 solution IM; salbutamol 5 mg nebulizer if wheezy; hydrocortisone 100–200 mg IV and chlorpheniramine 10 mg IV.

– Consider adrenal insufficiency, especially if the patient is on steroids or has a history of Addison's. Give hydrocortisone 100 mg IV (to cover the added stress of illness irrespective of the cause).

4 If you feel out of your depth, call for senior help immediately. Most often the cause is obvious but if not, do the following until help arrives:

- IV access.
- Face-mask O_2.
- ECG and mobile CXR.
- Bloods: FBC and clotting screen (INR and APTT), U&E, glucose, G&S (cross-match if suspect bleeding – see Upper gastrointestinal bleeds, above), ABGs or at least pulse oximeter, and blood cultures.
- Monitor urine output and consider catheterisation.

Hints

■ Post-op falls in BP are common and often due to opiate analgesia. If the patient is otherwise well with no evidence of bleeding, ask the nurses to continue to monitor the temp, BP and pulse and to call you if the patient becomes unwell or the BP substantially dips from its post-op plateau. The BP should rise as the anaesthesia wears off.

■ Always manually recheck the BP yourself, remembering to use a big enough cuff for large arms.

■ Bradycardia suggests a vasovagal or arrhythmia (e.g. complete heart block unless the patient is on beta blockers or has raised ICP).

■ If the patient is hypovolaemic, but there is no evidence of dehydration or bleeding, consider an occult bleed. Risk factors for occult bleeding include NSAIDs, stress ulceration, recent instrumentation/surgery, hidden fractures (especially in the elderly).

■ Dehydration is common in frail patients.

Insomnia

Avoid prescribing sleeping tablets without first considering why the patient cannot sleep. That said, it can be difficult to sleep on a noisy ward. Providing the patient does not take them home and develop dependency, short-acting sleeping tablets can be helpful.

Differential diagnoses and suggested management

1 Noise, light or too much daytime sleep. These are the commonest causes of insomnia in hospital and often the hardest to fix. Commonsense suggestions include:

- Suggesting that the patient need not worry about not sleeping at night. If they really need to sleep, they will.
- Avoiding stimulants before bedtime, such as cigarettes, tea or coffee.
- Wearing ear plugs and an eye visor.
- Ask the nursing staff whether it is possible to cancel the patient's early morning observations. Minimize noise from monitors.
- Resolve conflicts between patients (consider moving beds around).
- Move the patient to a side room if possible, or to a quieter corner of the ward.

2 Pain:

- Analgesia will facilitate sleep better than sleeping tablets.

3 Confusion, excessive anxiety or irritation, depression:

- Do not sedate the patient without excluding medical causes such as hypoxia, alcohol withdrawal, wrong drug dosages or electrolyte derangements (check fluid and drug charts).
- Depression is common in hospital patients (see Chapter 10, Depression). Be wary of inducing benzodiazepine addiction in such patients (who may be especially vulnerable). Seek psychiatric and pharmacological advice if in doubt.

4 Disturbed sleep pattern due to frequency of micturition, orthopnoea or PND:

- The patient may need better control of LVF. Avoid prescribing diuretics close to bedtime.

5 Disturbance in regular medication and bedtime habits:

- Often patients take an over-the-counter 'sleeping remedy' at home or have a supply of sleeping tablets which are not included in the GP's letter. The patient may not inform you about them unless specifically asked, and may suffer rebound insomnia in hospital.

Management with benzodiazepines

Benzodiazepines (e.g. temazepam 10–20 mg or oxazepam 15–30 mg) are the mainstay of therapy for insomnia, but some patients cannot tolerate them. Amitriptyline 25–50 mg nocte is useful when chronic pain accompanies sleep disturbance. Use lower doses of all sedatives in the elderly (consult the *BNF*). Beware co-prescribing with opiates.

If you prescribe a sedative, tell the patient to call the nursing staff if they need the toilet. Sedatives in an unfamiliar environment can cause falls.

Itching

Except in the unusual event of anaphylaxis, itching is rarely serious, but can be very distressing for the patient. Exclude simple dermatological problems before considering symptomatic treatment if the patient has skin lesions or a rash (see Rashes and skin lesions, below).

Differential diagnoses (if no visible skin lesions or rash)

- Dry skin
- Drugs or allergies
- Jaundice
- Early shingles

- Infestations (scabies, lice)
- Rarities: polycythaemia rubra vera (myeloproliferative diseases), Hodgkin's lymphoma

- Late renal failure

On the ward

1 Check the patient's skin for rashes or lesions. If present, see Rashes and skin lesions, below.

2 If there are no visible skin lesions, by far the most common cause of itching is dry skin, followed by drug reactions. Try to identify and replace the drug (seek pharmacological advice if unsure). Treat with emollient lotions after bathing (e.g. calamine lotion). Use cold compresses and moisturizers such as E45 for localized itching. Advise minimal use of soap and shampoo. Discuss alternatives with nurses.

3 If you are called at night and the patient is well, it is reasonable to treat symptomatically. Choose a sedating antihistamine at night (e.g. chlorpheniramine 4 mg tds) or a non-sedating one if preferred (e.g. terfenadine 60 mg bd).

Hints

Scabies is common and can cause intense itching anywhere on the body, except the head. The S-shaped burrows are easy to miss – look carefully around the itching site, particularly along the fingers and in the webs. Contrary to popular mythology, scabies does not imply that the patient is unhygienic. Consult the BNF for treatment of scabies and other infestations. Clothes and bedding need to be washed. Check with nurses that other nearby patients (or staff!) are not similarly infested.

Major trauma

It is unlikely that you will ever be solely responsible for patients with major trauma. However, if you are first to arrive at a trauma scene, it is worth having a mental plan of action. This is a simple format based on the Advanced Trauma Life Support (ATLS) protocol and is intended for initiating management of the person until senior help arrives.

On the ward (or A&E)

1 Do not be distracted by gruesome injuries. Start with a primary survey while senior help arrives. If you have time before the patient arrives, then don universal precautions and prepare the equipment you think will be necessary (airway adjuncts, cannulae and fluids, defibrillator and pads etc.).

2 Airway and cervical spine control: clear the airway of any blood, teeth and foreign bodies. Do not move the neck more than is necessary; get someone to

hold the neck still until a hard collar can be placed. Intubation requires skill, and in addition to moving the cervical spine it can cause cardiovascular instability and actually compromise oxygenation if performed incorrectly or carelessly. It is often best to start with an oropharyngeal airway.

3 Breathing and oxygenation: give 100% oxygen (by non-rebreathing bag) and check if the patient is breathing. If not, start basic life support (see Basic emergency routine, below).

4 Circulation and haemorrhage control: check for a carotid pulse and start basic life support. Get good intravenous access and start fluid resuscitation.

Hints

■ Once senior help arrives, continue with a specific task (e.g. intravenous access) and watch how the trauma team works. This is the best way to get experience.

■ Consider an Advanced Trauma Life Support (ATLS) course, particularly if you intend to pursue a career in trauma or surgery. Other excellent courses include Advanced Life Support (ALS) a more medically orientated course and Advanced Paediatric Life Support (APLS).

Minor trauma

Do not feel embarrassed about asking for help with minor injuries; the variety can make them more challenging than you might imagine. Despite this, you will learn quickly and common sense usually prevails.

The most common minor injury results from falls in hospital (see Falls, above). When answering your bleep, ask for:

■ BP and pulse.

■ Any analgesia the patient has received.

On the ward

1 Start by assessing airway, breathing and circulation.

2 When seeing the patient, ask about likely causes (see Falls, above).

3 Give analgesia if the patient is in pain. Paracetamol or ibuprofen are usually adequate.

4 Things to consider with any injury are:

● Skin break: a plaster or dressing is adequate in most cases. If there is a laceration, clean the wound. If the skin edges are opposed to each other and are not likely to be displaced, leave well alone. Otherwise a stereostrip or a suture may be necessary.

● Soft tissue injury: analgesia and rest is sufficient. For limbs or joints, consider a splint and ice. Advise early mobility of the affected area once swelling subsides.

• Fracture: if there is bony tenderness, consider performing a plain X-ray of the area. Two views are more useful than one (see Hints, below for X-ray guidelines).
• Organ injury: if concerned, reassess airway, breathing and circulation, and seek urgent senior help.

Hints

• The best person to ask about minor injuries is usually a senior nurse. They will have seen it all before.
• Fracture clinics are useful places to send well patients with fractures for follow-up after discharge.
• The 'Ottowa rule' for ankle injuries states that there is usually no need to perform an X-ray on an ankle if:
○ The person is weight-bearing after the injury and can weight bear for 2 steps.

○ No tenderness over the posterior or tip of the medial malleolus.
○ No tenderness over the posterior or tip of the lateral malleolus.
○ No tenderness over the calcaneum or navicular.
○ No tenderness over the base of the 5th metatarsal.
○ No tenderness of the proximal fibula.
Document these when tested and lower your threshold for reattenders.

The moribund patient

If you are called to see a 'flat' patient, don't panic. You usually have more time than you think. The priority is to buy time by supporting the vital functions while getting basic background information and examining as you go. Call your senior early and do not be afraid to call the crash team before the patient arrests. This is often advised but rarely undertaken. Think CASH (Table 7.8)! Stay calm and remain polite; if the doctor panics, so will everyone else.

Table 7.8 Differential diagnoses to a moribund patient (acronym: CASH).

Chest	Abdomen	Systemic	Head
■ Pulmonary oedema	■ Haemorrhage	■ Drug overdose (e.g. opiates)	■ CVA
■ MI	■ Perforated bowel		■ Post-ictal
■ Arrhythmia	■ Pancreatitis	■ Hypothermia	■ Hydrocephalus
■ Pneumonia		■ Septicaemia	■ SAH
■ Asthma		■ Hypoglycaemia	
■ Pulmonary embolus		■ Anaphylaxis	
■ Dissecting aneurysm		■ Major electrolyte derangement	
■ Pneumothorax			

On the ward

1 See the patient urgently. Check their ABC:

- Airway clear? Y/N
- Breathing? Y/N; Trachea central? Bilateral breath sounds?
- Circulation – Pulse? Y/N; If Y – BP?

2 Bring (or get somebody to bring) the crash trolley to hand and to call the crash team if an arrest looks imminent.

3 Give O_2.

4 Establish large bore IV access: 16G if possible. Don't rush. Consider inserting two cannulae at separate sites.

5 If BP <80mmHg, consider starting a rapid colloid infusion (Haemaccel, Volplex or Gelofusin) unless a cardiac cause is probable. Use saline, if sepsis is likely.

6 While the infusion is being set up, quickly assess preceding symptoms, PMH and current medications. Examine the chest and heart.

7 If a cardiac cause is likely:

- Do an ECG and request a mobile CXR. Do not delay treatment.
- Pulmonary oedema, arrhythmias or MI are the most likely causes. Consider pericardial tamponade.

8 Exclude hypoglycaemia or opiate overdose:

- If blood glucose is less than 2.5mmol/l, give 50ml of 50% glucose IV (flush vein with saline afterwards) or 1mg glucagon IV/IM/SC.
- Note the size of pupils. Give naloxone 400–800μg IV if the patient has pinpoint pupils and is on opiates. Repeat if necessary.

9 Listen to the chest. If markedly tachypnoeic in the absence of pulmonary oedema or pneumothorax, consider PE.

10 Feel the peripheries. If the patient has warm peripheries with hypotension, consider sepsis.

11 Consider anaphylaxis:

- New drug started recently, hypotensive, SOB, wheezy, swollen lips/eyelids, urticarial rash.
- Give 100% O_2; adrenaline 1ml of a 1:1000 solution IM/IV; salbutamol 5mg nebulizer; hydrocortisone 100mg IV and chlorpheniramine 10mg IV.

If the cause is not clear, do a brief neurological examination: level of consciousness (obeying commands), pupils and eye movements, limb tone, reflexes and plantars. Consider occult bleeding, post-ictal states and meningitis. Seek senior advice.

12 Urgent investigations:

- ECG.
- FBC and INR, U&E, glucose, amylase.

- ABGs.
- Mobile CXR, as erect as possible to check for free air under the diaphragm. View carefully for a pneumothorax, often missed in a panic.

Hints

■ Metabolic acidosis, confirmed by an ABG, can cause compensatory tachypnoea. If the patient has metabolic acidosis and hypotension, consider sepsis, ischaemic bowel or perforated viscus or pancreatitis and acute renal failure.

■ Relieve a tension pneumothorax by inserting a needle or Venflon into the second intercostal space, mid-clavicular line.

Nausea and vomiting

Any acute illness can cause non-specific N&V. Be wary, however, of prescribing anti-emetics without also investigating the cause. If the patient is distressed, it is reasonable to give an anti-emetic before examining them.

Differential diagnoses

1 Surgical conditions

- Intestinal obstruction (adhesion, hernias, tumours) and peritonism (perforation, pancreatitis, etc.)

2 Medical causes

- Local causes
- Oesophagitis
- Gastritis
- Peptic ulcer
- Central causes
- Raised ICP (tumour, meningitis, subdural haemorrhage, etc.)
- Migraine
- Systemic causes
- Infection (UTI, pneumonia, gastroenteritis)
- Metabolic (organ failure, electrolyte imbalance – Na^+, K^+, Ca^{2+})
- Drug reactions (opiates, digoxin, NSAIDs, dopamine agonists, chemotherapy)

3 Special causes

- Pregnancy

On the ward

1 Exclude severe dehydration (BP sitting and lying).

2 Rule out common surgical conditions – intestinal obstruction and peritonism.

3 Think about medical causes as above.

4 Special considerations:

- Is the patient pregnant? Do Beta-Human Chorionic Gonadotrophin (B-HCG) levels.
- In the elderly, an inferior acute MI can present with N&V in the absence of pain. Do ECG and serial cardiac enzymes.

5 When there is no obvious cause after history and examination:

- If the patient had a single episode of vomiting without associated symptoms or signs, ask the nurses to observe the patient and monitor temp, BP, pulse and urine output. Dipstick the urine.
- If N&V persists or there is systemic upset, consider MSU, FBC, U&E.

6 Further investigations to consider include:

- Ca^{2+}, Mg^{2+}, phosphate, amylase.
- ABGs if severe vomiting.

7 Management options to control symptoms: The two most commonly used drugs are prochlorperazine: 25 mg PR or 12.5 mg IM and metoclopramide 10 mg IM or IV (caution in young women due to risk of dystonic reactions like an oculogyric crisis). Alternatives include:

- Cyclizine lactate: 50 mg IM or IV.
- Domperidone: 30–60 mg PR.
- Droperidol: 1–10 mg IV or IM.
- 5-HT$_3$ antagonists (e.g. ondansetron, granisetron) are very effective but are expensive and usually reserved for chemotherapy-induced N&V. However, if they are the correct choice, you should prescribe them.
- Diphenhydramine counteracts extra-pyramidal side effects of phenothiazines.

Oxygen therapy

Methods of oxygen delivery

Face-masks (e.g. system 22 or Ventimasks) are good for the acute situation. Controlled percentage face-masks control the amount of O_2 the patient receives, and are graded 24%, 28%, 35%, 40% and 60%. You need to adjust the O_2 flow rate at the wall or cylinder, according to the rate printed on the mask – usually about 2 l/minute for 24% masks and 15 l/minute for 60% masks. It takes at least 15–20 minutes for blood gases to equilibrate after changing the percentage of inspired O_2. This is *not* a reason to delay giving oxygen; there is no justification in removing a patient from oxygen for a 'baseline' ABG.

Nasal specs are useful if the patient cannot tolerate a face-mask and for longer-term O_2 therapy. It is difficult to regulate O_2 delivery with nasal specs, so regular blood gas checks may be necessary. For standard size specs, a flow rate of 4–6 l/minute is usual for achieving an inspired O_2 percentage of 30–40%.

For patients with chronic obstructive pulmonary disease

Under normal conditions, the concentration of CO_2 in the blood is the primary stimulus of the respiratory drive. Some patients with severe COPD become insensitive to CO_2 levels and are dependent on low O_2 levels (mild hypoxia) to maintain their respiratory effort. If you give too much O_2, the hypoxic stimulus may be lost and they will hypoventilate, leading to CO_2 retention (hypercarbia). This can cause CO_2 narcosis and death. However, this is an unusual cause of death and simple hypoxia is a much more common killer.

Therefore, when non-emergency O_2 therapy is required in patients with COPD:

1 Start with a 24% face-mask and re-measure the ABGs after 1 hour to ensure that the CO_2 levels are not rising. You need to find a level that achieves a fine balance between improving oxygenation and keeping the CO_2 at a safe level. Ask for senior advice if the CO_2 level rises $> 1.5\,kPa$ above the previous ABG level or rises above $8\,kPa$.

2 If the CO_2 level does not rise but hypoxia is still a problem, increase the oxygen to 28% then 35%, etc., repeating the ABGs an hour after each change.

3 If you cannot increase the percentage O_2, despite persisting hypoxia, because of hypercapnia, a doxapram infusion or mechanical ventilation may be necessary – discuss with your team. Bipap is a common choice of non-invasive ventilation in type 2 respiratory failure due to COPD.

In emergencies, use 100% O_2, even when the patient is known to have moderately severe COPD (unless you know they are fitting from CO_2 narco-sis!). Hypoxia kills quickly (within minutes), whereas CO_2 narcosis kills slowly (over hours). You will have time to check the ABGs if there is a history of COPD. If the CO_2 is rising, you may need help but withholding oxygen from a patient with a falling O_2 is hard to clinically defend.

Hints

■ Use a humidifier with O_2 if possible.
■ Patients may be left on O_2 for longer than they need it. Always ask whether or not they really need it, as the face-mask and straps are uncomfortable.
■ Strictly, you are supposed to prescribe O_2 therapy on the drug chart.

Pulse oximetry

Pulse oximetry measures the percentage of blood O_2 saturation. It is not a direct assay of PaO_2 or $PaCO_2$. It is not as trustworthy as arterial blood gases, particularly in COPD patients, as they may retain CO_2 in spite of reasonable percentage O_2 saturation. Also, pulse oximetry may not detect low PaO_2 due to the steep sigmoid curve of the O_2 saturation curve. If in doubt, do ABGs.

Phlebitis

Phlebitis is indicated by pain and redness at IV sites, and is prevented by changing the IV site every 2–3 days (important if the patient has a structural cardiac abnormality or prosthetic valve).

Management

1 Remove the cannula and apply heat (e.g. damp, warm towel).

2 Elevate the limb.

3 Give mild analgesia if the site is very painful (e.g. a NSAID such as ibuprofen 400–600 mg tds).

4 Suppurative phlebitis is more worrying (pus at the IV entry site, induration, fever and enlarged draining lymph nodes). Try to express some pus and send a swab to microbiology for urgent MC&S. Prescribe IV antibiotics to cover *Staphylococcus aureus*. If the patient is well, flucloxacillin alone may suffice. The addition of penicillin or substitution with co-amoxiclav may be necessary. Discuss local protocols with a microbiologist. Surgical drainage is occasionally required.

Potassium

Hyperkalaemia

K^+ greater than 6.5 mmol/l needs urgent treatment, but first exclude false-positives from old or haemolysed samples. Repeat the sample if in doubt. In the hospital setting, by far the commonest cause of hyperkalaemia is drugs or renal failure. Differential diagnoses are:

- K^+ sparing diuretics – spironolactone, amiloride, triamterene (beware: if these are given with ACE inhibitors rapid, fatal rises in potassium can occur)
- ACE inhibitors
- Excessive K^+ supplements
- Metabolic acidosis
- Acute renal failure
- Diabetic ketoacidosis
- Cell lysis
- Massive tissue trauma
- Massive blood transfusion
- Mineralocorticoid deficiency
- Addison's disease

On the ward

1 See the patient. Repeat K^+ and check their renal function (U&E). In the meantime, if the initial K^+ was greater than 6.5 mmol/l:

2 Do an ECG urgently (look for widened QRS complexes and peaked T waves).

3 Get access and give calcium gluconate (or carbonate) 10 ml of a 10% solution IV over 10 minutes.

4 Do urgent ABGs. If acidotic, discuss with your senior. The use of bicarbonate (100 ml of a 4.2% solution) is highly controversial.

5 Give 10–15 units soluble insulin with 50 g of glucose 50% IV.

6 Set up a continuous 50% glucose infusion (50 ml/hour) with insulin according to 1–2-hourly glucose readings (insulin drives K^+ back into cells).

7 Consider polystyrene sulphonate resin (calcium resonium) 15 g 6–8-hourly PO or 30 g in methylcellulose solution PR. As this causes severe constipation, consider giving a laxative at the same time. This is only appropriate for chronic hyperkalaemia not an acute event.

Hypokalaemia

In the hospital setting, hypokalaemia is usually caused by diuretics, inappropriate replacement fluids or taking blood from the drip arm. Differential diagnoses are:

- Inadequate potassium replacement in IV fluids
- Renal losses
- Diuretics
- Other drugs – amphotericin B, carbenicillin, ticarcillin
- Excess mineralocorticoid (tumours)
- GI tract losses
- Diarrhoea
- Vomiting

- Intestinal fistulae, villous adenoma
- Intracellular potassium shifts
- Alkalosis
- Insulin and glucose administration

On the ward

1 See the patient. If the K^+ is less than 2.5 mmol/l, or less than 3.0 and the patient is taking digoxin, you need to replace K^+ urgently, as there is a risk of arrhythmias:

- Give 20 mmol/hour KCl at a concentration not exceeding 40 mmol/l (maximum 60 mmol/l in emergencies via a central line). Concentrated K^+ damages peripheral veins. Never give bolus KCl, which can cause fatal arrhythmias. If a central line is available, 20 mmol/hour in 50–100 ml of 5% dextrose can be infused, but ensure that the infusion rate is monitored. Central infusion is paradoxically safer due to the faster flow rates. 20 mmol/l of potassium will raise the serum value by around 0.25 mmol/l.
- Do an urgent ECG, looking for low, small T waves. Consider an ECG monitor. Patients with arrhythmias should be transferred to the CCU.
- Monitor K^+ 4-hourly until stable.

2 If the K^+ is between 2.5 and 3.0 mmol/l:

- Oral replacement therapy is usually sufficient (see below). However, if the patient is at risk for arrhythmias (e.g. recent MI or on therapy for arrhythmias), give cautious IV therapy (10–15 mmol/hour).

3 If the K^+ is greater than 3.0 mmol/l:

- Give oral replacement therapy unless the patient is NBM or vomiting. Prescribe 80–120 mmol K^+ in divided doses per day. There is a wide range of pills with varying amounts of K^+ in each. You can also advise the patient to eat K^+-containing foods such as bananas and chocolate.

4 Investigations to consider:

- Monitor K^+ every 1–2 days.
- Do ABGs if you suspect alkalosis (alkalosis causes intracellular K^+ shifts).
- Consider measuring Mg. Hypomagnesaemia may cause the hypokalaemia to be refractory to therapy.

A rough guide to calculating the total amount of potassium replacement required

In adults, a drop of plasma K^+ from 4 to 3 mmol/l represents a total body deficit of 100–200 mmol K^+. Each further 1 mmol/l drop below 3 mmol/l represents a deficit of an additional 200–400 mmol K^+.

Hints

- Avoid slow-K non-effervescent tablets, as they cause severe oesophageal and gastric irritation. Use the horrible tasting, but more effective, soluble effervescent tablets or syrups. The smaller 'slow K+' tablets have a sustained release profile but are easier to swallow.

■ In patients with normal renal function, it is difficult to overdose with oral K$^+$. However, DO NOT give K$^+$ if the patient is oliguric. Consult your senior.

■ Low plasma bicarbonate levels suggest that the patient has long-standing, intracellular K$^+$ depletion. K$^+$ replacement can take days.

■ Contrary to popular belief, hypokalaemia secondary to vomiting is due to metabolic alkalosis (which causes intracellular K$^+$ shift and renal excretion of K$^+$), not to loss of K$^+$ in gastric juices, which contain very little K$^+$.

■ Be careful in prescribing long-term oral K$^+$ supplements for patients to take home. It is usually wise to limit TTOs to 3 days with GP review.

Rashes and skin lesions

The algorithm below is designed to help you make an initial diagnosis of the patient's rash or skin lesion. By far, the commonest cause of new rashes in hospital is drug reactions, but psoriasis, shingles and other relapsing skin conditions can all flare up with the stress of illness. Dermatologists are usually helpful and keen for referrals. Seek their advice if in any doubt.

Questions to ask are:

1 Are the lesions filled with fluid?
● No → go to the next question.
● Clear fluid → (1) vesiculobullous diseases.
● Pus → (2) pustular diseases.

2 Are the lesions coloured but not red?
  Yellow → (3) yellow lesions.
  White → (4) white lesions.
  Brown → (5) brown lesions.
  Skin coloured → (6) skin coloured papules and nodules.

3 If the lesions are red, are they scaling?
● No scaling:
  – Macular/flat → (7) vascular reactions.
  – Papular/ → (8) inflammatory raised papules/nodules.
  – Scaling:
  – No epithelial → (9) papulosquamous disruption diseases.
  – Epithelial → (10) eczematous disruption reactions.

Disease categories 1–10

1 Vesiculobullous diseases:

● Vesicles: Herpes simplex; shingles; chicken pox; tinea pedis; scabies; dermatitis herpetiformis; dyshidrosis.

● Bullae: pemphigus; pemphigoid; bullous impetigo; erythema multiforme bullosum.

2 Pustular diseases:

● Acne; folliculitis; candidiasis; rosacea.

3 Yellow lesions:

• Xanthelasma; necrobiosis lipoidicum.

4 White lesions:

• Tinea versicolor; pityriasis alba; vitiligo.

5 Brown lesions:

• Macules – freckles and lentigines.

• Papules and nodules – junctional or compound naevi; melanoma; seborrhoeic keratoses.

• Patches and plaques – café-au-lait spots; giant pigmented hairy naevus.

6 Skin coloured papules and nodules:

• Rough surface – warts; actinic keratoses; squamous cell carcinoma.

• Smooth surface – condylomata acuminata; basal cell carcinoma; epidermoid cysts; lipomas; molluscum contagiosum.

7 Vascular reactions:

• Blanching lesions – macular and diffuse erythema (toxic erythema, e.g. skin rash of viral illness); urticaria; erythema multiforme; erythema nodosum.

• Non-blanching (purpuric) lesions – the vasculitides.

8 Inflammatory papules and nodules:

• Papules – insect bites; pyogenic granulomas; cherry angiomas; granuloma annulare.

• Nodules – furunculosis ± cellulitis.

9 Papulosquamous diseases:

• Plaque formation – psoriasis; lupus erythematosus; mycosis fungoides; tinea corporis; tinea cruris and tinea pedis.

• Predominantly papular – lichen planus, secondary syphilis, pityriasis rosea.

10 Eczematous reactions:

• Atopic dermatitis; dyshidrotic eczema; contact dermatitis; others.

Diagnosing skin tumours

▤ Melanoma

• Itching; crusting; bleeding; change in size, shape or colour of mole; weight loss; satellite lesions

■ Basal cell carcinoma

• Pearly nodule/ulcer with prominent blood vessels

■ Squamous cell carcinoma

• Non-healing; crusting ulcer with rolled edge

Hints

■ Generalized erythematous rash (or blistering) and fever should ring alarm bells as they may be associated with serious bacterial infections (e.g. streptococcal and staphylococcal).

■ Take very seriously any new rash in people who are immunocompromised (e.g. HIV, high-dose chemotherapy, leukaemia), as this could herald sepsis, which may be rapidly fatal.

■ Similarly, take seriously a new rash in people taking medication that may cause agranulocytosis (e.g. ticlopidine or carbimazole).

Shortness of breath

When answering your bleep
Ask the nurse to assess the respiratory rate, pulse, BP and, if possible, peak flows (essential in a comprehensive assessment of respiratory function) and pulse oximetry readings.

Differential diagnoses

- Acute LVF
- Asthma
- Pulmonary embolus
- Pneumonia
- Pneumothorax
- COPD exacerbated by acute illness

Rarely
- Pericardial tamponade
- Anaphylaxis

On the ward

1 See the patient. Check the T, BP and pulse and assess for respiratory distress (respiratory rate >30/minute ± cyanosis) and hypotension.

2 If the patient is hypotensive, consider: acute MI, large PE, tension pneumothorax, pericardial tamponade and anaphylaxis. Lower the patient's head and institute emergency treatment. Get senior assistance (see Hypotension, above).

3 If the patient is markedly tachypnoeic or cyanosed:

- Give O_2. Even if the patient has COPD, it is safe to give initial O_2 and reduce as soon as possible (hypoxia kills quickly, high CO_2 kills slowly) (see Oxygen therapy, above).
- Exclude pneumothorax with auscultation.
- Give salbutamol 5 mg stat using a nebulizer. Repeat as necessary.
- Examine quickly for acute pulmonary oedema (JVP, basal crackles or effusion). If present, sit the patient up, give furosemide 40–80 mg IV, diamorphine 5 mg IV slowly and an anti-emetic (e.g. metoclopramide 10 mg IV/IM). Consider MI or arrhythmia and do an urgent ECG.
- Request a mobile CXR.
- Do ABGs.
- Notify your senior. Get help early if the patient is deteriorating.

Important note: if you cannot distinguish between early pulmonary oedema, asthma or pneumonia (often difficult to differentiate), treat for all three (see [3] above). If there are no signs of heart failure or asthma, consider pulmonary embolus. Heparinize if in doubt (see p. 126) and confirm the diagnosis later.

4 If the patient is not acutely distressed: take a full history and examination. Do not forget to ask about chest pain or leg swelling, history of asthma or IHD and any recent changes in medication. Consider the differential diagnosis and treat accordingly.

5 Investigations to consider:

- FBC, U&E.
- ABGs.
- CXR (expiratory to show a pneumothorax better).
- ECG.
- Consider urgent ECHO or FAST scan if you suspect tamponade.

Hints

■ Hypoxia can cause euphoria, so do not be reassured by an apparently undistressed patient. Be guided by the signs.

■ A good way to assess respiratory rate is to breathe with the patient, as this also reveals abnormal breathing rhythms (not all dyspnoeic patients are tachypnoeic).

■ Patients at risk for pneumothorax include those with a central line, pneumonia, COPD or asthma. Pneumothorax is easy to miss on CXR; get an *expiratory* film.

■ Psychogenic SOB (hyperventilation) is suggested by peri-oral tingling, pins and needles, carpopedal spasm and especially alkalosis on ABGs. Treat by having the patient breathe into a paper bag. Diazepam may be necessary.

■ A fever suggests infection, but also consider PE or MI.

■ Check for pulsus paradoxus (drop in BP of greater than 10 mmHg on inspiration), which suggests an acute exacerbation of COPD, asthma or tamponade.

■ If possible, take an ABG sample before starting the patient on O_2.

Diagnosing the important common conditions causing acute SOB

■ Acute LVF
- Raised JVP
- S3 gallop
- Cold peripheries
- Basal inspiratory crackles

■ Severe asthma
- Pulse > 120/minute, rate > 30/minute
- Pulsus paradoxus (BP drop < 10 mmHg on inspiration)
- PEFR < 100
- Rising $PaCO_2$ (anything over 5 kPa is worrying in the face of tachypnoea)
- Exhausted patient barely able to speak

■ Pulmonary embolus
- DVT, pleuritic chest pain, pleural rub
- RV strain: raised JVP, RV gallop
- RV strain on ECG: prominent R waves in V_1–V_2 (common), inverted T waves in III and V_{1-4}, deep S wave in I, Q wave in III (less common)

■ Pneumothorax
- Chest hyper-resonant to percussion
- Markedly decreased vocal resonance (a very useful sign!)
- Decreased breath sounds
- Often funny noises or clicks with heart beat during respiration

The sick patient

The following is a checklist of things that you should consider when seeing any patient who is very unwell (modify in light of the specific system involved):

1 What are the temp, BP, pulse and respiratory rates?

2 Are ABC adequate?

3 Does the patient need:

- Analgesia?
- ABGs or pulse oximetry?
- Baseline bloods?
- CXR (mobile)?
- ECG or ECG monitor?
- IV access?
- IV fluids?
- O_2?
- Senior opinion?
- Urinary catheter?

Sodium

Hyponatraemia

Mild to moderate hyponatraemia is common in hospital due to excess IV (hypotonic) fluids. Hyponatraemia usually develops over days; replacement of Na^+ should be cautious. More urgent treatment is required if there are neurological symptoms which range from lethargy to severe confusion or coma, but symptoms should not be ascribed to hyponatraemia if the serum Na^+ is $>125\,mmol/l$.

Differential diagnoses

- Over hydration with IV fluids
- Renal/metabolic – Nephrotic syndrome, Addison's Disease, Interstitial renal disease, *SIADH*
- CNS
- Malignancy
- Drugs – chlorpropamide, haloperidol, thiazide diuretics
- Chest-infection, CCF
- Cirrhosis
- Severe hypothyroidism

On the ward

1 See the patient and assess their fluid balance (JVP, fluid chart, chest).

- If dehydrated, measure urinary Na^+.
- If urinary $Na^+ >20\,mmol/l$ with hyponatraemia, consider renal causes.
- If urinary $Na^+ <20\,mmol/l$, consider other causes.
- If not dehydrated, is the patient puffy?
- If yes, volume overload is likely but exclude nephrotic syndrome, CCF, cirrhosis and severe hypothyroidism.
- If no, but the urine is concentrated (osmolality $<500\,mmol/kg$ or high specific gravity), SIADH is most likely. Look for the cause (see Differential diagnoses, above).

2 Investigations to consider:

- Urinary Na^+, urine and plasma osmolality, U&E, liver chemistry. • CXR.
- Discuss others with senior according to clinical setting.

3 Management: Treat underlying cause. Urgent Na^+ replacement may be required if patient is severely symptomatic and $Na^+ <125\,mmol/l$. Seek expert guidance.

- If hyponatraemia is mild with no symptoms, and the patient is not dehydrated, treat by restricting fluid only. Start with 1.5l/day, and reduce by 50 ml/day if there is no improvement within a few days.
- If the patient is dehydrated with normal renal function, give 0.9% saline.
- Beware of correcting hyponatraemia too rapidly. This can cause central pontine myelinolysis with irreversible brain damage and locked in syndrome. IV hypertonic saline is rarely required unless the patient is fitting or unconscious. Discuss with your senior.

Hints

■ Hyponatraemia due to ectopic ADH secretion may be the first sign of a small-cell carcinoma of the lung.

■ SIADH can only be diagnosed if the patient is hyponatraemic and the urine is more concentrated than the plasma.

■ Mild hyponatraemia is frequently seen in severely ill patients ('sick cell' syndrome) but rarely needs treatment.

Transfusions

While blood transfusions are common in hospital, always be alert to transfusion reactions. Remember to reassure your patient that all blood is tested for HIV and other viral infections.

Blood transfusions

For chronic stable anaemia (see Anaemia, above)
Remember that these patients have had a low Hb for a long time. Providing there has been no additional acute fall in Hb, transfusion is not urgent and is seldom needed in the middle of the night. Ensure any blood tests (FBC, iron studies, B_{12} and folate, blood film, Hb electrophoresis) have been sent before transfusion. Transfusion should be slow, to avoid causing heart failure.

1 Estimate the red cell deficit (1 unit of packed cells raises the Hb by 1 g/dl).

2 In general:

- Transfuse the patient to >8 g/dl if they have a reversible cause of anaemia.
- Transfuse to >10 g/dl if they have an irreversible cause of anaemia (e.g. myelodysplasia).

3 Check the patient's pulse, BP, JVP and chest for basal crackles as a baseline before transfusing.

4 The rate of transfusion will depend on the clinical setting and the presence or absence of heart disease.

- Transfuse slowly (each unit over 4–6 hours) in the elderly.
- Give furosemide 20–40 mg PO before the first unit and then with alternate bags if you are concerned about heart failure.
- If the patient becomes fluid overloaded, give furosemide (frusemide) 40 mg IV (do not mix in the bag). Repeat as necessary.

5 If the patient has had a previous transfusion reaction, give hydrocortisone (100 mg IV) and chlorpheniramine (chlorphenamine) (10 mg IV) before the transfusion. This is often necessary in patients who have had multiple transfusions.

Hints

■ Do not transfuse a new patient with chronic anaemia without checking iron and TIBC, B$_{12}$ and folate (see Anaemia, above).

■ Do not transfuse blood through lines used for solutions containing dextrose, as this causes red cells to clump.

In the acute setting

1 Estimate how many units of blood the patient will need. In the acute setting, the Hb level lags the actual red cell loss by 12–24 hours.

2 Packed cells have few clotting factors and platelets. Therefore, for transfusions of more than 4 units, check the INR and APTT, and add 1–2 units of FFP for every 4 units of packed cells.

3 Transfuse to above 8 g/dl. Recheck the FBC daily.

Hints

■ In acute and subacute bleeds, the MCV is normal.

■ Remember hidden fractures in the elderly. The thigh can conceal 2 l of blood.

Platelet transfusions

Indications

■ Platelet count $<20 \times 10^9$/l, or $<40 \times 10^9$/l and the patient is at risk of bleeding (e.g. going for major surgery).

■ Thrombocytopenia or dysfunctional platelets with active bleeding.

To order platelets, you only need to know the patient's blood group; a crossmatch is not necessary. If the patient has had a previous platelet transfusion reaction (common), administer hydrocortisone (100 mg IV) and chlorpheniramine (chlorphenamine) (10 mg IV) before the transfusion. If the patient has had previous severe reactions, discuss HLA-matched platelets with the haematologist (they are very expensive).

Hints

Platelet clumping often leads to erroneously low platelet counts. You can ask the haematologist to confirm an unexpectedly low count by manual differentiation.

Transfusion reactions

■ *Slow rising fever <40°C*

A fever of <40°C is very common during transfusions. It is treated by slowing the transfusion and giving paracetamol (1 g 6-hourly) if the patient is otherwise well.

■ *Severe transfusion reaction*

If the patient has a rapid temp spike >39°C at the beginning of a transfusion, temp >40°C at any time, an urticarial rash or wheezing and hypotension (anaphylaxis):

1 Stop the transfusion immediately. Send the bag and line to the lab for analysis.

2 Give the patient hydrocortisone 200 mg IV and chlorpheniramine (chlorphenamine) 10 mg IV stat.

3 If the patient deteriorates or becomes hypotensive, call for immediate help and give 0.5–1.0 ml of a 1:1000 solution of adrenaline IM.

4 Monitor closely (risk of shock and acute renal failure).

Urine, low output (oliguria/anuria)

Oliguria is defined as a urine output of less than 500 ml in 24 hours. The minimum urine output is 0.5 ml/kg/hour (35 ml/hour in a 70-kg patient). Urgent assessment is required for an output of less than 20 ml/hour, a daily output of less than 500 ml or for painful urinary retention (see Table 7.9).

Table 7.9 Differential diagnoses of oliguria/anuria.

Pre-rental	Renal	Post-renal
Hypovolaemia /Hypotension	Nephrotoxic drugs	Blocked catheter
■ Occult bleed	■ Aminoglycosides	
■ Dehydration	■ IV contrast dyes	■ Urinary retention
■ Cardiac failure	■ Penicillins	■ Prostate enlargement
	■ Sulphonamides	■ Tumour
Apparent hypovolaemia	■ NSAIDs	■ Idiopathic
■ 'Leaky capillaries'		
■ Septicaemia	■ Systemic diseases	
■ Pancreatitis	■ SLE	
■ Post-major surgery	■ Malignant hypertension	
■ CCF, liver failure	■ Interstitial nephritis	
Renal artery occlusion		
■ Emboli		
■ Aortic dissection		

On the ward

1 Check first for post-renal causes:

● Palpate the patient's abdomen for a distended bladder. Catheterize if the patient is in urinary retention. This can easily be confirmed at the bedside with a bladder scan. Remember to do a PR in men and PV in woman once the bladder is relieved, to exclude prostatic disease and pelvic masses, respectively. If a PSA is needed, then this should be taken before rectal examination.

• If the patient is already catheterized, ask the nurse to do a small volume (100 ml) sterile bladder washout to make sure that it isn't blocked.

2 Check for hypovolaemia and sepsis:

• Check BP, pulse, temp and JVP.

• Assess fluid balance. Remember to include unrecorded losses (sweating, incontinence, etc.).

• Consider sepsis.

• If the patient is hypovolaemic, challenge with 500 ml IV normal saline over 30 minutes. If there is no urinary response, recheck their JVP and repeat the fluid challenge if it is low (and there is no risk of inducing CCF). In patients with poor cardiac function, give 200 ml challenges. Consider a central line to monitor the CVP if the patient is acutely unwell.

3 Check for CCF:

• Oliguria indicates very poor cardiac output. Management should be discussed with your senior.

4 If you are unsure of the cause, get senior advice and do the following urgently:

• U&E. A creatinine : urea ratio of less than 10:1 (i.e. urea disproportionately raised) suggests a pre-renal cause.

• Urinary Na^+. A urinary Na^+ of less than 15 mmol/l suggests pre-renal causes; more than 20 mmol/l suggests renal causes.

• Urine microscopy.

Hints

■ Remember to alter the doses of renally excreted drugs if the patient has prolonged oliguria. Patients with peripheral oedema may still be hypovolaemic.

■ Never use K^+-containing solutions for fluid challenges, as the impaired kidney may not be able to clear K^+.

■ In a patient with oliguria or anuria (with a near-empty bladder), catheters can be very uncomfortable. This is relieved by a bladder washout. A washout will also exclude a blocked catheter as a cause for poor urine output.

■ If a catheterized patient has passed absolutely no urine for many hours, the most likely cause is a blocked catheter. Palpate for a distended bladder. If a washout does not clear the catheter, try replacing with a new catheter.

Basic emergency routine

■ If the patient is flat or very ill, get help fast and don't hesitate to call the crash team if you feel the patient is deteriorating. Check ABC.

■ Briefly check for the 6 Hs:

1 Hypoglycaemia

2 Hypotension

3 Hypothermia

4 Hypovolaemia

5 Hypoxia

6 Arrhythmias (Heart)

Check the BP (lying and sitting) and JVP, look for cyanosis and measure the respiratory rate. A good way to do the latter is to breathe with the patient. Do a blood glucose stick, ECG, pulse oximeter reading and consider doing a blood gas and rectal temperature. Check urine output.

■ Ensure good IV access and consider a catheter and O_2. Monitor the patient's condition (quarter to half-hourly observations, ECG monitor, urine output) and do baseline investigations (see below).

■ If the patient is well or stable, you have time for a more thorough history and examination, although this does not mean a full CNS examination at 2 a.m. (unless the problem is neurological!) For stable patients, urgent investigations are usually unnecessary and impede technicians' processing real emergencies. Before ordering new tests in the middle of the night, look at recent baseline tests and consider how new information will change management. If a test is not urgent but you don't want to forget it, write the card for the morning and write it in the notes.

Obstetrics and gynaecology calls

Thanks to Dr Lyann Edwards-Gross for contribution to this section.

Talking to the patient

Many gynaecology patients will be shy and base their behaviour on yours. If you are shy, they will be shy too. If you are direct with your questioning and professional, they will be more forthcoming. History taking should also expand on the previous gynaecological and obstetric history. This should focus on:

1 Previous pregnancies and details (e.g. full term, miscarriages and terminations).

2 Ask directly about miscarriages and TOPs.

3 LMP, cycle information.

4 Cervical smear.

5 Sexual history – ask directly whether they are sexually active, what type of contraception and about any sexually transmitted diseases. Patients will not volunteer information if you don't ask!

● Find out what the patient has come for – even more important in O&G as many patients have unspoken concerns and an agenda. Don't forget to ask if pregnancy is planned. If not, ask her how she feels about it and who is entitled to know.

● Listen to the patient. Female patients with pelvic pain will often get mislabelled as gynaecology patients. Keep an open mind. Appendicitis referred to as an ectopic pregnancy is common.

● If taking GP referrals, always take clear details and think where and when is best to see the patient. Remember about any early pregnancy clinic (EPC) and Genitourinary Medicine (GUM) clinic, if appropriate. All patients should have a pregnancy test before being referred to you.

● Be specific about details of the presenting complaint, especially with PV bleeding (e.g. Is it definitely vaginal or could it be rectal? Is the blood just on wiping or on underwear? Needing to wear a pad? If so, how many? Any clots?).

- Always check the results of the last cervical smear and any contraception used.
- Take accurate PMH to assess suitability for theatre if necessary.
- Certain words are prone to being misunderstood by non-medical people, for example, many patients think all ovarian cysts or breast lumps are the same as cancer. Be sure to ask the patient what they understand about what you told them.
- Routine pre-op clerking is similar to any surgical pre-clerking. Patients tend to be younger than surgical patients so pregnancy and fertility are important issues.

Gynaecological examination

Examining the abdomen

■ Before you examine the patient, make sure you have a private area. Have a chaperone and document their presence afterwards. Make sure you have everything you need (e.g. swabs, slides) before you start, so you do not leave the patient half naked.

■ When examining the abdomen, don't forget surgical conditions. If the patient has RIF tenderness, don't forget appendicitis even if the location or presentation is somewhat atypical. If the patient is post-operative, check for bowel sounds.

■ Urinalysis is an easy test and can provide important clues, it is also sensible to confirm pregnancy (with consent) before any referral.

■ Listen to the ward sister or midwife. They are very experienced.

Bimanual (vaginal) examination

■ Many patients will not know what to expect. Explain what you are doing and what the patient should expect to feel. Talk to the patient while you are examining her and tell her what you are doing just before you do each step.

■ The cervix takes practice to feel. The cervix can be tender so warn the patient that it might hurt before you test for cervical excitation (pain in the adnexae when the cervix is moved to one side).

■ Both adnexae need to be examined and this often requires quite firm pressure. Once experienced, you will be able to feel the ovaries in many women. Warn the patient beforehand.

Using the speculum

■ Warm the speculum under warm water first if it is metal.

■ Use a lot of lubricant on the speculum.

■ Use a smaller speculum in post-menopausal women, as there will likely be some degree of atrophy.

■ It is easier to assess a cervical os with a speculum. Cervixes are in different positions in every person, so it will take a bit of practice to learn where to look and how to position the instrument. If the cervix is very posteriorly positioned, try using a larger speculum. Getting the patient to put her hands under her bottom can help to bring the cervix into view.

■ Do not rush. Never force the speculum. If the patient is in pain, be prepared to try a smaller speculum or abandon the procedure.

■ Observe for any discharge; you will soon learn to distinguish different types and learn what is normal. It is good practice to take triple swabs (high vaginal, low vaginal and endocervical) for all patients while the speculum is in. When you withdraw the speculum keep looking for abnormalities; not all will be visible with the speculum in.

Obstetric examination

■ Precise measurements are necessary. Use a tape measure to measure symphysis-fundal height.

■ Remember that medical and surgical conditions do not have classical presentation in pregnancy. Have a low threshold for suspicion for other pathologies. White cell counts are raised in pregnancy, so it is not a useful marker.

■ Listen for foetal heart or use a Doppler probe if available. Foetal heart sounds should be audible after 13–15 weeks' gestation. Reassure the patient that in early pregnancy, it may not be detectable. Check the maternal pulse at the same time to make sure the two are not mixed up.

■ Before you perform a vaginal examination on any person of more than 20 weeks' gestation, check the placental position on the 20-week ultrasound scan to exclude placenta praevia (especially crucial if presenting with PV bleeding). Speak to your senior if no scan is available as rupture of a praevia can be catastrophic.

■ When using a speculum, take triple swabs. Candidal infection is common in pregnancy. Remember that infection can cause uterine irritability and therefore induce (pre-term) labour.

■ Speculum examination can also be used to assess for pre-term rupture of membranes. A pool of liquor may be seen in the posterior fornix or liquor coming through the os.

Reading the CTG

Use the simple mnemonic (DR BRAVADO):
■ DR – define risk
■ BR – baseline rate
■ A – accelerations
■ VA – variability
■ D – decelerations
■ O – opinion

Being a male

Being a man in a woman's world can be a very disconcerting experience. It is ridden with medico-legal hazards and cultural obstacles but it can be extremely rewarding to view life on the other side.

■ Always be sensitive to the patient's feelings, wishes and privacy. It is best to offer to speak to the patient without the presence of relatives or partners.

■ Always ask permission before examining (or even touching) the patient. At each stage of examining a patient (i.e. normal physical, breast, genitalia, vaginal, rectal), check with them before proceeding.

■ Have a neutral chaperone (preferably of the same gender as the patient) with you. Do not rely on relatives. Document who was there by name and title.

■ It is advisable not to try any humour until you are confident.

Although most of the above tips are directed at male doctors, they also apply to female doctors (including the need for a chaperone).

Common gynaecological calls

Gynaecological problems should be considered when investigating common symptoms such as abdominal pain and anaemia. If you are confronted with a complex gynaecological or obstetric problem, do not hesitate to refer to the specialists.

Vaginal bleeding

Menstrual bleeding is common in hospital, but if the patient is post-menopausal or the bleeding is abnormal, carcinoma

of the cervix and uterus must be excluded. Differential diagnoses include:
■ Menstrual bleeding (illness can cause abnormal periods).
■ Break-through bleed on the OCP, especially if the patient is taking antibiotics.
■ PID, especially if IUCD is in situ.

■ Fibroids or endometriosis.
■ Tumours (e.g. cervical or uterine).
■ Threatened miscarriage or ectopic pregnancy – the later is a diagnosis you cannot afford to miss. In abdominal pain, *always* do a pregnancy test.

On the ward
■ Confirm that bleeding is vaginal, not rectal and that this is different to normal menses.
■ Exclude pregnancy-related bleeding (ask about the LMP, contraceptive use and recent sexual history). Always think of pregnancy in pre-menopausal women. Send urine to the biochemistry lab for testing if in doubt.
■ Consider PID, especially if low grade fever or tender abdomen. Do a PV examination for pelvic tenderness.
■ Get a gynaecological referral if the patient is post-menopausal, or pre-menopausal with persistent bleeding and no obvious cause.
■ Investigations to consider:
– Pap smear.
– High vaginal swab.
– FBC, clotting studies, ESR/CRP.

Hints

Anticoagulation does not cause abnormal PV bleeding but may unmask mucosal defects or tumours.

Dysmenorrhoea

This is a common and painful problem for menstruating women.

On the ward
■ Differentiate the pain from other causes of cramping, and lower abdominal pain. Most women will recognize period pain.
■ Ask what medication works for the patient and prescribe this if no contraindication. Mefenamic acid 500 mg tds or ibuprofen 400–600 mg tds are useful. Co-proxamol and codeine are perfectly acceptable alternatives. A hot water bottle also helps.

Termination of pregnancy (TOP)

As a junior doctor, you may be asked to be involved with TOPs in the following scenarios:

1 Counselling patients in clinic which will include taking consent and prescribing the agents for a medical TOP.

2 Assisting in theatre.

3 Dealing with any immediate or delayed complications of TOP.

If you have any moral objections, just make them known to your consultant at the beginning of the job and you will not be expected to be involved. However, whatever your ethical beliefs, it will be expected that you will deal with any patient who is unwell after a TOP.

General tips

■ Although a delicate issue, if the patient is under-aged you should try to ascertain the age of the father as there may be child protection issues.

■ Always discuss contraception – most forms of hormonal contraception should be started on the day of the TOP.

■ If unsure of gestation, get an ultrasound scan. The TOP may not be legal.

■ It is normal for a pregnancy test to remain positive for up to 2 weeks post-TOP. But if β-HCG levels are persistently positive, this could imply retained products or failure of TOP.

Chapter 8
DEATH AND DYING

Terminal care

About 65% of people die in hospital in the UK. Caring for dying people is stressful. Evidence suggests that medical students and junior doctors come to terms with mortality much younger than most people.

There are five elements to good terminal care: communication, pain control, symptom control, good prescribing knowledge and self-care.

Communication

Breaking bad news

Breaking bad news is difficult but important. Contrary to popular opinion, people often remember how bad news was related to them. While every situation demands a unique approach, the following may be helpful:

■ If you are uncertain about how to start, talk to the patient's nurse. It is generally a good idea to ask nurses what they think the patient knows before seeing the patient. Take a nurse with you to the bedside.
■ If possible, take the patient to a private room to tell them bad news.
■ Have tissues handy.
■ Try to hand your bleep to a nurse or colleague for at least 15–20 minutes.
■ If you are unsure about how to proceed, it can be helpful to ask the patient 'What have you been told?'

■ Do not be afraid to give information. Studies show that people almost always want more information than doctors give them.[1]
■ Watch and listen to the patient carefully for clues about how much information they want. If they indicate that they do not want to know everything at once, you may be more effective by feeding them information over several days. It is acceptable to ask the patient "how much do you want to know?"

Useful questions to assess how much someone wants to hear

1 What have you been told?

2 Are you the sort of person who wants to know exactly what's going on?

3 Would you like me to tell you the full details of the diagnosis/results/ treatment options?

4 Do you want me to go on?

---

[1] In 1961, 90% of doctors thought that patients were better off not being told about terminal disease, compared with 3% in 1979. Martin J. (1993) Lying to patients: can it ever be justified? *Nursing Standard* **7**, 29–31.

The Hands-on Guide for Junior Doctors, Fourth Edition. Anna Donald, Michael Stein and Ciaran Scott Hill. © 2011 Anna Donald, Michael Stein and Ciaran Scott Hill. Published 2011 by Blackwell Publishing Ltd.

■ Tell the truth and answer questions directly if asked (the patient may have been waiting all week to talk to you). Be ready to answer questions and to admit uncertainty. People are usually willing, even in the face of their own death, to cope with honest uncertainty. Have all investigations and findings to hand.

■ Avoid using medical jargon.

■ Write down relevant information and consider drawing diagrams to explain what you are saying more clearly (about 60% of spoken information is lost). Be prepared to repeat yourself many times.

■ Ask the patient to write down questions they might have over the next few days. Give them your name or that of a colleague so that they can contact a doctor if they need to.

■ Find out if the patient wants you to break the news to their relatives.

■ Write in the notes what you have told the patient. This saves embarrassment for the team and sets a baseline for future explanations.

■ It is very important to communicate to the nurses what you have told the patient. They can follow up with further information and support.

■ Consider other people who can help with breaking bad news: other doctors, nurses, chaplain or religious support worker (about 25% of families in the UK accept chaplaincy support),[2] GP, nurse, police, social worker or support groups.

Ongoing communication with dying patients

■ Pay a quick visit to the patient's bedside the next day (or at night if you're on call). Ask them how they're feeling and if they have any questions.

■ Pain causes fear and anxiety, which may lead to the patient being withdrawn or aggressive. If you are not getting very far with a patient, remember to ask if they are in pain, or if they are frightened that they might develop severe pain. Reassure them that pain can be controlled; it is one of the most important contributions you can make to a dying patient.

■ If someone's English is poor, ask the nurses or switchboard to help you to find an interpreter. Most hospitals have a list of employees who can interpret for you.

■ Be alert to attention-seeking symptoms, such as headaches and insomnia, which are probably better treated with TLC than pills. A direct approach is usually the best one. A colleague once had a patient who had 22 symptoms in 24 hours and kept calling the nurses. The patient had been told that she had metastatic cancer that week. The doctor asked her outright 'How are you feeling about having secondaries?' She burst into tears and told her she was terrified of dying – and stopped calling the nurses.

■ Maintaining continuity of care, despite ward staff changes, is especially important for dying patients. Tell patients and relatives that you are going home for the weekend or on holiday, and the name of the doctor who will replace you.

■ Elisabeth Kubler-Ross suggested five stages of dying in her 1969 book *On Death and Dying*. These were denial, anger, bargaining, depression and acceptance. Pitch your information and communication to wherever the person is today. (This is easier said than done – remember to consider where you are at today too!)

■ Do not be surprised by dying patients' aggressive or abnormal behaviour. This is when they need acceptance

[2] Burgess K. (1992) Supporting bereaved relatives in A&E. *Nursing Standard* **6**, 36–39.

the most. Do your best not to take it personally – and check that there is no physical cause (e.g. pain, hypoxia). Managing dying patients is not easy, it is a difficult skill and sadly you are unlikely to always say the right thing when you are starting out.

■ Many dying people say that the most hurtful and distressing thing for them is avoidance and silence. Although it is often hard to do, allow patients to discuss dying with you (see below).

Five questions to ask dying patients

1 What have they most enjoyed in their life? Ask them to describe it to you.

2 What would they like someone to hear, that they have never said?

3 What would they most like to say to people they love that they have never said? Ask them if there is any way they can communicate this (e.g. write a card, phone them from the ward, ask them to visit).

4 What are they most frightened of? You may be able to reassure them about pain and symptom control.

5 What do patients need to do (in practical terms) before they die? Talk to support staff (nurses, Macmillan nurses, social workers) and relatives about making this happen. It is very difficult for people to do things from a hospital bed. Remember that some industrial diseases are eligible for financial support and that this is dated from the time of application, for example, Mesothelioma (call the Department for Work and Pensions Benefit Enquiry Line on 0800 822 200).

■ Look patients in the eye when you talk to them.
■ Reassure people that pain and other distressing symptoms can be treated.
■ Check that the patient does not have awful images of dying patients from films!

Hint

Woolley and colleagues (1989) interviewed parents about their experiences of the way in which they were told of their children's life-threatening illnesses. This article is well worth reading and pinning to your wall, as it gives an excellent, boxed outline of how to impart really difficult news. The reference is: Woolley H., Stein A., Forrest G.C., Baum J.D. (1989) Imparting the diagnosis of life threatening illness in children. *British Medical Journal* **298**, 1632–1636.

Difficult situations

■ Try turning difficult questions for you back to the patient. For example, you can ask them: 'What makes you ask that question?'[3]
■ If family members make it clear to you that they don't want the patient to know that they are going to die, ask your senior or nurses for help. The relatives are not your primary responsibility, although obviously you have to work with them. You can point out that it is your duty to inform patients of their condition unless it will cause them undue harm, this is rarely the case.
■ Write down relatives' concerns in the patient's notes.

[3] Macguire P., Faulkner A. (1988) Communicate with cancer patients: Handling bad news and difficult questions. *British Medical Journal* **297**, 970–974.

Mistakes we've made: avoid them!

■ Do not underestimate how much caring for dying patients can affect you. If you feel irritable or low, don't give yourself a hard time.

■ Avoid medical jargon.

■ Do not overwhelm patients and families with big doses of information at once. Try to give information in bite-size chunks.

■ Write things down and draw clear diagrams for patients to look at after you've gone.

■ Do not leave patients waiting. If you promise to return, do so. People stay awake waiting for doctors to return. If you can't visit when you said that you will then call the ward and ask for the patient to be informed that you will be late.

■ Never say 'Nothing can be done' or give the patient the impression that the medical staff have lost interest in them. Symptoms and distress can always be alleviated. Someone can always be present.

■ Contrary to intuition, dying patients do not need to eat. It can be cruel to force them to do so.

■ Never give patients a 'date or time of death'. You will probably be wrong. Also, it is awful for all concerned if the patient lingers on after they 'should have died'.

Pain control

(see Chapter 12, Pain control)

Pain is one of the things that dying patients are most afraid of. You can help them enormously, but you may need help:

■ Use the pain clinic and ask for senior advice sooner rather than later if pain control is difficult.

■ Remember the person may not admit to being in pain (check their pulse).

■ Reassure patients that severe pain can be controlled, however severe.

Symptom control

(listed alphabetically in Chapter 7)

The *BNF* has a fabulous, two-page section on symptom control in terminal care (look under 'Terminal care' in the index) which we have not tried to replicate for fear of being too quickly outdated.

Prescribing for the dying

■ Many drugs are available as suppositories, which are useful if the patient cannot swallow or is vomiting.

■ Keep drugs as simple as possible. Discontinue when close to death.

■ Keep analgesia continuous. IV or SC opiate infusions are useful for this as are PRN doses to back up regular doses of analgesia. Nurses will usually set up infusions for you. In dying patients, the ultimate aim is pain control and quality, not quantity of life. Discuss pain management with the nurses so that they do not simply stop infusions to avoid respiratory depression.

■ Consider Patient Controlled Analgesia (PCA). Discuss with the ward pharmacist.

■ Consider withdrawing IV fluids but discuss with seniors and relatives first.

■ Infusion pump troubleshooting:

1 Light not flashing – pump not plugged in; battery inserted wrongly.

2 Infusion running too fast or too slowly – syringe incorrectly inserted, rate wrongly set, tubing kinked or blocked; needle site tissued.

Support for the dying and for you

Hospice (NHS or non-NHS); chaplain; hospital bereavement officer (if you have one).

CRUSE (widowed people caring for the newly bereaved), Cruse House, 126 Sheen Road, Richmond, Surrey TW9 1UR, Go to http://www.crusebereave mentcare.org.uk/LocalCruse.html for a list of local telephone numbers.

Macmillan Nurses (nurses specially trained for palliative care), part of Macmillan Cancer Relief, Anchor House, 15–19 Britten Street, London SW3 3TZ, Tel: 0808 808 00 00 (free phone).

Marie Curie Cancer Care, Marie Curie Memorial Foundation, Head Office, 28 Belgrave Square, London SW1X 8QG, Tel: 020 7599 7777 (England); 01495 740 888 (Wales); 0131 561 3900 (Scotland); 028 9088 2060 (NI).

Some questions to ask yourself if *you* feel excessively miserable caring for dying patients

■ Make a list of five 'significant losses' you have experienced. Write down positive outcomes that arose from those situations, and identify ways in which you developed as a result.

■ Do the same exercise for 'necessary losses' – those which you had no control over.[4]

Death

If the patient dies, don't panic. While sad, death is often merciful when people have been suffering – for them, their relatives and ward staff. You can make a big difference to relatives if you handle the paperwork efficiently, allowing them to proceed with the funeral.

What to do when a patient dies

1 See the body.

2 Confirm death: fixed and dilated pupils, no respiratory effort for 3 minutes, no pulse, no heart sounds for 1 minute. If you are unsure, do an ECG or look at the fundi. The blood in the retinal veins separates into discrete blotches after death.

3 Write in the notes: 'Called to confirm death. No vital signs'.

4 Sign your name clearly with your bleep number. It is important that coro-ners and bereavement officers can con-tact you if necessary.

5 Note date and time of confirmation of death.

6 If possible write down the cause(s) of death.

7 NOTE WHETHER OR NOT THE PATIENT IS FITTED WITH A PACE-MAKER OR RADIOACTIVE IMPLANT. If the patient is to be cremated, pace-makers and radioactive implants *must* be

---

[4] Hasler K. (1994) Bereavement counselling. Continuing Education article series (article 306). *Nursing Standard* **7**, 31–35.

removed or they blow up in the incinerator at considerable cost to yourself. It is easiest to check for these while you still have the patient and the notes in front of you. If you do not check this now you will have to chase the body and the notes in the morgue in order to sign the cremation form.

8 Liaise with nurses about calling next of kin. Nurses usually tell the next of kin and meet them on the ward, but relatives may want to see you.

9 Note the GP's telephone number and name. You should call him or her at the earliest opportunity to let them know so they don't make a faux pas when they next see the relatives ('So how's so and so doing in hospital?')

10 Write 'GP informed' in notes.

11 Ask your senior early whether or not a PM is desirable, and what cause(s) of death should be written on the death certificate.

Telling relatives about the patient's death

1 Wherever possible, inform the relatives that their loved one is close to death. Ask relatives whether they want to be contacted in the middle of the night, establish the next of kin and how they can be contacted.

2 After death, ask the nurses whether they have told the relatives about the patient's death. They will often do so – sometimes before you make it to the ward.

3 If it is up to you to inform relatives, make sure you contact the patient's designated 'next of kin'. Ask the nurses

who this is, or look in the nursing or medical notes.

4 It is usually best to tell the next of kin what has happened over the phone (rather than just asking them to come in urgently). Sometimes people don't want to see the body or would rather wait until morning.

5 If you receive the relatives, take them to a private room. If they have come a long way they might be grateful for a cup of tea.

6 Try to establish:

- If the body is to be cremated or buried. If the former, you will need to fill out a cremation form (see below).
- If the relatives will consent to a post mortem (see below).

Religious practices on death

Some awareness of religious or cultural customs on death is invaluable to prevent misunderstandings and often also allows the relatives to deal with their grief.

- Buddhism: no special arrangements on death.
- Christianity: no special arrangements on death.
- Confucianism: no special arrangements on death.
- Hinduism: cremation of the body.
- Islam: burial intact by the next sunset.
- Judaism: body should not be left alone. Consult with relatives for additional requirements, such as speed of burial.
- Sikhism: do not move the body. Cremation of the body.
- Zoroastrianism: no special arrangements on death.

Post mortems

- Preferably before the patient dies, ask your colleagues if they want a PM so that you can ask the relatives when the patient dies.

■ PMs requested by the coroner are mandatory by law. Otherwise, you cannot force a next of kin to agree to a PM. Many people will oblige if you explain why you want one, particularly if it is a limited PM.

■ Send case notes (complete with recent investigation results), the next of kin's consent form and a brief synopsis of the patient's history and hospital progress to the PM room, together with your name and bleep number.

■ Request that the pathologist bleeps you or your senior with the results.

Death certificates

Only doctors who have seen the patient within 14 days before death are legally allowed to sign a death certificate. The next of kin must take this to the Registrar of Births and Deaths within 5 days (8 days in Scotland) in a sealed envelope. Give the signed death certificate to either the nurses, the ward clerk or the family.

If there is no next of kin, you must ensure that the death certificate is sent to the registrar.

Writing the death certificate

Make sure you fill in the death certificate correctly or you may be recalled by the registrar and delay the funeral. The bereavement office may help you with the details but don't be too hard on yourself if you do make mistakes, as it is not the simplest document to fill out.

1 Part one: Fill in the sequence of conditions that caused the patient's death.

1a) is the condition that caused death. Causes of death are recognized pathological states, such as myocardial infarction. The cause of death must not

be too general. For example, organ failure is not an acceptable cause. Other unacceptable causes are tabulated below. Ask your senior or ring the registrar if you are unsure about how to describe the cause of death.

Unacceptable 'causes' of death	
Asphyxia	Hepatic failure
Asthenia	Hepatorenal failure
Brain failure	Kidney failure
Cachexia	Renal failure
Cardiac arrest	Respiratory failure
Cardiac failure	Shock
Coma	Syncope
Debility	Uraemia
Exhaustion	Vagal inhibition
Heart failure	Vaso-vagal attack

1b) and c) are diseases underlying this condition. For example, if the cause of death was MI, the underlying disease might be ischaemic heart disease, or chronic hypertension.

2 Part two: Fill in other diseases that were not directly linked with the cause of death in 1a), but which may have contributed to the patient's overall demise.

3 Sign the death certificate on the relevant part of the form.

4 Print your name, hospital and most recent medical qualification on the relevant part of the form.

5 Print the name of the patient's consultant on the relevant part of the form.

6 Fill in the counterfoil ('cheque-butt') part of death certificate. This retains the basic details of the death when the relatives have taken the main certificate.

7 Fill in the 'note to informant'. This is given to the next of kin.

- If you are unsure about any part of the death certificate, call the registrar's officer or talk to a colleague or bereavement officer. The registrar's office is in the phone book under 'Registrar of Births and Deaths'.
- Do not use abbreviations on the death certificate.
- If your hospital has a bereavement officer, he or she will usually discuss the request for a PM with the relatives and will help you with the death certificate.
- It is courteous to relatives to write the cause of death in lay-language (e.g. 'heart attack' as well as myocardial infarction).
- If your patient was a war pensioner or serviceman/woman, you can influence whether or not their spouse continues to receive war widow(er)'s pension by what you write on the death certificate. This is especially important if the person died from war-related causes.
- Doctors must record diseases that may have been due to previous employment.

Referring to the coroner (Scotland: procurator fiscal)

1 To contact your local coroner or procurator, ask your senior, switchboard, the police station or directory enquiries for the phone number.

2 It is the statutory obligation of the Registrar of Births and Deaths, not you, to report suspect deaths to the coroner or procurator fiscal. However, it saves time if you know what these are and can send the death certificate directly to the coroner. They are:

- Unknown cause of death.
- The patient was not seen by a certifying doctor within 14 days of death.

- Death was caused by medical treatment (e.g. dying in theatre, or within 24 hours of an anaesthetic).
- Death was suspicious in any way.
- Death occurred within 24 hours of admission to hospital without a firm diagnosis being made.
- Death was caused by a road traffic accident, an industrial disease or accident, a domestic accident, violence, neglect, abortion, suicide or poisoning (including acute alcohol ingestion).
- Death occurred during legal custody.
- Where there is any claim for negligence against medical or nursing staff.
- Death may have occurred from industrial injury or employment.
- Death of a foster child, patient under Mental Health Act (1983), mentally disabled people, Service Pensioners.

3 The coroner can request:

- The issue of a normal death certificate.
- A post mortem (see Post mortems, above).
- An inquest.

Cremation forms and fees

You receive £73.50 for every cremation form you fill out; this is charged to the funeral director by the hospital who then passes the bill on to relatives. The charge is made because this is considered outside of a doctor's contracted NHS duties. 'Crem forms' are legal documents to establish beyond any doubt the deceased's identity, as incinerated bodies cannot be exhumed. If you have not seen the patient since death, you must pay a quick visit to the cold room so that you know you are signing the form for the right person. The body cannot be released until this form is filled out.

Cremation forms are straightforward to fill out, provided you are certain there are no radioactive or pacemaker implants in the body.

■ Ensure you fill in the same cause(s) of death on the cremation form that you did on the death certificate or you will be chased by the coroner.

■ If in doubt, call the coroner's office or ask a medical colleague.

■ If the family is poor you can forgo the cremation fee. In some hospitals this is standard policy. If you choose not to accept cremation fees, you need a tax exemption form from the morgue director or bereavement officer so that you don't get taxed for fees you haven't taken.

■ Keep details of cremation fees you have taken as you need to declare them in your tax forms. Increasingly the Inland Revenue is checking up on doctors for non-declaration.

To check for pacemakers

■ Feel the chest.

■ Look through the notes for history of implantation of pacemaker or radioactive implant.

■ Look for ECGs that will demonstrate an active pacemaker by small, regular vertical lines throughout the trace.

■ The only sure-fire way to exclude a pacemaker is to see a recent chest X-ray. Make sure you see it before the radiology department removes it from the inpatient file.

Further reading

There are many excellent books and articles on death and dying. Ask your librarian. Here are some useful articles for starters:

Buckman R. (1992) *How to Break Bad News. A Guide for Health Care Professionals*. Papermac, London.

Continuing Education article series on bereavement counselling. (1994) *Nursing Standard*.

Cooke M., Cooke H., Glucksman E. (1992) Management of sudden bereavement in the accident and emergency department. *British Medical Journal* **304**, 1207–1209.

Egan G. (1990) *The Skilled Helper. A Systematic Approach to Effective Helping*, 4th edn. Brookes-Cole, Pacific Grove, CA.

Macguire P., Faulkner L. (1988) Communicate with cancer patients: Handling bad news and difficult patients. *British Medical Journal* **297**, 907–909.

McLauchlan C. (1990) Handling distressed relatives and breaking bad news. *British Medical Journal* **301**, 1145–1149.

Raphael B. (1996) *The Anatomy of Bereavement: A Handbook for the Caring Professions*. Hutchinson, London.

Thayre K., Hadfield-Law L. (1993) Never going to be easy: Giving bad news. RCN Nursing Update; Continuing Education article series. *Nursing Standard* **8**, 3–13.

Worden W. (2002) *Grief Counselling and Grief Therapy. A Handbook for the Mental Health Practitioner*, 3rd edn. Springer, London.

Chapter 9
DRUGS

Don't worry if pharmacology seems a long time ago. Prescribing and giving drugs is easier than it may seem!

General

■ The single most useful pharmacology tip is: always refer to the *BNF* if in any doubt about any drug. As a junior doctor, you will rarely be expected to prescribe drugs that are not in the *BNF*. Also, it's worth reading the *BNF* for entertainment during long ward rounds; it contains lots of useful information and time spent familiarizing yourself with the layout will seldom be wasted. For example, it contains prescribing guidelines for the elderly, the terminally ill and children.

■ Make the most of your ward pharmacist. Not only are pharmacists happy to discuss patient management and find alternatives for problematic drugs (or patients), but they are often willing to find recent articles and other information about specific drugs for you. This can be useful for clarifying unusual side effects and for academic talks.

■ For easy reference, make yourself a chart of common drugs and doses used on the wards and stick it on the front of your folder or Filofax. It is particularly useful to do this for antibiotics and infusion dosages, which can be painstaking to look up every time you make up an infusion. We have refrained from providing such lists in this book because every hospital's protocol is different and drug

doses vary over time. As always, check the *BNF*.

Prescribing drugs

Drug charts

Drug charts are straightforward to fill out. Basically, there are four parts to a drug chart:

1 A place for regular drugs.

2 A place for 'PRN' or 'when required' drugs.

3 A place for one-off drugs.

4 Fluids and infusions.

For each section of the chart, you need to fill in the date, the generic name of each drug, its dose, how frequently it should be prescribed, and your signature. Abbreviations for prescribing are shown in Table 9.1.

Tips for filling in drug charts
■ Write legibly. Other people have to administer drugs that you prescribe. Slips of the pens can have huge consequences.

■ In particular, take care in writing dose amounts and units. Micrograms (abbreviated mcg or μg) can easily be mistaken for milligrams (mg); the *BNF* advises that 'micrograms' and 'units' be written in

The Hands-on Guide for Junior Doctors, Fourth Edition. Anna Donald, Michael Stein and Ciaran Scott Hill.
© 2011 Anna Donald, Michael Stein and Ciaran Scott Hill. Published 2011 by Blackwell Publishing Ltd.

Table 9.1 Abbreviations for prescribing drugs.

Abbreviation	Meaning
ac (ante cibum)	before food
pc (post cibum)	after food
bd (bis die)	take twice daily
mane	take in the morning
nocte	take in the evening
od	take once daily
prn (pro re nata)	take when required
qds	take 4 times a day
stat	take straight away
tds	take 3 times a day
T.	1 tablet/dose
T.T.	2 tablets/doses
T.T.T.	3 tablets/doses
x/7	x days
y/52	y weeks
z/12	z months

full. (A doctor was sued when a patient was given 125 mg of digoxin by a nurse who misread the scrawled 'mcg'. She had to open many packets of the drug to give such a dose, so also ended up in the dock for failure of common sense.) Using 'u' for 'units' is also very susceptible to be misread as an additional zero.

■ Develop a good relationship with the ward pharmacist. They review all drug charts, albeit often after the drug has been given a number of times, and will hopefully bleep you if you prescribe anything idiotic – this is something you should encourage! Similarly, nurses, who administer many drugs, will usually let you know if you have made a prescription error.

■ Hospital pharmacists usually use green ink. To avoid confusion, use a different colour when writing on drug charts.

■ If drug administration is complicated, write additional instructions on the drug chart. There is no harm in writing extra notes to nurses and doctors on the drug chart. In fact it is legally advisable to do so.

Writing prescriptions

FY1 junior doctors are only permitted to write prescriptions for the hospital pharmacy. However, if you do need to write a prescription on plain paper the essential ingredients are:

■ Date
■ Name of patient
■ Date of birth
■ Address of patient
■ Generic drug name and amount
■ Dose/day
■ Your signature
■ Your GMC registration number

Controlled drugs

Prescriptions for take-home controlled drugs have to be written in a particular way, otherwise the pharmacy will send the prescription back. This wastes a spectacular amount of time. To write a controlled drug prescription:

The prescription must be in your handwriting – don't use sticky labels. Include:

■ Date
■ Name of patient and their date of birth
■ Address of patient
■ Generic drug name and amount (e.g. '10 mg')
■ Dose/day
■ **Total** number of tablets in **both** numbers and letters (e.g. '10/ten tablets')
■ Your signature and printed name

For example:
5/4/02
Mr TSD
2 Tatelman Street
Wolfchester WC5
MST continuous tablets 10 mg
10/ten tablets
10 mg twice daily for 5 days
(Your signature and printed name)

Verbals

It is now legally suspect to prescribe drugs for patients 'verbally' over the phone to nurses. However, in certain instances it still occurs. Typical verbal requests might be 'Mr Smith has a headache. Could he have two paracetamol please?' The nurse writes your prescription in the drug chart, with a small note saying 'Dr X will sign this'. Verbals are fine for relatively harmless drugs, such as one-off doses of paracetamol or aspirin, or for doses of necessary drugs when you have been held up and coming to the ward is monumentally inconvenient.

■ Check hospital policy. Increasingly verbals are not allowed by Trusts. They should only be used in exceptional circumstance that could not have been predicted. Some trusts only allow them if the medication is already prescribed and in use but a dose change is necessary. Verbals are never acceptable for controlled drugs.

■ It is important to sign verbal requests on the drug chart as soon as possible. Should any problems arise in the interim, the nurse who took the verbal is liable. Because of this, some nurses refuse to take verbals altogether and insist you come to the ward to sign the drug before it is given. This is a reasonable stance for a nurse to take and you should think twice before you criticize it.

■ Nurses will rightly usually refuse to accept verbals if they think the patient should be seen by a doctor before taking the drug. While this can be frustrating, remember that nurses' scruples provide a big safety net for you. Everyone remembers times when they were glad that nurses forced them to question what they were doing.

■ Some hospitals allow a limited number of drugs (e.g. paracetamol, sublingual nitrate, lactulose, antacids) to be prescribed by nurses after calling the duty doctor. While you need not see the patient, it is prudent to check the reasons for the request. You may be required (depending on local policy) to sign for the drugs later.

Giving drugs

Nurses give oral drugs, suppositories, subcutaneous and intramuscular drugs. In most hospitals nurses also give intravenous drugs. However, certain drugs do require a specially trained nurse or a doctor. These vary between hospitals.

■ Do not feel rushed when making up a drug or administering it. Being rushed, particularly when doing something unfamiliar, is when mistakes happen.

■ Glass vials are designed to snap at the neck in the direction of the blue dot on their neck. The dot is the 'weak spot'.

■ Use a metal file to open difficult glass drug vials by scratching the neck with the file, and snapping it off. Nurses may have a file stashed somewhere on the ward.

■ Wear gloves or use your nondominant hand when opening multiple vials. Your dominant hand's index finger can get chaffed with minute glass splinters if you snap open many glass vials consecutively. It is common to see new doctors in areas like anaesthetics with a constant plaster around their dominant index finger!

■ Avoid using normal saline as a dilutant for drugs in patients with liver failure – the extra salt load can precipitate ascites; 5% dextrose is usually adequate.

■ Avoid dextrose in patients with diabetic coma. Give normal saline instead. Refer to the *BNF* for alternative dilutants for different drugs.

■ When making up cytotoxic drugs, always wear gloves, apron and goggles (and keep your mouth closed!) Wash your hands afterwards. Follow local and national protocols and do not do anything you are uncomfortable with.

■ The plastic containers with prefilled syringes (e.g. adrenaline) in cardiac arrest trolleys are easily opened by holding the box with both hands and twisting it. Make sure you do this at least once before you attend your first arrest.

Drug infusions

Continuous infusions are easy to make up, but they are a complete pain at 4 a.m. While it was traditional to make up midnight infusions like morphine, dopamine and GTN infusions before going to bed, this is now considered bad practice and the advance preparation of medicines is frowned upon. The exception is where an infusion is drawn up and attached to the patient – clearly this does not need to necessarily run continuously.

To make up an infusion

1 Find the vial of drug in the drug cupboard. Check the dosage and the expiry date.

2 Open the vial and draw up the drug into a suitably large syringe, usually 50 ml.

3 Draw into the syringe the required amount of dilutant fluid. Usually normal saline, water for injections or 5% dextrose, drawn from unopened (sterile) containers.

4 Label the syringe with a large sticky. Specify on the sticky:

● Date and time you made infusion up.
● Name of patient.
● Amount of drug in amount of dilutant (e.g. 50 mg GTN in 50 ml normal saline).
● Rate at which solution should run (e.g. 2 ml/hour).
● Your signature.

Prescribing drug infusions

1 Prescribe infusions on the fluid section of the drug chart. In some hospitals this is a separate sheet at the end of the patient's bed.

2 Write: '*a* units of *b* drug in *x* ml of *y* dilutant to run at *z* ml/hour'. For example, 500 mg of aminophylline in 500 ml of normal saline. Run at 35 ml/hour.

3 To avoid confusion, convert the amount of drug/hour to the amount of infusion to be given every hour (i.e. ml/hour, not mg/hour). To do this, ask yourself the following questions:

● How many units of drug should the patient get per hour?
    For example, 35 mg/hour (0.5 mg/kg for a 70 kg male).
● How many units of drug are there per ml of infusion?
    For example, 500 mg/500 ml infusion = 1 mg/ml.
● Therefore, how many ml do I need to give so that the patient gets the right amount of units per hour?
    For example, 35 mg/hour ÷ 1 mg/ml = 35 ml/hour.

4 You can always write additional instructions on the drug chart regarding infusion administration.

For example, 50 mg GTN in 50 ml N/saline; run at 1–10 ml/hour titrated against chest pain but maintain a systolic blood pressure > 100 mmHg etc.

5 It is often easier to calculate by making up the drug to a concentration of 1 mg/ml as in the example above.

6 Be mindful of the volume of drug infusions, as they are in addition to normal intravenous fluid infusions.

Administering infusions

If the nurses are willing to administer infusions, all you have to do is let them know that you have made up the infusion, and where they can find it. Many nurses will make up the infusions themselves and administer them. The safest stance though is to presume they don't until you confirm otherwise with them.

■ If you have to run the infusion yourself then get a nurse to show you how to set up a pump (e.g. Vickers). It is not difficult. Basically you insert the syringe into the pump with the drug label facing outwards, set the rate on the machine, plug it in and turn it on. You also have to remember to connect the patient to the syringe.

■ Infusions can run through central or peripheral lines. Many infusions can run concurrently with other drugs through three-way taps or multiple-tap ('traffic light') giving sets. These are simple to set up with initial nurse supervision.

■ Some infusions cannot be mixed with others. The most problematic are those containing chelating ions, such as Ca^{2+}. Unfortunately these require a second Venflon or need flushing with heparinized saline (Hepsal) or saline before another drug is administered through the same line.

■ Place the syringe driver or infusion bag *below* the level of the patient's head to avoid the risk of siphoning.

Intravenous drugs

If you are in a hospital where nurses do not administer IV drugs, which is now thankfully rare, then you need to mix them with dilutant and give them yourself. This can mean doing an IV drug round 3–4 times daily. In reality you are unlikely to be asked to inject any medicines except for controlled drugs such as morphine and midazolam.

1 Ensure the patient really needs the drug IV. Most drugs may be given PO, PR, SC or IM. It is time-consuming for you and expensive for the NHS to give drugs through IV. It is often a fallacy that IV drugs are more effective. Many medications have only a marginally reduced oral bioavailability.

2 Read the instructions in the drug packet. Some drugs can be injected directly into the patient's vein. However, they usually need to be diluted first.

Liquid drugs not requiring dilution

If the drug can be given without dilution, draw it up with a small syringe and inject it over the recommended time. Some drugs must be given slowly to avoid anaphylaxis or pain in the patient's arm which they won't thank you for. Most drugs can be given quite quickly (over less than 30 seconds to 1 minute). Read the *BNF* and the drug's instructions – take these seriously, complications from incorrect methods of administration (including those due to lack of knowledge) do occur.

Liquid drugs requiring dilution

If the drug comes in liquid form which needs diluting, this is easily done by drawing the drug into a suitably large syringe (e.g. 10 or 20 ml), and then

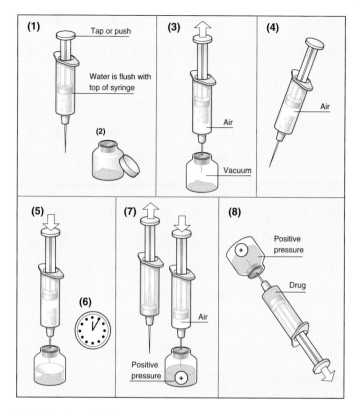

Fig. 9.1 Preparing powdered drugs.

drawing in sterile saline or water for injection (available in small, sterile vials in the drug cupboard). Always use sterile fluid when diluting drugs; patients can get septic from once-sterile fluid that has been lying around unsealed.

Powdered drugs

If the drug comes in a vacuum container as a powder, you need to dissolve it with a solute, such as water for injection. Most antibiotics come this way. To avoid giving yourself and the ward a drug shower (Fig. 9.1):

1 Draw the required amount of water for injection into a suitably large syringe through a needle. Tap or push the end of the syringe to expel any air, so that the water is flush with the top of the syringe.

2 Remove the flip-off plastic top of the drug vial.

3 Push the needle through the rubber top of the drug vial and withdraw some air to create a vacuum inside the vial.

4 Tap or tilt the syringe upwards so that the withdrawn air moves through the water to the back of the syringe.

5 Inject the water into the vial, with the assistance of the vacuum you have just created. You may need to repeat this several times.

6 When you have injected enough water, shake the vial (or leave it to dissolve while you do something else).

7 Withdraw the needle. Draw some air into the syringe. Reintroduce the needle into the vial through the rubber top and inject some air to create positive pressure inside the vial.

8 Turn the vial upside down and withdraw the dissolved drug from the vial with the assistance of the positive pressure.

9 Don't worry if on first attempts you spray yourself, the desk and unwary passers-by with the drug. You will soon be able to do the whole thing perfectly in your sleep. Practice makes perfect!

Specific drug topics

Antibiotics

■ Check your hospital drug guidelines with seniors, pharmacists or ideally the consultant microbiologist. Each hospital has particular protocols which are usually published. The variation in advice between hospitals is not random – the incidence of organisms is in constant flux and advice is based on regional surveillance data.

■ Always ask patients if they have known antibiotic (e.g. penicillin) allergy before prescribing any drug but in particular penicillin or cephalosporin antibiotics. Erythromycin is usually a reasonable alternative to ampicillin and related drugs. Also be alert to pseudomembranous colitis a dangerous

condition that is particularly associated with ciprofloxacin and some of the cephalosporins. Send stool specimen for *Clostridium difficile* if the patient develops diarrhoea and fever.

■ Common antibiotic side effects include diarrhoea and vaginal (and other) candidiasis (thrush). If the patient is high risk it may be worth prescribing an anti-candidiasis pessary or cream on the PRN side of the drug chart.

■ Warn women taking the oral contraceptive pill that antibiotics (and other drugs affecting liver metabolism) reduce its efficacy.

■ Consider giving at least 24 hours IV treatment if the patient is very unwell.

■ Check the *BNF* and local guidelines for the most current treatment.

■ Gentamicin and vancomycin need regular peak and trough levels (see the *BNF* or phone pharmacology).

Standard treatments for common infections are listed in Table 9.2.

Anticoagulation

Foundation doctors are often required to anticoagulate patients following unstable angina, heart attacks, DVTs and PEs. Ask your colleagues for local protocols. These generally involve giving a low molecular weight heparin and warfarin together, then stopping the heparin once the INR is high enough (i.e. when the warfarin begins to work and is 'within range').

1 Check that the patient has no bleeding disorder. Check FBC, INR and APTT.

2 If using *unfractionated* intravenous heparin (usually indicated where rapid reversal of anticoagulation may be required):

Start the patient on a heparin pump (usually 25,000 units in 50 ml of normal

Table 9.2 Standard treatments for common infections (please refer to the protocols in your local trust for more information as regional variations exist).

Type of infection	Treatment
Community acquired pneumonia	Oral amoxicillin (erythromycin if penicillin allergic)
	Second choice or atypical pneumonia: erythromycin or ciprofloxacin
Severe or hospital-acquired infection	IV cephalosporin, e.g. cefuroxime
Aspiration pneumonia	Amoxicillin and metronidazole
UTI	Oral trimethoprim or nitrofurantoin or ciprofloxacin
Tonsillitis	Penicillin
Cellulitis	Flucloxacillin and penicillin or co-amoxiclav
	Consider metronidazole if the wound smells strongly of anaerobes
Septicaemia	IV cefuroxime and gentamicin (see hospital policy)
Clostridium difficile diarrhoea	Oral metronidazole or oral vancomycin

saline), run at 2.8 ml/hour (1400 units/hour). Check the APTT at least once a day and adjust the heparin according to a sliding scale (see the *BNF*). Ideally, the APTT should hover around 1.5–2.5 depending on the indication. The heparin should be stopped if the APTT is more than 7.

3 If using low molecular weight heparin:

- Prescribe daily subcutaneous low molecular weight heparin. Each hospital has its own preferred brand; check with your formulary and weight-adjust the dose as per *BNF* guidelines. Dosing regime will vary with brand and indication. APTT need not be checked. If a check is required then monitoring is with factor Xa activity. Note that they undergo renal excretion and reduced doses are often required if renal clearance is impaired.

4 Start the patient simultaneously on warfarin. Note that initially giving warfarin is *pro*-thrombotic due to its differential effects on clotting factor activity (it reduces protein C firstly); this can lead to warfarin necrosis. This is the reason why it is paramount that heparin cover is instituted before warfarin. The *pro*-thrombotic state obviously quickly reverses with time as the other vitamin K dependent factors fall. The standard loading protocol is:

- Give 10 mg of warfarin on the first day, 5 mg on the second and third, then adjust according to the INR. This protocol may need to be modified for the elderly, frail, those with liver disease and on liver-stimulating drugs. If you dose every patient like this you will quickly encounter problems. A starting dose of 5 mg is usually more reasonable but in those with sensitivity this may still be too high.

Be particularly cautious with postoperative patients who are at risk of bleeding. Check with your senior if you are unsure.

• You need to check the INR daily from the first dose. Reduce the warfarin dose if the INR rises too quickly or too high (e.g. above 5). Remember that the peak blood level is 36–48 hours after the dose so the INR you see will usually be 'on the way up'.

> The INR needs to be checked:
> Every day for 1 week.
> Every week for 3 weeks.
> Every month for 3 months.
> Every 8 weeks after that.

Always inform the GP in the discharge summary that the patient has been started on warfarin. Most hospitals and some GP surgeries have anticoagulation service which manages the patient's INR.

• You are usually aiming for an INR of 2–3 (but this varies depending on the condition – it may be higher in metallic valves, for example; check the *BNF*).

• Clearly explain the potential side effects of warfarin to the patient and that they must inform their GP and any other health professional that they are taking warfarin. It is also advisable to tell the patient to keep tablets well hidden from small children. Advise patients to let their pharmacist know that they are taking warfarin before buying over-the-counter medications.

• If the INR or APTT are too high, simply stop the warfarin and/or heparin. If the INR is greater than 10, or the patient is bleeding, give 4 units of FFP and recheck the clotting. A small dose (1–2 mg) of vitamin K will reverse the clotting in a few hours. Beware of giving higher doses as this prevents further anticoagulation for weeks. Always consult with a haematologist and colleagues if a patient is in danger of bleeding. Beware of anaphylaxis (be prepared to treat with O_2 and adrenaline, see p. 91). FFP can also be given stat to decrease a bleeding tendency.

• The half-life of unfractionated heparin is quite short (approximately 90 minutes), so stopping the infusion is usually sufficient. Alternatively, heparin can be reversed with protamine sulphate. Use 1 mg protamine sulphate/100 iu of heparin, to a maximum of 50 mg. This should work within half an hour.

Anti-emetics
(see Chapter 7, Nausea and vomiting)

Digoxin

Digoxin is commonly used to slow down the ventricular rate in atrial fibrillation. It is potentially dangerous with many side effects, such as fatigue, confusion, N&V, anorexia, diarrhoea and arrhythmias. Digoxin also interacts with many drugs (see the *BNF*). In particular, beware of drugs which lower K (e.g. diuretics), as hypokalaemia predisposes to dangerous digoxin toxicity.

How to digitalize (discuss with your senior first):

1 In the non-acute situation:

• Give the patient 125–250 µg (micrograms) of digoxin twice daily for 1 week. No loading dose is required.

• Reduce dose to once daily for maintenance. Digoxin maintenance dosage varies according to age, weight and renal function. In general:

> Normal dose 125–375 µg.
> In the elderly 62.5–125 µg.

If in renal impairment, reduce the dose and discuss with pharmacologist.

• If the patient experiences side effects like sepia vision (xanthopsia) or halos,

Table 9.3 Therapeutic drug levels and sampling times.

Drug	Sampling time	Therapeutic range
Amiodarone	Any time when levels are stable (after 1 month)	0.6–2.5 mg/l
Carbamazepine	Peak 3 hours after dose	Single therapy: 8–12 mg/l
		Multiple therapy: 4–8 mg/l
Digoxin	At least 6 hours after dose	0.8–2 µg/l
		Check U&E and Ca^{2+}, as toxicity is potentiated if Ca^{2+} is high or K^+ is low
Gentamicin and tobramicin	Peak 1 hour after dose	5–10 mg/l
	Trough (just before new dose)	<2 mg/l
Lithium	12 hours after dose	0.4–1.0 mmol/l
Phenytoin	IV peak 2–4 hours after dose	10–20 mg/l
	Oral peak 3–9 hours after dose	
Sodium valproate	Plasma levels are not a good guide to efficacy	
Vancomycin	Peak 1 hour after dose	25–40 mg/l
	Trough (just before new dose)	1–3 mg/l
		Check U&E for renal toxicity

nausea or delerium, then measure digoxin levels for toxicity and look for prolongation of the PR interval and an atrial tachycardia. Digoxin-specific antibodies are available as an antidote to digoxin poisoning.

2 In the acute situation (for more rapid control of the ventricular rate):

• Give 500 µg of digoxin 8-hourly until the rate is controlled (usually takes 3–4 doses), then give the maintenance dose (see above), *or*
• Give 500 µg IV and 500 µg orally at the same time, then continue with maintenance doses. This method is faster.

Night sedation
(see Chapter 7, Insomnia)

Be wary of giving night sedation without making sure that the patient does not need further medical attention or better day management.

Therapeutic drug levels

Junior doctors are sometimes required to check the blood levels of several commonly used drugs (Table 9.3). This involves liaising with the nurse giving the drug so that you can take blood for levels at the appropriate times (e.g. at peak and trough dosage times). Ask the biochemistry technicians which tube to use (usually a biochemistry tube).

Steroids (see Chapter 10, The patient on steroids)

Miscellaneous tips

■ Metronidazole can be given easily and cheaply as a suppository. This is particularly useful after an appendicectomy, if the patient does not need a drip.

■ If a drug risks causing anaphylaxis (e.g. phytomenadione), ensure that you have adrenaline ready and a resuscitation trolley available. *Do not leave the ward for 5 minutes after giving these drugs.*

■ Any drug which is protein-based can cause anaphylaxis.

■ Always consider prescribing laxatives and anti-emetics prophylactically with opiate analgesia (at least on the PRN side).

■ Steroid conversion (also see Chapter 10, The patient on steroids): 0.75 mg dexamethasone = 5 mg prednisolone = 20 mg hydrocortisone.

■ Consider pre-emptive prescribing (i.e. prescribing certain drugs on the PRN side of the chart for all patients without contraindications) to prevent nurses bleeping you and your colleagues: paracetamol, cyclizine, laxatives.

Chapter 10
HANDLE WITH CARE

Some patients need special attention as they are especially vulnerable from physical or mental frailty, and stigma.

Alcoholism

Many more of your patients will be addicted to alcohol than you realize. To assess alcoholism, do the CAGE questionnaire,[1] which is remarkably reliable for picking up alcoholism:

1 Have you ever felt you should **C**UT down on drinking?

2 Have people made you **A**NGRY by asking about your alcohol intake?

3 Have you ever felt **G**UILTY about your drinking?

4 Do you ever drink first thing in the morning (or take an **E**YE OPENER)?

Answering 'yes' to two or more of the above questions gives the patient an 80% chance of having an alcohol problem.

• Ask the patient for a typical day, with the amount and type of alcohol taken at each time.

• Tactfully ask relatives or friends about the patient if you suspect denial of alcoholism.

• Do an MCV (with FBC) and GGT. Both rise with prolonged use of alcohol, and the former can take approximately 2–3 months to return to normal following abstention (the later usually reduces in days to weeks depending on the degree of liver damage). If these are raised, discuss the findings with the patient and your colleagues regarding further treatment. Note that there are other causes of a raised GGT like benzodiazepines, phenytoin, obesity, gallbladder and pancreatic disease.

• Women should not drink more than 14 units/week; men 21 units/week. One unit contains 8 g of alcohol. Drinks containing 1 unit of alcohol include a half pint of beer, a small glass of red or white wine, a single bar serving of spirits or sherry or fortified wine.

• Consider a nutritional screen and vitamin supplements (especially B, D and K groups).

• Offer the patient local alcoholic support services. Try not to be judgemental, alcohol dependence is a complex multifactoral disorder and you should approach it as such.

Alcohol withdrawal

Some patients will be admitted specifically to withdraw from alcohol; others will have their alcoholism unmasked in hospital. Always consider alcohol (and nicotine) withdrawal if your patient suddenly becomes unexpectedly ill or agitated.

[1] Mayfield D., McLeod G., Hall P. (1974) The CAGE questionnaire: validation of a new alcoholism screening instrument. *American Journal of Psychiatry* **131**, 1121–1123.

The Hands-on Guide for Junior Doctors, Fourth Edition. Anna Donald, Michael Stein and Ciaran Scott Hill.
© 2011 Anna Donald, Michael Stein and Ciaran Scott Hill. Published 2011 by Blackwell Publishing Ltd.

Table 10.1 Prescribing chlordiazepoxide. Do not treat with chlordiazepoxide for more than 9 days.

Day	Dose of chlordiazepoxide	Tablet timing
Days 1–2	10–20 mg	Four times daily
Days 3–4	10 mg	Thrice daily
Days 5–6	10 mg	Twice daily
Day 7	10 mg	Once daily

■ Ask your senior for local protocols.

■ Watch for hypotension, dehydration, hypoglycaemia and electrolyte imbalance. Ensure 4-hourly observation and regular U&E, glucose, FBC.

■ Benzodiazepines such as chlordiazepoxide, clomethiazole and lorazepam are all used; chlordiazepoxide is the most commonly used. See Table 10.1 for dosing regimen of chlordiazepoxide.

■ Consider IV clomethiazole if the patient is vomiting. A 0.8% infusion of clomethiazole at 3–7.5 ml (24–60 mg)/minute, reducing to 0.5–1 ml (4–8 mg)/minute, should keep the patient lightly sedated. Consult with your senior before administering IV clomethiazole. A resuscitation trolley must be available and frequent observations performed, as the patient may become too deeply sedated. Similarly as it impairs the rate of alcohol breakdown if the patient drinks while receiving the medication, the results can easily be fatal.

■ Be careful with any benzodiazepines. Patients should not drive for 48 hours after taking the last dose. Sedation may mask hepatic coma. Avoid prolonged use and abrupt withdrawal. Dependence becomes a problem after about 9 days.

■ Randomized controlled trials suggest that patients are likely to do better if they are initially detoxified in hospital, as opposed to being managed solely in the community.[2]

Children

You may work with children as a surgical junior doctor, although you are not expected to provide full paediatric care. These tips may help:

■ If you normally power dress you may wish to consider outfits that are a little more casual; it helps to avoid doctor phobia and unnecessary formality.

■ For children under 14, get consent from parents/guardians while they are on the ward, or you will have to call them in from home.

■ Minors between 14 and 16 can legally sign for themselves, but it is usually a good idea to get parental or guardian consent unless there is an emergency.

■ Ask the anaesthetist to insert cannulae when the child is asleep for theatre, to minimize needle trauma and phobia. Young children are usually induced with

[2] Walsh D.C., Hingson R.W., Merrigan D.M. et al. (1991) A randomized trial of treatment options for alcohol-abusing workers. *New England Journal of Medicine* **325**, 775–782.

volatile agents and so do not require IV access as a prerequisite.

■ Paediatric bottles from the paediatrics ward minimize the amount of blood needed.

■ Use local anaesthetic cream before inserting cannulae and taking blood in young children.

■ Be cautious when prescribing IV fluids and drugs – different-sized children have very different fluid and drug needs. Consult the *BNF for children* if in doubt, this is preferable to asking colleagues.

■ In emergencies, intraosseous access is preferable to a delay in finding intravenous access. You ideally need to practice this on a model before doing it for the first time. Although scalp veins may be easy to access in those under 10 months (and can even be used to site central cannulae), you are advised to seek a senior opinion before you attempt to access them. If doing so, an elastic band can act as a useful tourniquet. Be strict with your asepsis; infections of the scalp can lead to meningitis.

Depression

People in hospital are often depressed – with good reason. Hospitals can be scary, lonely places even if you are well, let alone facing serious illness or death. A week working in hospital may seem like a long time but it is *much* longer if you are a patient!

■ Be alert to sudden mood changes and negative conversation. Ask patients about their fears. You may be able to help immediately with reassurance or liaison with social workers, nurses, psychiatrists and medical colleagues.

■ Interestingly, many elderly patients suffering from acute conditions such as MI or strokes have been recently bereaved. Your patient may be grieving.

■ If your patient seems low, they may be suffering from occult pain, hypoxia, alcohol or drug withdrawal, electrolyte and thyroid imbalances, as well as concerns about employment, home care and other likely worries.

■ Alert psychiatrists and colleagues if you think a patient is in danger of attempting suicide (see Chapter 4, Overdose).

Elderly patients

Like children, elderly patients can present with non-specific, understated symptoms. Elderly patients are often stoical and may hide quite severe pain.

1 Monitor vital signs. Count respiratory rate or breathe with the patient to exclude quiet tachypnoea. Consider checking core temperature.

2 Go through a checklist of systems to make sure you're not missing something serious. In particular, watch for:

• Fractures: old people often don't complain of pain. Look at the limbs (especially the hips, legs and wrists) and feel for crepitus.

• Hypoxia: people may present with euphoria. Measure the respiratory rate and do pulse oximetry or blood gases if concerned.

• Fluid overload and electrolyte imbalance: check IV fluids, electrolytes and slow down or stop fluids if necessary. Monitor electrolytes daily and regularly reconsider whether the patient needs IV fluids.

• A basic IV fluid regime for a small elderly person who is not septic would look something like this:

> 500 ml of normal saline with
>   20 mmol KCl over 6 hours
> 500 ml of normal saline with
>   20 mmol KCl over 6 hours
> 500 ml of 5% dextrose with
>   20 mmol KCl over 6 hours
> 500 ml of 5% dextrose with
>   20 mmol KCl over 6 hours

■ Hypothermia: consider checking rectal temperature.

■ Malnutrition: look for flaky skin, poor gums, unhealed bruises or scratches. Consider a nutritional screen; vitamin deficiencies occur relatively commonly in the elderly and can have serious sequelae.

■ K^+-wasting with diuretics. Check K^+ and supplement orally if necessary. Be careful not to produce hyperkalaemia. If you send the patient home with K supplements, be sure to notify both the patient and the GP, so K^+ can be monitored – it is usual to only prescribe 3 days worth to avoid hyperkalaemia.

■ Infantilization of elderly patients. Remember that 80% of elderly patients live at home. Only 14% of people over 75 have any form of dementia. Be careful not to treat elderly people like children.

Haemophiliacs

All in all, haemophiliacs get a bad deal. Adult UK haemophiliacs are not uncommonly Hep B/C and/or HIV-positive. Haemophilia can be crippling, as members of various royal families can testify. People with haemophilia often have many bad hospital experiences. More than most, this group needs open and honest communication. Because of the high rate of infectivity, you need to take the following precautions.

Taking blood

■ Minimize taking blood. Question your colleagues if they have requested frequent routine bloods.

■ Phone a haematologist or ideally the nearest haemophiliac service; usually they will take blood for you. Ask the haematologist where the nearest service is.

■ Paediatric bottles from the paediatrics ward can be used to minimize the amount of blood needed.

■ Don't use a vacutainer; its 18 gauge needle is too big. Use the smallest possible needle or blue butterfly on small veins. Knuckle veins can be useful.

■ Never use a tourniquet. It causes excessive bruising and occasionally major bleeds from pressure trauma to blood vessels. If you need pressure to find a vein, very gently inflate a blood pressure cuff, but release the pressure as soon as you are in the vein, or you will cause major bruising. A good alternative is to get a nurse to gently squeeze the arm.

■ Never give or prescribe drugs IM.

■ Always use standard precautions for taking blood samples. Many UK haemophiliac adults have Hep C and HIV.

■ Always alert the lab to the haemophiliac status of a patient and their hepatitis/HIV status if known.

■ Tell patients why you are taking blood and that you are taking care to avoid any unnecessary tests. These patients are often loath to have more blood taken.

For theatre

■ Do a full clotting screen (INR, bleeding time, APTT, fibrinogen) preoperatively and a screen for antibodies. Liaise with the haematologist. Any deficiency of factors VIII or IX must be corrected before theatre. If the deficiency is corrected, the patient can be treated like other patients post-operatively, except:

■ Factor VIII levels should be tested post-operatively twice per day (factor IX levels once per day). Make sure the first level is taken before the patient is bathed and the wound dressed.

■ Delay suture removal beyond the usual 10 days, as haemophiliacs are prone to bleeding about this time. Get senior advice.

HIV/AIDS

It goes without saying that these patients need special care. They face both death and stigma. You face potentially dangerous needlestick injuries. Time, care and an honest, open approach are essential.

Taking blood

■ It is completely fine to touch HIV/AIDS patients without gloves just about anywhere – just not in a major artery! It is really awful for such patients if health professionals are scared to treat them normally.

■ However, do always wear gloves when taking blood. Always have plenty of space for your tray and sharps. Use a nursing trolley if possible and have separate cardboard trays for sharps.

■ Don't do things in a hurry. Leave plenty of time for procedures and explanations.

■ Label blood samples with high-risk stickies (not in front of the patient). These are available from the labs if they are not already on your ward. It is your responsibility if a lab worker contracts HIV from an unlabelled sample.

■ Use two specimen bags for high-risk samples.

■ Always warn theatre staff if a patient has HIV or AIDS.

■ Treat oral *Candida* with nystatin lozenges (mild) or ketoconazole/miconazole (see the *BNF*).

■ Be aware that HIV/AIDS patients may suffer from depression and may consider suicide. Consider referring to the psychiatrists or social workers. Discuss concerns with the nursing staff – and the patient, of course!

■ AIDS patients may suffer from multiple serious medical problems which may require urgent or aggressive therapy. Common problems include: fever, atypical pneumonia, diarrhoea, skin sores and drug reactions. For reasons that are as yet poorly understood, allergies are much more common in patients with AIDS. If you find yourself looking after an AIDS patient in a general ward, get expert advice from infectious disease staff.

■ If necessary, reassure non-medical ward staff that they cannot catch HIV from an AIDS patient, so that they don't emit an aura of apprehension that the patient will quickly detect.

■ If you get a needlestick injury, don't panic. Only a tiny minority of needlestick injuries (even from HIV patients) transmit an infection (1 in 250), and even fewer do after prophylaxis. Wash out the injury and get rid of the sharp; bleeding the wound is controversial and not currently recommended by the Centre for Communicable Disease (CDC). Call occupational health to arrange for prophylaxis or testing. If it is out-of-hours, get hold of the on-call medical team or A&E.

HIV testing

Patients need counselling and preparation for HIV tests. Discuss doing HIV tests with seniors; they can advise you on hospital policy. The genitourinary specialist nurse may be able to help you with this.

■ Explain HIV/AIDS. Being HIV-positive is not the same thing as having AIDS. At present 50% of asymptomatic HIV-positive patients get AIDS after 10 years.

■ Explain the benefits of the test. If the patient is HIV-positive, you can monitor T-cell function, treat infection better, and he or she can practise safe sex and protect his or her partner; 24-hour support is available for people with HIV.

■ Explain the problems of the test. Some life insurance companies may discriminate against the HIV-positive person (this is being phased out). A way around this is to get tested anonymously at a genitourinary medicine clinic.

■ Arrange with a virologist to have the blood tested as soon as possible (so the patient is not stewing for days).

■ Label the sample carefully and take all precautions when taking it.

■ Tell the patient at what time the result will be back. If there is any delay, let the patient know and reassure him or her that it is not due to the sample being infected.

Jehovah's Witnesses/ Christian Scientists

■ As with any person, you cannot force a Jehovah's Witness or Christian Scientist to accept treatment (e.g. a blood transfusion). Make sure they sign a statement acknowledging refusal of treatment. Most hospitals have policy documents and suitable consent or exemption forms. Discuss the case with your seniors.

■ In an emergency, you can legally instigate treatment to save someone's life unless it is clear that the patient has given an informed refusal of that treatment which remains in force. Again, get nursing and senior advice and, if necessary, advice from your defence organization. The GMC has issued guidance on this subject 'Personal beliefs and medical practice'.

Pregnant women

■ Get senior advice about X-rays in pregnancy (see Chapter 14, Pregnancy). Make sure you notify the radiologist that the patient is pregnant – write it clearly on the form and preferably speak to the radiologist yourself.

■ Always ask women of child-bearing age the date of their LMP and whether or not they are likely to be pregnant. Most will agree to a urinary pregnancy test if asked.

■ Pregnant women have hyperdynamic, volume-expanded circulations. Their JVPs are usually slightly raised. This is okay, but it also means that they can lose a lot of blood before they exhibit signs of hypovolaemia.

■ Most drugs are potentially toxic. Check the BNF guidance. Make sure you know the trimester and always get senior or pharmacist advice before prescribing.

■ Fetuses are like enormous tumours. They consume folate, iron, Ca and other vitamins that would normally go to the mother. Ensure that pregnant women have adequate nutrition and supplement if necessary.

■ Be wary of pregnant women with abdominal pain. Organs such as the appendix get displaced, and inflammation can present in bizarre ways. For example, appendicitis may present as chest pain if it irritates the diaphragm. Always seek senior advice. Consider notifying an obstetrician.

Sickle cell anaemia

Be alert to sickle cell anaemia in any black, Arabic, Indian or Mediterranean patient within the UK with acute pain in the spine, joints, chest or abdomen. Within the UK, all patients of African descent need a sickling test before surgery. Heterozygous patients are only likely to suffer severe symptoms when hypoxic, as may occur during anaesthesia or at high altitudes. However, in homozygous patients, sickling crises are precipitated by hypoxia, infection, cold and other common stressors. Sickling crises can develop with alarming rapidity and can be fatal without prompt treatment. The patient will often know when they are going into crisis.

1 Symptoms of a sickle crisis include severe bone pain, acute abdominal pain, SOB and neurological symptoms such as fits and cranial nerve palsies.

2 Basic management includes prompt analgesia (pethidine 100–200 mg IM 2 hourly as required) – do not be shy with this! Also, O_2 therapy, rehydration (ensure fluid intake of at least 3 l/day) and antibiotics if pyrexial or evidence of infection. Make sure the patient is warm. Seek urgent, expert help especially if they do not improve quickly – these patients can deteriorate within hours! Lung involvement is particularly worrying.

3 Investigations: the patient will need urgent IV access and baseline bloods, cross-match, FBC, reticulocyte count and film, blood cultures, MSU and chest X-ray. Include ABGs if there is any CXR-shadowing, respiratory symptoms or infection. Measure Hb daily.

4 If the patient needs surgery, make sure a suitable experienced anaesthetist is involved; this may require seeking specialist advice.

The patient on steroids

Patients on steroids are vulnerable to infection and other side effects, and may require additional steroid cover while ill. Steroids affect the immune system, fluid balance, carbohydrate, lipid and protein metabolism. Anti-inflammatory steroid equivalent doses are shown in Table 10.2.

Side effects of steroids

Mineralocorticoid effects:
■ Na and water retention, hypertension.
■ Hypokalaemia.
Glucocorticoid effects:
■ Diabetes.
■ Changes in fat distribution.
■ Changes in protein mobilization: osteoporosis, skin atrophy, striae, muscle wasting, delayed wound healing.
■ Mental changes. These occur in most patients. They vary from subtle changes to frank paranoid psychosis. Warn the patient (and relatives and friends!) that they may become easily irritable or

Table 10.2 Anti-inflammatory steroid equivalent doses.

Steroid	Dose (mg)
Dexamethasone and betamethasone	0.75
Methylprednisolone and triamcinolone	4
Prednisolone	5
Hydrocortisone	20

'difficult' and that they should inform the doctor if this causes problems. Initial euphoria and increased appetite are common.

■ Infection:

– *Candida* infection: oesophageal (dysphagia) or vaginal (itching).

– Disseminated viral infection: measles, varicella zoster and herpes zoster.

– Bacterial infection. The inflammatory response is suppressed hence late presentation and rapid systemic spread of infection. Be alert to the 'silent' abdomen, septicaemia and TB.

Other effects:

■ Peptic ulceration: severe dyspepsia is common although the link to ulceration is less well understood.

■ Acne is common.

■ Withdrawal reactions (see below).

Managing ill patients on steroids

Illness (acute stress, especially surgery or infection) increases steroid requirements. Decide if your patient needs additional steroids or not. Prescribe hydrocortisone 25–100 mg tds (or equivalent) in addition to existing steroid dose if required. See Chapter 15, Steroid-dependent patients, for surgical steroid cover. Always be aware of 'silent' infections in a patient on high-dose steroids (see side effects).

Treating common side effects

1 *Candida* infection. Prescribe nystatin lozenges or miconazole oral gel for oral/oesophageal infection, and clotrimazole (Canesten) cream/vaginal pessaries for vaginal infection. Fluconazole 50 mg PO daily is useful as prophylaxis for high-dose steroids.

2 If the patient is known to suffer from cold sores or shingles, tell the patient to start high-dose acyclovir at the earliest sign of recurrence.

3 Heartburn. Prescribe ranitidine 150 mg nocte, lansoprazole 30 mg or equivalent.

Withdrawing steroid therapy

The longer the patient has been on steroids, the more gradual the reduction of steroids needs to be. Abrupt withdrawal may cause acute adrenal insufficiency or Addisonian crisis. Therapy for longer than 2 weeks can lead to adrenal suppression.

You can reduce steroids from high doses by 5 mg of prednisolone (or equivalent)/week until you reach the equivalent of 10 mg prednisolone/day. Thereafter, reduce by 2.5 mg/week until you reach 5 mg/day. After this, the rate of reduction depends on the preceding length of therapy. If this was greater than 3 months, reduce slowly, for example, by 1–2 mg/week.

Withdrawal reactions include Addisonian crisis (hypotension, dehydration, hyperkalaemia, hyponatraemia), arthralgia, conjunctivitis, mood change, rhinitis, skin rashes (itchy nodules or acne) and weight loss. Morning irritability can be prevented by taking the daily dose bd; note, however, that taking steroids on a bd basis is less physiological and more likely to cause Cushingoid symptoms.

Chapter 11
APPROACH TO THE MEDICAL PATIENT

A major task during medical posts is clerking patients. This section provides a practical approach to history and examination of the medical patient, and optimizing your time in getting to know the patient and getting a feel for their problems.

With the introduction of shift work, it is inevitable that you will find yourself looking after a patient you did not admit and do not know. It is well worth the effort to re-clerk these patients, albeit briefly, as soon as possible. It takes less time than you think and will allow you to develop a better relationship with the patient. While your night-shift colleagues are unlikely to miss an obvious sign, it is remarkable how much more information is yielded by a history taken in the light of day.

An approach to history taking comprises two essential parts, which enable management to be tailored to the individual patient and his or her disease:

1 Getting to know the patient (the person and their medical background).

2 Getting to know the disease (the presenting problem).

Getting to know the patient as a person
■ Patient ID – age, sex, etc.
■ Work.
■ Lives with and the family environment.
■ Social support – family, friends, finances.
■ Mobility.

■ Home help.
■ Problems as perceived by the patient: worries, fears.

The medical background
■ Past medical history.
■ Past surgical history.
■ What operations and any anaesthetic complications.
■ Allergies, drug history.
■ Family history.

Getting to know the disease
Presenting complaints. Identify as clearly as possible the reason for the patient presenting now and think of the possible causes for the symptoms so that you establish an early ranked differential diagnosis. Do not take a history blindly without this kind of forethought. Be aware of the diagnostic possibilities based on the background and the presenting complaint so that you ask questions that strengthen or refute a specific possibility. At this stage it is useful to stop, think and construct a ranked differential diagnosis before the next phase of the history taking.

The present history. This is what the patient tells you about their present illness. Listen

The Hands-on Guide for Junior Doctors, Fourth Edition. Anna Donald, Michael Stein and Ciaran Scott Hill.
© 2011 Anna Donald, Michael Stein and Ciaran Scott Hill. Published 2011 by Blackwell Publishing Ltd.

History / Getting to know the patient as a person

Patient ID – age, sex, etc.

Work .... Mobility ....

Lives with .... Home help ....

Social support – Problems as perceived by the patient,

family, friends .... worries, fears ....

Finances..

The medical background

Past medical history

1 CVS – IHD, rheumatic fever, hypertension, other..

2 RS – asthma, smoker, TB, exposure to irritants..

3 Diabetes, thyroid disease, other medical illnesses ....

Past surgical history

What operations ....

Any anaesthetic complications ....

Drug history and allergies

Current medication ....

Relevant past medication ....

Allergies ....

Family history ....

Hobbies and pets ....

Getting to know the disease

Presenting complaint/s ....

....

(STOP–THINK–CONSTRUCT A RANKED DIFFERENTIAL DIAGNOSIS)

The present history and the specific directed enquiry

(What the patient tells you about their illness and directed questions to define the differential.)

Systematic (or functional) enquiry

1 General – loss of appetite, loss of weight, fever, night sweats, any lumps, itch and rashes.

2 CVS/RS – chest pain, dyspnoea, orthopnoea, PND, cough, haemoptysis, sputum, ankle oedema, intermittent claudication.

3 GIT – dyspepsia, nausea, vomiting, diarrhoea, change in bowel habit, blood or mucus PR.

4 GU – dysuria, frequency, urgency, nocturia, haematuria, polyuria, incontinence.

5 Gynaecology – vaginal discharge, menses, first day of last period (LMP), menarche, menopause, pregnancy.

6 CNS – fits, blackouts, headaches, visual disturbances, sensory disturbances, weakness/paralysis, falls, loss of hearing. Higher mental function.

7 MSK/skin – joint pain/swelling, stiffness.

Refined differential diagnosis

....

....

Fig. 11.1 Approach to history taking.

carefully and ask clarifying questions. Attempt to live the patient's life from the onset of the symptoms so that you become aware of important details that will refine your differential diagnosis. Next, try to refine your differential diagnosis and identify those features of the most likely diseases that have emerged thus far. Ask about these features now – the specific directed enquiry – and write down your differential diagnosis and problem list before the examination.

The systematic (or functional) enquiry. This is usually the least useful part of the history. While it provides a convenient list of symptoms, it encourages thoughtless history taking that overworked junior doctors don't need! It should therefore be left until last and although it can sometimes be shortened it is inadvisable to omit in its entirety. For the detailed list of symptoms see Fig. 11.1.

The examination

The same general examination for all patients should be followed by a directed systemic examination, based on the diagnostic possibilities elicited in your history. For example, you would make a careful check for signs of infective endocarditis in a patient with a history of valvular heart disease and recent decrease in exercise tolerance. Note the important negative findings, for example, no splinter haemorrhages, no vasculitic skin lesions, no splenomegaly. Fully document your findings.

We provide an outline of the general and systematic examination of the medical patient in Fig. 11.2. While it is structured in the order for 'routine' examination, few patients are 'routine', and you should examine some systems in more detail according to your differential diagnosis.

Summing up

At the end of your history and examination, it is a good idea to sum up for presenting on ward rounds.

1 Patient ID and salient medical background. (Mention only that which is pertinent to the present problem.)

2 Presenting complaint.

3 Current problems – medical, pharmacological, social.

4 Investigations.

5 Plan for discharge – how the team is going about solving the patient's problems and the likely time of discharge from hospital.

History and examination

Figures 11.1 and 11.2 provide an outline of the above approach to history and examination. Retype and photocopy if you want.

Clinical stalemate

Your patient sits in bed day after day, and no progress is made. What do you do?

1 Decide if the patient is sick or not, and getting better or getting sicker day by day. Sometimes you should let well alone.

2 If the patient is ill or getting worse, then rapidly identify the main problems and make a management plan, for example, is the renal function, mental state or pulmonary function deteriorating?

3 Having addressed obvious problems, review the case. It can be helpful to 're-clerk' the patient, especially as this clerking will have the benefit of hindsight, and the use of previous notes, the patient's drug chart, etc.

- Main complaint.
- History of main complaint.
- PMH.
- Drugs, allergies, habits, travel, etc.

4 Repeat a complete examination. Like the history, the examination will benefit from hindsight and recent investigation

Examination	In order of examination

1 Appearance. Does the patient look ill? General nutrition

2 Temperature

Working up the arm:

3 Hands, nails

4 Pulse

5 Respiratory rate

6 While doing the above, consider evidence of endocrine disease (pituitary, thyroid, Addisons), Paget's; body hair, skin pigmentation, skin lesions

7 BP

8 Eyes – pallor, jaundice

9 Mouth and tongue – cyanosis, smooth or furred tongue, any lesions?

10 Examine the neck – nodes, goitre

CVS examination with patient at 45° :

11 JVP and cartoid pulses

12 Praecordium – inspect, palpate, auscultate

13 Sacral oedema? Ankle oedema?

RS examination with patient at 90° :

14 Chest – inspect, palpate (trachea, expansion), auscultate

15 Breasts and axillary nodes

GIT examination with patient lying flat:

16 Abdomen – inspect, palpate (tenderness, visceromegaly), auscultate (bowel sounds)

Legs:

17 Swelling, pulses

CNS examination:

The detail of this examination will depend on the differential diagnosis. The essentials include:

18 Cranial nerves – pupil responses; fundi; corneal reflexes; 'Open your mouth; stick out your tongue; show me your teeth; shut your eyes tightly; raise your eyebrows; shrug your shoulders'

19 Peripheral nerves and motor function – wasting; sensation (vibration, light touch); tone; power; gait

20 Speech and higher mental functions

21 Do PR and FOB test. Consider PV

22 Dipstick urine and consider microscopy

23 Summarize findings and list your plan for solving the patient's problems:

- Patient ID and salient medical background
- Presenting complaint/s ....
  ....
- Current problem/s ....
  ....
- Investigations ....
  ....
- Plan for discharge ....
  ....

Fig. 11.2 Approach to examination.

results. Examine test results critically – are they reliable or spurious? Are they up to date?

5 Now formulate a list of problems, differential diagnoses, and investigations to be requested. You may not come up with blinding new answers immediately, but you will know the case a lot better and avoid the embarrassment of having over-looked key pieces of information in the history, examination and investigations.

6 Now write a summary in the notes of your findings at this stage. If appropriate, use tables for important serial data.

Preparing patients for medical procedures

During your placement you will prepare patients for many different procedures. This section explains what needs to be done and what complications to expect. It is important to realize that, while most procedures are routine for you, they are usually frightening for patients. Probably the scariest thing is not knowing what will happen next, so lots of information can make a big difference. A list of patients' common concerns about pro-cedures includes:

1 What does the procedure entail?

2 Why are they having this done?

3 How long will the procedure take?

4 Do they need a general anaesthetic?

5 Will the procedure be painful?

6 What should they do if they have pain or other symptoms after the procedure?

7 When can they eat/drink/drive/talk/ have sex?

8 Will they have any scars/permanent after-effects?

9 Who is doing the procedure?

The GMC guidance on consent now states that it should only be undertaken by someone who fully understands the procedure and its alternatives/ complications, and ideally be taken by one who is capable of doing the proce-dure themselves but as a minimum has training in taking consent. This is usually the consultant in charge of the patients or a nominated deputy.

Cardiac catheterization

Preparation

1 Consent (if angioplasty or stenting is planned in addition to diagnostic cathe-terization, this should be explained. There are variants of the procedure, for example, left and right heart catheters, coronary angiography, electrophysiologi-cal studies, depending on the indication. Ask the cardiologists what they intend. If unsure how to consent accurately, ask them for help). Informed consent is ide-ally only obtained by the person doing the procedure, although you can make their job easier by explaining the proce-dure to the patient.

2 Make sure the patient has stopped oral anticoagulants at least 3 days prior to the procedure. In some cases, for instance, when a patient has a metal valve replacement, the patient should be admitted for heparinization, since this can be discontinued a few hours prior to the procedure.

3 Request FBC, INR, APTT, G&S, U&E and creatinine to check renal function.

4 Secure peripheral venous access.

5 Check all peripheral pulses (this acts as a baseline, since rarely, cardiac cathe-terization can cause peripheral arterial thromboembolism).

6 If the patient has renal impairment or diabetes, seek senior advice.

Consider telling patient

1 Why they require cardiac catheterization.

2 The procedure will be done under local anaesthetic and sometimes mild sedation, via the blood vessels in the groin (although sometimes a brachial approach is used via the antecubital fossa, particularly where the patient is anticoagulated).

3 The procedure takes place in a special unit (the 'cath lab'), under X-ray guidance.

4 The process may be diagnostic (coronary arteriogram, left ventriculogram and sometimes right ventriculogram, which requires an additional, transvenous approach) or therapeutic (angioplasty or stent).

5 Afterwards, the patient will need to lie flat for about 4–6 hours.

6 In some centres, routine diagnostic angiography is done as a day case. Check, and let patients know when they are likely to be allowed home.

7 Afterwards, there may be some bruising, and sometimes an ache in the groin, but this should subside.

Complications

1 Bleeding/bruising at groin puncture site.

2 False aneurysm in groin.

3 Stroke, death, MI (risk is < 1/100, but varies with the details of the procedure and baseline characteristics of the patient – ask the cardiologists what risk you should quote for the procedure intended).

Following the procedure

1 Patients are usually taken over by cardiologists following therapeutic cardiac catheterization of a general medical inpatient.

2 Patients must lie flat for several hours.

3 Check groin wound is clean, and there is no evidence of false aneurysm before discharge.

Elective DC cardioversion

Preparation

1 ECG (check that patient is still in fast atrial fibrillation (or have another indication), and that there are no ventricular abnormalities, for example, frequent ectopy).

2 INR (check that INR is currently >2.0, and has been for the last month).

3 U&E (check that serum potassium >3.5 mmol/l, and that other electrolytes are in the normal range).

4 Patient has been NBM for 4 hours prior to attempted cardioversion.

5 If patient is taking digoxin, exclude symptoms of digoxin toxicity (nausea, diarrhoea, visual disturbance, confusion).

6 Peripheral venous access.

7 If the patient has renal impairment, seek senior advice.

8 Inform the anaesthetist and the staff who are required for the procedure. In some centres, the procedure is carried out in theatre recovery or in the induction room, in which case the theatre manager needs to be informed. In other places, it is done on the cardiac day ward, in which case the ward staff should be informed.

9 Obtain informed consent (ask a senior if you are unsure what risks to quote for a particular patient).

10 Ensure that the skin overlying the right sternal border and the cardiac apex is shaved.

Other information to tell the patient

1 Why they require DC cardioversion.

2 It is done under a brief general anaesthetic.

3 What the procedure involves (see below under practical procedures).

4 There is no guarantee that it will cause reversion to sinus rhythm, but that successful cardioversion should bring symptomatic benefit. (The probability of success is highly variable. In young people with no structural heart disease and fairly recent onset, the chances of success are very high; in older people with structural abnormalities and chronic AF, the chances are slim.)

5 Procedure is usually a day case. The patient can go home once the anaesthetic has worn off, but should be taken home by somebody else, and should not drive or operate machinery for the rest of the day.

Complications

1 Small risk of major complication (thromboembolism, life-threatening arrhythmia, aspiration).

2 Skin burns where pads were applied.

Following the procedure

1 Check ECG.

2 Inform patient that the procedure was successful/unsuccessful. If successful, warn patient that effects may not be sustained indefinitely, and that AF may reoccur.

3 Continue medications and arrange outpatient clinic appointment. You may need to check these arrangements with a senior colleague.

4 Wait for 2–3 hours before discharging. Ensure that patients do not go home on their own, and that there is somebody at home to supervise them for the rest of the day.

Upper gastrointestinal endoscopy

Preparation

1 Consent.

2 NBM for 4 hours. If you suspect gastric outlet obstruction, allow only water for 8 hours and NBM for 4 hours.

3 FBC and INR (in case of biopsy).

4 Insert cannula (usually 21G, although 23G sometimes suffices) in the arm that will make endoscopic manoeuvring easiest (usually the right arm).

5 Barium can block the suction channel of the endoscope, so delay for 24 hours following upper GI barium studies.

Consider telling the patient

1 What endoscopy is and why they are having it.

2 That the procedure takes about 5–10 minutes, although it may seem longer.

3 During the procedure, they will be given IV sedation, but not a general anaesthetic, to make them drowsy. They shouldn't drive until the following day. Also, their throat will be sprayed with local anaesthetic so that they won't feel the endoscope too much.

4 An endoscope (tube) the thickness of a little finger is passed into the food pipe and into the stomach. It is uncomfortable but should not be painful.

5 The doctor might take a tiny sample of the inside of the gullet or stomach to examine under a microscope. This is painless.

6 The patient can eat and drink after the local anaesthetic has worn off, which should take about half an hour. They might have a sore throat, which should get better within 1–2 days.

Complications

1 Transient sore throat and possible numbness.

2 Rarely oesophageal perforation (about 1 in 1000).

3 Mild bleeding (and rarely haemorrhage) following a biopsy.

Colonoscopy

Preparation

1 Consent.

2 Low residue diet for 36 hours and fluids only for 12 hours before the procedure.

3 Two Picolax sachets (sodium picosulphate and magnesium citrate) or equivalent 24 hours before the procedure. Use one sachet for frail, elderly patients. Do not give to patients with inflamed colonic mucosa (UC, Crohn's, etc.).

Consider telling the patient

1 What colonoscopy is (a way of looking directly at the bowel) and why they are having it.

2 Warn that Picolax causes explosive diarrhoea. They need to drink plenty of clear fluids to maintain hydration (2–3 l/day: three to four jugs of squash).

3 IV sedation is given that will make them drowsy, but it is not a general anaesthetic.

4 A flexible tube is passed into their back passage.

5 The whole thing takes about 20–30 minutes, and the patient can go home accompanied as soon as the sedation has worn off – usually in about 2 hours. They should not drive until the following day.

Complications

1 Mild abdominal discomfort during and after the procedure is common due to a small amount of gas that is pumped in to aid vision through the colonoscope during the procedure.

2 Incomplete examination, requiring a second examination or barium enema, occurs in up to 10% of cases.

3 Perforation occurs about 1 in 500, more commonly in acute colitis or extensive diverticulosis. If this unlikely event happens, the person usually will need to have their bowel repaired under a general anaesthetic.

4 Serious haemorrhage post-biopsy or polypectomy is rare.

Flexible sigmoidoscopy

Preparation

1 Two phosphate enemas.

2 Explanation as for colonoscopy except sedation is not usually needed.

Liver biopsy

Preparation

1 Consent.

2 Bloods: FBC, INR and APTT, liver biochemistry and G&S.

3 Abdominal US advisable to check anatomy (ask the person performing the procedure).

4 Mild pre-med, such as pethidine (50 mg) and prochlorperazine (12.5 mg). Temazepam (10 mg) can also be given if the patient is not at risk of hepatic failure or jaundiced.

5 IV access with at least a green cannula.

Consider telling the patient

1 What a liver biopsy is and why they need one.

2 The procedure is performed on the ward or in an operating theatre. The biopsy itself is very quick (a few seconds) but the whole procedure might take up to 30 minutes – and may seem longer than this. They will have to stay in hospital overnight.

3 The procedure does not usually involve heavy sedation or a general anaesthetic.

4 The site of the biopsy is on the patient's right side, between the 8th and 10th ribs. The patient will need to help by holding their breath during the biopsy.

Complications

1 Shoulder tip or local abdominal pain for a few hours (up to 2 days) is common but relieved by paracetamol 1 g 6-hourly.

2 Bleeding possibly requiring transfusion (about 1 in 50).

3 Infection, abscess, pneumothorax (rarely requiring drainage) and biliary peritonitis are uncommon (<1:100).

Following the procedure

1 The patient should lie on their right side for at least 2 hours and remain in bed (absolute bed rest) overnight.

2 Observations: BP and pulse every 15 minutes for 1 hour, then every 30 minutes for 2 hours, then hourly for 6 hours. Ask to be informed if the BP falls (>15 mmHg) or if the pulse starts rising (>15 bpm).

3 Ensure that an IV line is secure and that analgesia is written up (ask the operator which they prefer).

4 Check the patient 4 and 8 hours following the biopsy for pain and vital signs.

Pacemaker insertion

Preparation

1 Informed consent.

2 FBC and INR.

Consider telling the patient

1 What a pacemaker is and why he or she needs one.

2 A very small wire is threaded via a large vein (the subclavian) into one of the chambers of the heart under X-ray screening. The wire is gently inserted into the wall of the heart. The other end of the wire is connected to a machine called a pacemaker that generates heart beats, which is placed into a small pocket fashioned in the fatty tissues of the chest. Its battery will not run out! The pacemaker causes a small lump under the skin on the upper thorax, but nowadays the generators are so small these are hardly noticeable.

3 The procedure is performed under local anaesthetic, sometimes with mild sedation.

4 The procedure is mostly painless. It takes 30–60 minutes.

5 In future, the patient will need to carry a card that says they are fitted with a permanent pacemaker, in case they ever need emergency treatment. A Medicalert bracelet is recommended.

6 Caution in pregnancy, as X-ray screening is used during the procedure.

Complications

1 As for central line placement – pneumothorax, bleeding.

2 Dislodgement of the wire leading to pacing failure. Electrical faults are uncommon.

Following the procedure

1 The patient will need a CXR to check lead placement and to exclude pneumothorax.

2 A pacemaker check ECG to make sure the pacemaker is capturing correctly.

Renal biopsy

Preparation

1 Consent.

2 Bloods: FBC, INR, G&S.

3 Abdominal US is essential to check that two kidneys are present.

4 Mild pre-med, such as pethidine (50 mg IM) and prochlorperazine (12.5 mg IM).

5 IV access with at least an 18G (green) cannula.

Consider telling the patient

1 What a renal biopsy is and why they need one.

2 The procedure is usually done in theatre and takes a few minutes. Sedation is usually required (but not a general anaesthetic).

3 The biopsy is taken through the left or right flank. The patient will need to hold their breath briefly during the biopsy.

4 The patient should drink a lot of fluids after the biopsy, to flush the kidneys and avoid renal colic.

Complications

1 Local pain (prescribe analgesia) and mild haematuria are common.

2 Haemorrhage requiring transfusion is less common (about 1 in 30–60). Surgical intervention for massive haemorrhage is rare.

3 Renal colic from clots may occur.

Following the procedure

1 Patient should lie on the side of the biopsy for at least 2 hours and remain in bed (absolute bed rest) overnight.

2 Observation: BP and pulse every 15 minutes for 1 hour, then every 30 minutes for 2 hours, then hourly for 6 hours. Ask to be informed if the BP falls (>15 mmHg) or if the pulse starts rising (>15 bpm).

3 Check for gross haematuria.

4 Ensure IV access is OK and that good analgesia is written up.

5 Check on the patient 4 and 8 hours following the biopsy for pain, unstable vital signs and gross haematuria or bleeding.

Specialist referrals and investigating the medical case

Most consultants have their own favourite investigations. Be guided by ward protocols, but ask someone if you do not understand the rationale for a particular investigation. Protocols often become outdated and nobody takes the time to inform the new junior doctor.

If a patient is unwell enough to be admitted, you should have the following results as a minimum:

1 Weight.

2 Temperature, blood pressure, pulse, respiratory rate and oxygen saturations.

3 Urine dipstick.

4 FBC +/− CRP and ESR.

5 Biochemistry – at least U&E.

When indicated (for most medical patients):

6 CXR.

7 ECG.

Below, we provide a list of further investigations to anticipate, listed under system headings for commonly encountered pathologies. In addition, these are a useful checklist when making specialist referrals. You will greatly impress the visiting consultant if you have useful results to hand. If in doubt, bleep their junior doctor to discover which investigations are flavour of the month.

Cardiology

Essential investigations before referral to a cardiologist include ECG and rhythm strip and CXR. In specific situations, see below.

Suspected acute MI

1 Serial ECGs (at *least* every hour if equivocal and then for three consecutive days).

2 Serial serum cardiac enzymes (including Troponin assay which, when taken after 12 hours, offers a more specific and sensitive marker of MI).

3 If within 6 hours of onset of chest pain, you can check lipid profile (levels are unreliable after this).

Ischaemic heart disease

1 ECG (preferably both during an episode of chest pain and when pain free).

2 Serum cholesterol and triglycerides.

3 Formal blood sugar (ward test is not good enough).

Heart failure (recent onset)

1 ECHO: this is urgent if there are murmurs of aortic valve disease or you suspect SBE (consider transoesophageal ECHO if available) or pericardial disease.

Hypertension

1 Cholesterol and triglycerides.

2 MSU for MC&S if blood or protein on urinary dipstick.

3 Ensure there is a recent record of an ECG, CXR and serum biochemistry.

4 US of the kidneys if symptoms are suggestive of clinical renal disease (history of nephritis, renal problems in childhood, family history of renal disease) or sudden onset or poorly controlled BP.

5 Fundoscopic examination.

Infective endocarditis

1 Blood cultures; at least three sets – ideally from different sites.

2 CRP, U&E and LFT.

3 Rh factor.

4 Urine dipstick and microscopy.

5 Blood film, serum haptoglobins and urinary haemosiderin.

6 Consider transoesophageal ECHO.

7 Document peripheral stigmata of infective endocarditis.

Endocrinology

Except for DM, endocrine disorders are relatively rare. Special tests are required according to the differential diagnosis before referral.

1 Flow chart the patients blood glucose readings and glycosylated Hb (HbA$_{1c}$) if available.

2 Renal function.

• Flow chart of creatinine and urea levels.

• 24-hour urine collection for creatinine clearance and protein.

3 Careful fundoscopy and ophthalmology referral.

4 Peripheral nerve examination.

5 Cholesterol and triglycerides.

6 ECG – have old ECGs to compare.

7 Arrange follow-up in diabetic clinic, arrange diabetic dietary advice by dietician, and involve the diabetic specialist nurse if available.

Investigation of Cushing's disease/syndrome

Consult a specialized lab for advice. Different labs prefer different tests.

Standard tests done in most labs include those listed below.

1 Midnight (or at least after 10 p.m.) and 9 a.m. cortisol levels. The night level is usually lower than the morning level, but this diurnal cycle is lost in Cushing's. The midnight level is often called a 'sleeping level' that can be done soon after waking the patient, not while they are actually asleep!

2 Shortened low-dose dexamethasone suppression test: 1 mg dexamethasone PO at 11 p.m. and measure the cortisol level in the morning at around 9 a.m. In Cushing's, the cortisol levels are not suppressed, whereas in pseudo-Cushing's (e.g. depression, severe obesity and alcoholism), the cortisol level is suppressed.

3 High dose dexamethasone suppression test: 0.5 mg dexamethasone 6-hourly for 48 hours. Next, measure the morning cortisol level at 24 and 48 hours. This suppresses cortisol levels in pituitary-dependent Cushing's *disease*, while it does not suppress cortisol levels in adrenal adenomas and ectopic ACTH (Cushing's *syndrome*).

4 Measure urinary-free cortisol (24-hour urine collections).

Investigations for phaeochromocytoma

Consult a specialized lab for advice. Different labs prefer different tests. Standard tests done in most labs include those listed below.

1 Three 24-hour urine collections for catecholamines (adrenaline, noradrenaline metabolites (HMMA/VMA) or total metadrenalines). Requires a special urine bottle. Tell the patient to avoid vanilla, bananas and aspirin.

2 Consider CT or MRI scan of chest and abdomen (phaeochromocytomas can arise anywhere along the sympathetic chain), and/or special isotope (MIBG) scan, if the urine test is positive.

Thyroid disease

1 Hypothyroidism: raised TSH, low T_4.

2 Secondary hypothyroidism (rare): low T_4 and T_3 but TSH is not raised; look for pituitary failure.

3 Hyperthyroidism: suppressed TSH and raised T_4 or T_3. In 10% of patients with hyperthyroidism, only the T_3 is raised.

Gastroenterology

Always do a PR before referring to a gastroenterologist. Gastroenterologists often request some unusual tests so investigate according to the differential diagnosis.

Upper GI symptoms

1 Barium meal or gastroscopy.

2 FBC.

GI bleeds (see Chapter 7, Upper gastrointestinal bleeds; Lower gastrointestinal bleeds)

1 Cross-match.

2 Hb, platelets and clotting studies.

3 Check LFTs, U&E.

4 Endoscopy.

5 Consider surgical consultation.

Chronic diarrhoea

1 Warm stool for MC&S including ova, cysts and parasites ($\times 3$), *Clostridium difficile* toxin and culture.

2 FBC (including MCV).

3 LFTs (albumin).

4 Ca^{2+} and phosphate.

5 Thyroid Function Tests (TFTs).

6 Amylase.

7 24 hours 5-Hydroxyindoleacetic Acid (5-HIAA) or chromogranin A (Carcinoid syndrome).

Chronic lower GIT symptoms

1 Faecal occult bloods – used as a screening tool, mainly in outpatients, but *not* diagnostically.

2 FBC and MCV.

3 Flexible sigmoidoscopy.

4 Consider barium enema or colonoscopy, depending on local expertise.

5 Consider a small bowel meal.

6 Consider other sources (e.g. GU tract) for symptoms.

Ascites of unknown origin

1 History of alcohol consumption.

2 Bloods for LFTs, hepatitis serology. Consider checking anti-mitochondrial antibodies (for primary biliary cirrhosis) and anti-smooth muscle cell antibodies (for chronic active hepatitis).

3 Aspirate the ascites (see Chapter 13, Peritoneal tap (paracentesis)). Re-examine following aspiration, especially for female pelvic organs. A PV is essential if the cause of ascites is unclear.

4 US the abdomen and pelvis (consider aspiration under US guidance if there is a small or loculated collection). US is most useful after aspiration. Specific points on US: Is the portal vein patent? Size and texture of liver and spleen? Porta hepatis nodes?

5 Consider a CT scan.

6 Consider a barium swallow or endoscopy for varices.

7 Consider peritoneoscopy – may be dependent on local expertise.

8 Consider a laparotomy.

Liver disease

1 INR, platelets, bleeding time (full clotting studies).

2 Liver function tests and general biochemistry.

3 Urine for bilirubin and urobilinogen.

4 Hepatitis screen – B and C (A if acute).

5 Iron/TIBC, caeruloplasmin, alphafetoprotein.

6 US abdomen.

7 Stool chart.

8 Consider liver biopsy.

9 Consider random alcohol level on this or next admission. MCV and GGT.

Haematology

Essential investigations before referral include FBC, differential, film and ESR.

Suspected DIC

1 Fibrin degradation products (FDPs).

2 INR and APTT.

3 LFTs.

4 Urine dipstick and microscopy.

5 Blood cultures.

(DIC is not an end diagnosis – you must find the cause.)

Anaemia (see Chapter 7, Anaemia)

1 Reticulocyte count and sickle cell status.

2 Serum bilirubin, LDH (a marker of haemolysis), serum haptoglobins.

3 Iron studies, vitamin B_{12}, serum and red cell folate.

4 CRP, ESR.

5 Consider Hb electrophoresis.

6 Consider bone marrow biopsy.

Suspected paraprotein/myeloma

1 ESR and viscosity.

2 Serum and urine electrophoresis, urine collection for light chains (15% of patients have urinary light chains only).

3 Skeletal survey.

4 Bone marrow biopsy.

Neurology

A thorough history and detailed examination are by far the most important things before you consider any referral.

Meningism

1 Do a LP (see Chapter 13, Lumbar puncture) if there are *no* signs of raised ICP (rising BP, papilloedema, depressed LOC) or contraindications like bleeding disorders. If possible, it is prudent to perform a CT prior to performing LP, to rule out compression of intracranial structures like the basal cisterns.

- LP pressure with a manometer.
- MC&S, cell count, xanthochromia.
- Consider Indian ink stains for *Cryptococcus*, ZN for AFBs, viral PCR.
- Glucose.
- Protein.

2 Consider serology for *Cryptococcus*, syphilis and viral causes of meningitis.

Unexplained coma

Before referral you should:

1 Ensure that the patient's ABC are adequate.

2 Obtain a history from relatives, friends and GP, especially regarding epilepsy, possible drug overdose or recent travel abroad.

3 Do a secondary neurological examination for clues. The neurological exam would initially have been restricted to the Glasgow Coma Scale and hard localizing signs.

4 Have the following results clearly documented (if available):

- Blood glucose stick that was done immediately on admission.
- FBC, U&E, Ca, phosphate, blood glucose.
- Liver biochemistry.
- Urine dipstick and MC&S.
- ABGs and toxicology screen.

5 Arrange an urgent CT scan head followed by LP.

6 Send a serum sample for storage (serology).

Unexplained weakness

Before referral you should:

1 Send off the following initial tests:

- FBC, U&E, CK, LFT.
- ESR, Ca^{2+}, Protein electrophoresis.
- Vit B_{12}, folate, blood glucose, thyroid function test.

2 Consider an Electromyography or nerve conduction study.

Renal medicine

Renal physicians rely heavily on biochemistry to manage their patients, so have a flow chart of the patient's U&E and creatinine results. Get their help early if a patient's renal function is deteriorating.

Renal failure/nephrotics/nephritics

1 BP.

2 Fresh urine for microscopy (do on ward) and send sample for MC&S.

3 Daily weights.

4 Fluid intake/output chart.

5 Serology.

- Virology: CMV, Hep B and C and HIV if candidate for haemodialysis/transplant (remember to counsel the patient).
- Bacteriology: VDRL and atypical serology.
- Immunology: CRP, Igs and serum electrophoresis, complement and auto-antibodies; ANA initially, but also consider ANCA, anti-GBM and cryoglobulins.

6 Biochemistry: in addition to renal and hepatic indices request: Ca, total protein, albumin, phosphate.

7 24-hour urine collection – protein and creatinine clearance.

8 Renal US – do early to exclude obstruction, especially if the renal function is deteriorating.

9 Consider renal biopsy.

Renal biopsy (see Renal biopsy, above)

Recurrent UTIs

1 BP, MSU.

2 Creatinine clearance.

3 Abdominal X-ray and/or non-contrast CT stone search to look for calculi. Consider an IVU or CT Urogram (looking for structural anomalies).

4 US kidneys (document the size).

5 Consider a micturating cystogram (reflux) – this is mainly used in children and is only usually requested in a specialist setting.

6 PR and proctoscopy.

7 PV and speculum examination.

8 Consider a urology referral.

Respiratory medicine

Essential investigations before referral to a respiratory physician are CXRs, ECGs and results of lung function tests and ABGs.

Pneumonia

1 CXR.

2 Sputum for MC&S, cytology and AFB.

3 Physiotherapy if bronchopneumonia or exacerbation of COPD – arrange ASAP. Physiotherapy is not indicated for lobar pneumonia.

4 ABGs are mandatory for any severe respiratory illness.

5 Send a serum sample for storage if you suspect an atypical pneumonia (*Legionella*, *Mycoplasma*, etc).

If you suspect TB

1 Sputum for AFB. (Hypertonic 5% saline nebulizer will encourage productive coughing if sputum is difficult to obtain.)

2 3+ early morning specimens of urine for AFB.

3 Mantoux test (see Chapter 13, Mantoux test).

Obstructive lung disease

Lung function tests pre- and post-bronchodilators.

Respiratory failure

ABGs and acid–base. (Raised bicarbonate or base excess is a useful indicator of chronic CO_2 retention.)

Pleural effusion

1 Send aspirate for:

- Protein, LDH.
- MC&S, AFBs and TB culture.
- Cytology.
- Glucose.

2 Consider pleural biopsy.

3 Consider tuberculin skin test.

Rheumatology

'Look, feel and move' all salient joints; FBC, ESR and CRP; X-rays of relevant joints. A hand X-ray can often be illuminating.

Polyarthritis

1 Urate.

2 Fresh urine for microscopy.

3 X-ray affected joints.

4 CRP.

5 ASOT, serum sample for storage.

6 Latex fixation for Rheumatoid factor.

7 Auto-antibodies screen – ANAs.

8 Consider joint aspiration ± synovial biopsy.

Chapter 12

PAIN

This section is designed to help you manage pain on the general wards. The first section provides a general approach to pain control and summarizes commonly used analgesics, categorized by method of administration (such as inhalational, oral, IM/IV). The boxed section is written by a pain relief specialist. It gives an overview of the crucial and often overlooked aspects of pain control. Finally we provide tables for managing pain according to its severity and underlying clinical conditions.

Pain control

Pain control is critical to good clinical practice, yet is often poorly managed and poorly understood. Never be afraid to seek senior or specialist advice. Uncontrolled pain is one of the worst things patients can experience. The resistance of some clinicians to involve specialist pain teams is difficult to justify.

General

■ When first presented with a patient in acute pain, you need to decide whether it is safe to treat the pain symptomatically or whether you should further investigate its cause before masking the symptoms. Do not just treat pain – where possible, find the underlying cause.

■ Analgesics are much more effective when used prophylactically. Frequent, mild analgesia may control pain much better than one-off hits of stronger preparations. It is worth explaining this to patients, particularly when they tell you that paracetamol 'doesn't work for me'.

■ Anticipate common side effects of analgesics, listed in Tables 12.2–12.4. Also

be alert to idiosyncratic drug reactions such as rashes and blood dyscrasias.

■ You will greatly alleviate acute physical pain by addressing the patient's fear and anxiety. Reassure the patient that the pain can and will be lessened. Next, prescribe an appropriate analgesic (see Tables 12.5 and 12.6).

Specific analgesics

Inhaled drugs
(see Table 12.1)

Entonox (50% nitrous oxide, 50% oxygen).

Oral drugs

Paracetamol (see Table 12.2)

Non-steroidal anti-inflammatory drugs (see Table 12.3)
■ Aspirin – enteric-coated preparations are designed to reduce dyspepsia. Good for migrainous pain although there are newer and more effective agents for migraines (consult the *BNF*).
■ Naproxen – low incidence of side effects, highly effective for inflammatory pain.

The Hands-on Guide for Junior Doctors, Fourth Edition. Anna Donald, Michael Stein and Ciaran Scott Hill.
© 2011 Anna Donald, Michael Stein and Ciaran Scott Hill. Published 2011 by Blackwell Publishing Ltd.

Table 12.1 Entonox (50% nitrous oxide and 50% oxygen).

Pros	Cons
Simple, fast and relatively safe	Does not work in all patients
Excellent for one-off or routine painful procedures where the stimulus and response are predictable	It cannot be used continuously or excessively because it causes bone marrow depression in a dose-dependent manner

Note: Never strap the mask in place; you may suffocate the patient. The patient should hold the mask.

Table 12.2 Paracetamol.

Pros	Cons
Few adverse effects	Hepatotoxic in overdose
Useful for mild pain	

Table 12.3 Non-steroidal anti-inflammatory drugs (NSAIDs).

Pros	Cons
Excellent for treating pain associated with inflammation	NSAIDs share many side effects, commonly dyspepsia and nausea
Antipyretic	Occasional GI bleeding or ulceration, diarrhoea
The use of ulcer prophylactic drugs (e.g. proton pump inhibitors) has made the use of NSAIDs safer	Hypersensitivity reactions (angio-oedema, bronchospasm, urticaria); headache; dizziness; vertigo; tinnitus; renal impairment Caution in the elderly or if volume depleted (low GFR). Can precipitate acute renal failure, especially if there is pre-existing renal impairment There is considerable variability in individual patient response to a particular drug

■ Diclofenac – see naproxen. Highly effective. The PR preparation is often used as the analgesic of choice in renal colic.

■ Diflunisal – see naproxen. Longer half-life allows for twice daily doses.

■ Ibuprofen – fewer side effects than other NSAIDs though less anti-inflammatory activity.

■ Tenoxicam – similar to naproxen. Long half-life allows once daily administration.

■ Selective inhibitors of cyclooxygenase type-2 (COX-2 inhibitors) – as effective as conventional NSAIDs, but not free of GI adverse effects as claimed by manufacturers. NICE recommends that they be used in preference to normal NSAIDs only in patients at high risk of developing GI side effects.

Crucial and often overlooked aspects of pain control

There are two types of pain: acute and chronic. Furthermore, each type of pain has two components: physical (sensory or 'stimulus-dependent') and emotional (Fig. 12.1). In addition, some pain cannot be reduced to physical or emotional components. This is known as 'stimulus-independent' pain. Finally, the relative importance of each component can change, so each patient's pain needs to be assessed daily. Bear in mind that the emotional component is often missed, but may be the most significant contributing factor.

Physical (stimulus-dependent) and stimulus-independent pain

In both acute and chronic pain, the stimulus and the response may not always be directly related. There is often background pain independent of the stimulus. Indeed, in chronic pain there may be no relationship between the stimulus and the pain perceived. This 'stimulus-independent' pain is often referred to as neuropathic pain, may be strongly affected by emotion (but not necessarily) and can be extremely difficult to treat. Such pain requires a different approach than

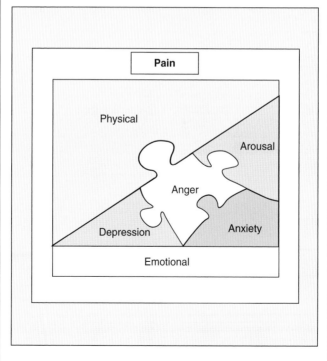

Fig. 12.1 Emotional and physical components of pain.

stimulus-dependent pain. An example of this is the pain of post-herpetic neural-gia. These patients have altered pain perception: they may be numb to a pin-prick but find light touch extremely painful. The most successful treatment for this pain is antidepressants, typifying the enigma of the neuropathic component of pain.

Emotional component of pain

There are four basic mood factors: arousal or awareness, anxiety, unhappiness or depression and anger (Fig. 12.1). The experience of pain is affected – and often heightened – by these different factors.

In *acute pain*, fear and anxiety heightens pain perception. These are usually reduced by treatment with regular painkillers together with reassurance that pain is to be expected and can be controlled. Occasionally, the emotional response is so intense that it is necessary to use a sedative such as midazolam. For example, arousal (awareness) during procedures is very unpleasant. In endoscopy, opiates are given in combination with sedatives (e.g. pethidine and midazolam) thus deal-ing with both the physical and emotional responses to the stimuli.

In *chronic pain*, the emotional response can include chronic anxiety, depres-sion and anger or frustration to varying degrees. The clinical significance of these responses needs to be identified and treated. Patients with chronic pain are often angry that the medical profession cannot cure them and may inad-vertently vent their frustration on junior staff. Such patients are best referred for treatment at the local pain clinic. Chronic pain patients frequently need help from people very experienced in pain control and in understanding their distress.

Contrary to widespread belief, NSAIDs can have GI adverse effects even when given via non-oral routes. This is because it is the anti-inflammatory inhibition of prostaglandins by cyclooxygenase that also causes a reduction in protective stom-ach mucus and leads to increased acid secretion.

Opiates (oral)

For pros and cons, see Table 12.4 for IM/IV opiates.

■ Codeine – mild to moderate analge-sia. High incidence of constipation and drowsiness. N&V are unusual.

■ Dihydrocodeine – similar to codeine.

■ Morphine (oral) – usually prescribed as slow release preparation (MST). Used for chronic pain in terminally ill patients. High doses are often required as tolerance (tachyphylaxis) develops quite rapidly.

IM/IV opiates

Bolus injection

■ This involves slow IV injection over 2–3 minutes.

■ Morphine – most commonly used, standard opiate for bad pain (see Table 12.5).

■ Pethidine – much weaker analgesic properties than morphine. Most often used as pain prophylaxis for procedures.

Table 12.4 IM/IV opiates.

Pros	Cons
Potent analgesics	Nausea, vomiting, constipation and drowsiness. An anti-emetic is usually required
Excellent for pain relief in the terminally ill	Respiratory depression and hypotension at higher doses Addictive if used chronically (tolerance also develops)

Side effects tend to be dose-dependent though there is variability between individual patients. Naloxone is a highly effective antidote for opiate overdose (hypotension, respiratory depression). Give in incremental doses of 100–20μg IV every 2 minutes. Beware of overtreating and throwing the patient into severe pain.

Table 12.5 Recommended analgesics for different levels of pain (this is based on the WHO pain ladder).

Mild pain

1 Paracetamol 500–1000 mg 4–6-hourly. Max dose in 24 hours is 4 g

2 Ibuprofen 400–600 mg 8-hourly. Max dose is 2.4 g daily

Moderate pain

4 Co-codamol paracetamol (500 mg) and dihydrocodeine (8 or 30 mg) in each tablet. Dose 1–2 tablets 4–6-hourly. Max eight tablets daily

5 NSAIDs: Diclofenac 50–150mg PO daily in two divided doses; should be taken with food. Dose by IM injection: 75 mg once daily for a max of 2 days. (Max dose 150 mg daily by any route)

6 Codeine 30–60mg PO/IM 4-hourly. Max dose 240 mg daily. Constipation is common so prescribe a prophylactic laxative (see Chapter 9, Miscellaneous tips)

Severe pain

7 Morphine sulphate 10 mg IM 4-hourly or 2–5 mg IV 4-hourly. (Use 15 mg IM for heavier, well-muscled patients)

8 Diamorphine 5 mg SC/IM 4-hourly or 0.5–2.5 mg/hour IV/SC as an infusion. (Use up to 10 mg IM/SC for heavier, muscular patients)

9 Pethidine 25–100mg IV/IM/SC repeated after 4 hours. Max dose in 24 hours is 400 mg. Opiates are usually administered with a prophylactic anti-emetic such as prochlorperazine (10 mg PO, 30 minutes before giving the opiate, or 12.5 mg IM)

■ Diamorphine – similar analgesic properties to morphine. A dose of 5 mg is equivalent to 10 mg of morphine. It is more soluble than morphine, so easier for SC infusions.

■ Papaveretum – mixture of morphine, codeine and papaverine. Most commonly used by anaesthetists for perioperative analgesia.

■ Tramadol – this provides analgesia through an opioid effect and an enhancement of the serotenergic and adrenergic pathways. It has less opioid side effects but its efficacy is weaker than some other opioids, particularly in the young.

Infusions (SC and PCA)

Morphine and diamorphine are commonly given as continuous infusions, particularly post-op or in the terminally ill. They can be administered as SC, continuous infusions or by PCA. Different hospitals use different pumps; ask nursing and medical colleagues how to set up opiate infusions for your patients. Also consult the *BNF* and see Chapter 12, Pain.

Opiate antidote

Naloxone is a highly effective antidote for opiate overdose (small pupils, hypotension, respiratory depression). Give in incremental doses of 100–200 μg IV every 2 minutes. Beware of overtreating, as analgesia may be reversed. Remember that naloxone has a short half-life, so check on the patient later and ask nurses to keep an eye on the patient to ensure they do not slip back into an over-opiated state. Alternatively, you could give naloxone as a slow IV infusion.

Other

Nerve blockades are rarely given by junior doctors. The technique for local blockade is described on see Chapter 9, Giving Drugs. Epidural and spinal blockades are specialist procedures.

TENS (transcutaneous electrical nerve stimulation). Small portable machines are usually available to local pain teams or physiotherapy teams. They work by Melzack and Wall's 'Pain Gate' theory that states that mechanical stimulation is carried in preference to nociception (think about how you might rub your knee when you hit it).

Acupuncture has an evidence base that is still in flux. It appears that it can be very effective for certain types of pain but not for others.

Pain control by severity and underlying condition

It is useful to categorize the patient's pain as mild, moderate or severe, and to

Table 12.6 Clinical conditions and commonly used analgesics.

Simple headache	Paracetamol
Severe post-op pain	Morphine, pethidine or papaveretum (IM/PO)
Colicky abdominal pain	Hyoscine butylbromide (Buscopan) (PO/IV/IM)
Renal colic	Diclofenac (PR/IM)
Acute MI	Morphine or diamorphine (slow IV injection)
Pleuritic pain	NSAID, e.g. naproxen or diclofenac
Metastatic bone pain	Slow release oral morphine plus NSAIDs
Sciatica	Co-codamol (mild pain), diclofenac or naproxen (severe pain)
Phantom limb pain	Gabapentin or carbamazepine (consult pain relief clinic)
Diabetic neuropathy	Carbamazepine (consult pain relief clinic)

become familiar with the use of two or three preparations in each category. Our favourite analgesics are listed in Tables 12.5 and 12.6.

Hints

■ Many of the compound analgesics contain small doses of codeine or other opiate analgesics. The *BNF* reports that these doses are of little clinical benefit while having the potential side effects of opiates. However, some patients swear by them and will only be happy if these are prescribed for their ailment. A common example is co-codamol (paracetamol 500 mg and codeine phosphate 8–60 mg).

■ Ward stocks of compound analgesics may be limited to one or two brands you are not familiar with. Nursing staff will often be able to advise which preparation is the most effective. They will have been dispensing the drug to patients for years. Don't be shy to ask their opinion.

Chapter 13
PRACTICAL PROCEDURES

Even those with absolutely no hand–eye coordination can master most practical procedures. Most importantly, practice makes perfect. Remember that mistakes are inevitable, so don't be too hard on yourself when you screw up – everyone does. Just be cautious at first and never be afraid to ask for help – if you feel uncomfortable about something, there is probably a good reason! This section is aimed to guide you through most procedures you will encounter as a foundation doctor. You will no doubt soon develop your own tricks to perfect your performance.

General hints

■ Always obtain consent from the patient – often verbal consent will suffice.

■ Never do a procedure unless you have been supervised at least once.

■ Order and space make procedures much easier. Before starting a procedure, get everything you need ready on a trolley. Make room for used sharps. Take a sharps bin to where you are working or have a kidney dish ready. Make sure you have enough local anaesthetic, needles and gloves. If it is an aseptic technique, then it is *very* helpful to have an assistant as you will invariably have forgotten something.

■ Consider taking the patient to a side room for the procedure, rather than performing it at the bedside which can be embarrassing for the patient and others on the ward. At least draw the curtains.

■ A warm, confident approach is most useful even if you are a barrel of nerves inside. It relaxes the patient and in turn will relax you. Try to avoid negative comments before a procedure: 'you look like you have difficult veins, this may

be a struggle'; this is far from preparing the patient for a stormy-time and instead just diminishes their confidence in you. It is, however, acceptable to warn them that there is no guarantee that you will be successful the first time. No one should ever make that promise.

■ Never be afraid to ask for help. It is really stupid to risk your reputation and the patient's well-being in order to prove bravado. People will trust you much more if they can rely on you to ask for help when necessary. In any case, seniors and nurses love showing off their skills; try and foster an environment around you where it is okay to ask for help and doesn't diminish a person's value – keep this approach with you as you become more senior.

■ Wear gloves. You will soon become accustomed to them and you will stop noticing a loss of sensation. Remember that the most unlikely people have Hep B.

■ Nurses can help in positioning and reassuring the patient.

■ Use local anaesthetic for all but the smallest procedures.

■ Keep a vial of atropine and a syringe to hand for procedures that involve

---

puncturing serosal linings (pleura, peritoneum), as vasovagal events are reasonably common. Give one ampoule (0.6 mg) IV stat if the patient feels faint.

■ Remember that you always have more time than you think, even during emergency procedures. If necessary, hand your bleep to a nursing or medical colleague while 'scrubbed up'. Less haste more speed is a good maxim for invasive procedures.

■ Use every single opportunity to be assessed. Bring an assessment form and a supervisor. When it comes to end of year assessments or job applications, you will sorely regret it if you haven't done so!

Arterial blood gases

Bleeding tendency is a relative contraindication for taking ABGs. Ask a senior for advice if you are in doubt about whether or not to proceed. Always apply pressure for at least 5 minutes after taking ABGs from patients on warfarin or heparin.

Arteries in order of preference

1 Radial – check collateral blood supply from the ulnar artery (especially if there is a history of wrist trauma) by asking the patient to make a tight fist and applying pressure over the radial artery. Ask the patient to relax the hand. If it remains white after 10 seconds, try the other arm (this is Allen's test).

2 Femoral – the problem here is that it is easy to hit the vein by mistake. Also, you really need to apply strong pressure to the puncture site for at least 5 minutes after taking blood. In obese patients it can be hard to find the artery.

3 Brachial – use this as a last resort. Use a 20–22G needle. The femoral is easier as it is much larger and less likely to thrombose.

Have ready

1 Lidocaine 1% *without* adrenaline.

2 One 2 ml syringe.

3 One 23–25G needle.

4 Heparin (1000 U/ml).

5 Povidone or iodine swabs or alcohol swabs.

6 Sterile swabs/cotton wool balls.

7 Syringe cap. Many hospitals supply special heparinized syringes, for example, 'Pulsator' for taking ABGs.

8 Plastic bag or carton with a few ice cubes at the bottom.

The procedure
(see Figs. 13.1 and 13.2)

1 Ask your colleagues where the blood gas machine is and how to read it before taking blood (it is often in ITU or A&E).

2 Most ABG syringes come with heparin already in them that can be easily expelled before use. If not, then draw up 0.5 ml of heparin into a 2 ml syringe, withdrawing the plunger fully to coat the syringe walls. Expel the heparin completely – classical teaching states that excess heparin will cause an erroneous acidosis; however, in reality this is only minimal and most effects are dilutional with a rise in $PaCO_2$ and a fall in PaO_2. You only need a few molecules of heparin to prevent the blood from clotting.

3 Wrist punctures are painful. It is a good idea to clean the skin and infiltrate superficially with a small bleb of local anaesthetic if there is no emergency.

4 Hold the syringe at a 60–90° angle to the skin and slowly advance the needle. Keep very still and the syringe will usually fill due to arterial pressure with 1–2 ml of bright red blood. If this is not

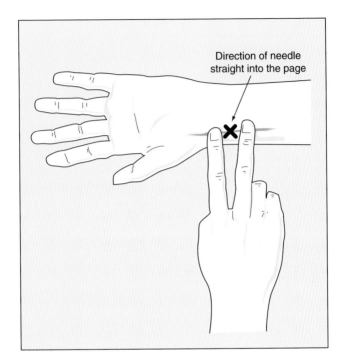

Direction of needle
straight into the page

Fig. 13.1 Radial arterial puncture.

forthcoming you can gently aspirate 1–2 ml; however, this often indicates a venous puncture that will be confirmed by the results.

5 Withdraw and apply pressure for at least 3 minutes (5 minutes if the patient is anticoagulated).

6 Expel all air from the syringe, tapping air bubbles towards the nozzle. Cap the syringe carefully, gently roll between your hands and either take to the ABG machine immediately (within 15 minutes) or place on ice and read as soon as possible (1 hour). Ice in a specimen bag is helpful to have ready, so that you are not in such a panic to get to the ABG reading machine.

7 Note the oxygen concentration that the patient is on. This is important for interpretation. Take the gas at least 10 minutes after a change in oxygen concentration. It is not acceptable to take a hypoxic patient off oxygen for a 'baseline' blood gas.

If you fail

■ Withdraw the needle to a point near the skin, redirect the needle and try again. The artery is usually only a few millimetres under the skin; it is not unusual to transect the artery. Try aiming the needle at a more shallow angle. This allows a steadier approach. Withdraw and try again.

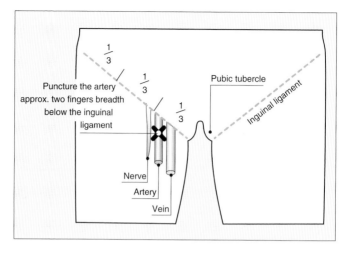

Fig. 13.2 Femoral arterial puncture: inguinal canal anatomy may be remembered using the mnemonic 'NAVY' – nerve, artery, vein, Y-fronts (!)

■ Try to avoid bones and tendons. If you hit bone, withdraw while gently aspirating.

Hints

■ It is important to expel all the air from the sample. Once this is done, ice only serves to slow cellular use of O_2 which is negligible over 60 minutes.

■ Do not expect immediate ABG changes after adjusting someone's O_2 supply. It takes up to 20 minutes for the ABGs to equilibrate to a change in inspired O_2 concentration. If a reading looks suspiciously high or low, repeat it.

■ You can tell the difference between arterial and venous blood by its percentage saturation: 50% or less suggests venous blood, while 80% or above is certainly arterial.

Interpreting arterial blood gases

Normal ABG values are shown in Table 13.1.

Table 13.1 Normal ABG values.

pH	7.35–7.45
PCO_2	4.3–6.0 kPa
Base excess	±2 mmol/l
PO_2	10.5–14.0 kPa
Serum HCO_3^-	22–26 mmol/l
O_2 saturation	95–100%

Points to consider when interpreting arterial blood gases

For a full explanation of acid–base disorders consult any good medical textbook.

PO_2 and $PaCO_2$

First ask yourself: does the patient have abnormally low O_2 for them? What is their baseline PaO_2 value? Many patients with chronic respiratory disease live quite happily with a PaO_2 of 7.5 kPa, so don't get too flustered by an apparently terrible PaO_2 value. Check the results of

Table 13.2 Interpreting acid–base disorders.

	pH	PCO_2	HCO_3^-	K^+
Acidosis				
Metabolic – early	↓	Normal	↓	Usually ↑
Metabolic – compensated	Normal	↓	↓	Normal or ↓
Respiratory – early	↓	↑	Normal or ↑	↑
Respiratory – compensated	Normal	↑	↑↑	
Alkalosis				
Metabolic – early	↑	Normal	↑	↓
Metabolic – compensated	↑	Normal	↑↑	↑
Respiratory – early	↑	↓	Normal or ↓	↓
Respiratory – compensated	Normal	↓	↓↓	Normal or ↑

Reproduced from Zilva J.F., Pannall P.R., Mayne P. (1989) *Clinical Chemistry in Diagnosis and Treatment.* Lloyd-Luke (Medical Books) Ltd, London.

previous ABGs when the patient was well to see how much they have decompensated. (If you do not have previous results to hand you may need to seek senior advice on how to proceed.)

Next check if the patient is retaining CO_2. This will determine the amount of O_2 therapy you can give (see Chapter 7, Oxygen therapy) and will guide you as to the degree that a respiratory component is determining their blood gas. The body never overcompensates; hence if $PaCO_2$ is high, then we know the patient is not ventilating adequately. The pH will tell us whether this is the primary problem (if there is an acidosis of respiratory origin) or if it is compensatory (if there is an alkalosis of metabolic origin and the patient is hypoventilating to try and raise their acid load).

Remember that the O_2 saturation curve for Hb is a steep sigmoid curve that starts to plateau around a PaO_2 of 9.1 kPa (70 mmHg). This means a patient may have a PaO_2 of 8.5 kPa and still have

better than 90% O_2 saturation. However, in the steep part of the curve (PaO_2 of 6–8 kPa), small changes in PaO_2 dramatically affect O_2 saturation and are very clinically significant.

pH

Is it normal or is there an acidosis (pH < 7.35) or an alkalosis (pH > 7.45)? If either exists, decide if it is metabolic or respiratory and whether or not it is compensated (see Table 13.2).

A compensated acid–base disorder suggests more chronic disease, over days to weeks, while an uncompensated acidosis or alkalosis suggests a more acute disorder. In general, the body compensates for changes in pH by altering the respiratory rate (e.g. in metabolic acidosis, CO_2 is 'blown off') and regulating renal excretion of HCO_3. Except in acute illness, most acid–base disorders are compensated to some extent. Respiratory compensation occurs much quicker than renal.

Serum electrolytes
(Na$^+$, Cl$^-$ and HCO$_3$)

If the patient is acidotic, you will need to calculate the anion gap ([Na + K] − [Cl + HCO$_3$]) in order to refine the differential diagnosis. A raised anion gap is due to addition of unmeasured acid to the system, for example, MUD PILES − methanol, urea, diabetes (ketones), paraldehyde, izoniazid, lactic acid (in anaerobic metabolism), ethanol and salicyclic acid. A normal anion gap acidosis is usually due to loss of base.

Hints

■ When interpreting ABGs, do not forget to note whether the patient is on O$_2$ and how much.

■ A patient with a mixed picture or who is well compensated may have a normal pH. Check all the parameters of the ABG analysis, not just the pH and PO$_2$.

■ If the results of the ABG analysis are very poor, you may have sampled venous blood. This is likely if the percentage saturation is 50% or less. Percentage saturation of arterial blood is usually over 80%.

■ Patients with decompensated organ failure (e.g. cirrhosis, CCF, respiratory or renal insufficiency) may have developed acid–base and electrolyte disturbances over weeks. Do not be tempted to correct them in a day. Rather, try to get the patient a little better each day and review according to the time frame over which the patient's illness developed.

Respiratory disease and arterial blood gases interpretation

Type 1 respiratory failure 'one thing wrong' (pink puffer):
■ PaO$_2$ less than 8.0 kPa (60 mmHg).
■ PaCO$_2$ less than 6.0 kPa (45 mmHg).

If stable, their ABGs will reveal a compensated respiratory alkalosis.

Type 2 respiratory failure 'two things wrong' (blue bloater):
■ PaO$_2$ less than 8.0 kPa (60 mmHg).
■ PaCO$_2$ greater than 6.0 kPa (45 mmHg).

If stable, their ABGs will reveal a compensated respiratory acidosis.

Patients with type 1 failure progress to type 2 as they tire.

Bladder catheterization

Ask an experienced colleague to supervise your first attempt and ensure that you know the procedure before your first night call. Female nurses usually (but not always) catheterize women; you will certainly end up catheterizing men (whether you are a man or a woman).

Men

Have ready

1 Catheterization pack – kidney bowl, gauze swabs, sterile towels, etc.

2 Sterile gloves.

3 Cleaning solution.

4 Sterile tube of lidocaine jelly.

5 10 ml syringe and 10 ml sterile water.

6 Several Foley catheters. For the first attempt, 14G is the usual size. Use a silastic catheter (which is firmer) for problematic catheterizations or when longer term catheterization is anticipated.

7 Urine bag and stand.

The procedure

1 Get a clean trolley that has been swabbed with an alcohol swipe and place the catheter pack on it. Also get a catheter stand.

2 Wash your hands thoroughly.

3 Wheel the trolley to the patient's bedside, draw the curtains and fully expose the patient's penis. Make sure there are no bedclothes in the way that might dirty the working area. UTIs are easy to induce with catheterization.

4 Tell the patient what you are about to do and why you are doing it.

5 Without touching the sterile contents themselves, open the catheter pack, sterile gloves, tube of lidocaine jelly, syringe, water and catheter onto the catheter tray (or a sterile surface). Pour the cleaning solution (some hospitals use sterile saline alone) into a receptacle.

6 Put on gloves.

7 Drape the sterile towels or paper sheets to leave only the patient's penis exposed.

8 Gently retract the foreskin and clean the urethral opening with cleaning solution, keeping one hand clean for inserting the catheter.

9 Gently squeeze the contents of the tube of lidocaine jelly into the urethra, massaging the underside of the penis to work the jelly towards the bladder.

10 Open the catheter wrapping at the tip end only and insert the catheter into the urethra, withdrawing the plastic covering in stages as you go. This is the trickiest part of the procedure. Make sure the end is in the kidney bowl to collect urine. You should get some urine back when you reach the bladder from all but the most dehydrated patients.

11 If you feel resistance, gently pull the shaft of the penis upwards. In some cases, pulling the penis down between the legs is more useful. *Never* use force.

12 Once fully inserted, inflate the catheter balloon with 5–10 ml of sterile water by placing the syringe directly over the proximal opening (no needle) and pushing hard. Stop immediately if the patient experiences pain, as the balloon may be in the urethra. Once inflated, gently pull the catheter until you feel resistance of the balloon so that you are sure that it is stable in the bladder.

13 Always remember to gently replace the foreskin over the penis tip and document this in the notes. If you cannot, gently try again. If the foreskin genuinely gets stuck and starts to swell, get senior help immediately. Paraphimosis is a medical emergency.

14 Connect the end of the catheter to the bag and mount on a catheter stand.

15 Briefly document the procedure in the notes and record any significant volume of urine (>10–20 ml) that was collected in the kidney dish in the patient's fluid chart, particularly if the patient is in renal failure.

16 Send a sample of urine for MC&S.

If you fail

■ The catheter may be blocked with jelly. Aspirate the catheter with the syringe or gently massage the bladder above the pubic bone to encourage urine flow.

■ The patient may have a large prostate or penile stricture. For strictures, a smaller size catheter should be used – proceed with care and be ready to abandon the procedure! For large prostates, *larger* catheters are useful, particularly stiff, silastic ones.

■ If after several attempts with different size catheters you cannot access the bladder, never be shy of calling for help. Even the most senior urologists have trouble sometimes and can show you tricks for really difficult urethras.

Suprapubic catheterization is a useful last resort. Again, ensure supervision before attempting this alone as you risk perforating bowel. It is also useful to perform a bladder scan to get an idea of the bladder volume before such a procedure.

Women

Have ready

Same equipment as for the men.

The procedure

1 Position the patient as for a vaginal examination. Ask her to lie flat on her back, knees bent, feet together and to allow her knees to fall down in full abduction.

2 Part the labia minora and clean the area with cleaning solution.

3 Locate the urethral opening just posterior to the clitoris and introduce a well-lubricated catheter tip. Female catheterization is usually much less problematic than for males because they have no prostate and a really short urethra.

As you will probably only be asked to catheterize women that the experienced nurses cannot manage, get taught how to do this before you get called. Be aware of underlying causes for the problem such as tumours. If concerned, do a PV and do not be shy to call for help.

Blood cultures

If you are going to the trouble of doing blood cultures, it is better to do two sets from different sites, particularly if accurate diagnosis is very important. Three sets should be taken at 2–3-hourly intervals for suspected infective endocarditis.

Have ready

1 1 or 2 sets of culture bottles (some hospitals now use a single type of culture

bottle for both aerobic and anaerobic cultures – particularly in paediatric samples).

2 Two 20-ml syringes and needles or a vacutainer system.

3 Lots of alcohol swabs.

The procedure

1 Select a vein.

2 Clean the skin with alcohol, from the centre out. Allow to dry.

3 Without relocating the vein, cannulate and withdraw at least 10 ml of blood for each set of cultures.

4 Withdraw and inject at least 5 ml into each bottle.

5 Place in incubator as soon as possible.

Hints

■ It is not necessary to change needles between taking blood and inserting it into the culture bottles. There is increased risk of needlestick injury and little increase in contamination.

■ It is also unnecessary to clean flip-cap culture bottle tops. Try to avoid getting air in the anaerobic bottle.

■ The above technique is fine for easy veins. If not, use a dressing pack, iodine, swabs, etc., and scrub up after you have got the patient ready. Keep your gloves sterile, as this will allow you to palpate for veins.

Venepuncture

Have ready

1 Tourniquet.

2 Needles (green or blue).

3 Syringe(s) of adequate size for the bloods you need to take.

4 Alcohol swab(s).

5 Cotton wool ball or small plaster.

6 Blood tubes.

7 A sharps container.

Vacutainers are much quicker to use than needles and syringes but have no 'flashback' to let you know when you have entered the vein. Therefore it can be useful to use syringes and needles at first, although the apparent increase in needlestick injuries sometimes makes it against local policy.

The procedure

1 Put on gloves.

2 Tell the patient what you are doing and why.

3 Choose the preferred arm – not a drip arm; tighten the tourniquet above the elbow and find a vein (see Choosing a vein, below). Visualize which way the needle will slide along the vein.

4 Swab the insertion area.

5 Put the needle on the syringe. Holding the patient's skin taut around the vein (tether it distilly), gently but firmly advance the needle through the skin and subcutaneous fat into the vein. After breaching the skin with the bevel up, make sure the needle is very shallow. With practice you feel the vein give way when you are through. You should get a small 'flashback' in the base of the syringe.

6 Holding the syringe and needle in the arm very still, steadily draw back the syringe until you have enough blood.

7 Undo the tourniquet *before* withdrawing the needle.

8 Apply pressure to the puncture site with cotton wool or have the patient do so.

9 Taking care not to needlestick yourself, insert the needle into the blood tubes and allow the vacuum to withdraw

the blood. Some labs recommend that you remove the needle from the syringe, uncap the tube and gently squirt the blood directly into the tube. This prevents needlestick injuries. In practice, very few junior doctors we know use this technique and it is not without risk as any mucous membrane splashes are as risky as needlesticks. Never squirt blood into the tube through small needles as this risks haemolysis and false readings. The main benefit of vacutainer systems is avoiding this high risk transfer of blood.

10 Tidy up, especially sharps.

11 Send blood to the lab.

Choosing a vein

Ask the patient for his or her preferred arm. Usually the left arm is best for right-handed patients. Obvious forearm or cubital fossa veins are good. In dialysis patients, never use their AV fistula arm. Likewise, never use an arm with lymphoedema, or one that has had its lymph nodes removed or irradiated.

If you can't find a vein

1 Hang the arm over the edge of the bed, 'milking' it or tapping the back of the hand. Hitting the skin releases histamine and brings up the veins, watch an anaesthetist do this and you will see that it has to be done quite vigorously to be effective.

2 Use a sphygmomanometer; it is better than a tourniquet. Pump it up to diastolic pressure; you are aiming for the artery to fill the limb in systole but prevent venous drainage. Also, ask the patient to pump their hand. For problematic patients, use a sphygmomanometer from the start. An experienced assistant who squeezes the arm may be equally effective.

3 Immerse the arm or hand in a bowl of warm water for 2 minutes; pump the sphygmomanometer up with the arm in the water; dry the arm and quickly look for veins.

4 Pump up the sphygmomanometer to above systolic pressure, asking the patient to exercise the hand until it aches (1–2 minutes), then release the pressure to diastolic level. The lactic acid produced as a result of anaerobic metabolism is a potent vasodilator. This method is painful. Use as a last resort.

Hints

■ Always gently invert filled tubes containing anticoagulant so that no clotting occurs (e.g. haematology tubes).

■ For the same reason, don't over-fill heparinized tubes – they will clot.

■ Paediatric tubes, which only require a few drops of blood, can be used for patients with very difficult veins (though your lab-based colleagues may disagree and question you when they note the date of birth!).

■ Find out from the labs how much blood is really necessary for standard tests at your hospital. Often you need very little, particularly for biochemistry. Clotting is usually the exception and requires a full bottle.

■ Try removing the rubber stopper of the bottle if you need to put more blood in the bottle and you have lost the vacuum. Gently squirt blood from the syringe directly into the bottle having removed the needle (to avoid haemolysis).

Cannulation (Venflon/ Line insertion)

(see Fig. 13.3)

No matter how much of a klutz you think you are, you will soon be inserting cannulae with the best of them.

Practice really is the only way to be good at this. Here we outline the basic procedure with a trouble-shooting guide; the best way to learn the procedure is to get someone with good technique to show you.

Have ready

1 Tourniquet or sphygmomanometer.

2 Appropriate size cannula (see Table 13.3).

3 Cannula dressing (wing-shaped).

4 5–10-ml syringe.

5 Saline flush.

6 Alcohol swab(s).

7 Cotton wool ball/small plaster.

8 Bandage and tape.

The basic procedure

1 Put on gloves and make sure you have all the equipment you need. Especially gauze to mop up any blood!

2 Tell the patient what you are doing and why.

3 Choose the preferred arm. Tighten the tourniquet above the elbow and find a vein (see below). Visualize which way the needle will slide along the vein. Vein choice is key (see below).

4 Swab the insertion area and allow the alcohol to dry (or it will sting).

5 Firmly advance the needle through the skin and subcutaneous fat into the vein. With practice, you feel the vein give way when you are through. You should get a small 'flashback' of blood in the base of the cannula. The flashback is an indication that the *tip* of the cannulae has entered the vein (but not necessarily the plastic of the cannulae); with the cannulae flat, advance the needle a millimetre or two more. The gap

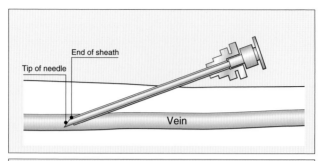

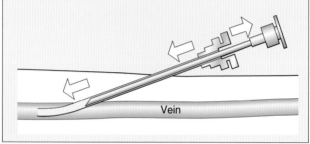

Fig. 13.3 Cannulating a vein.

Table 13.3 Cannulae sizes.

Colour	Size	Use
Yellow	24G	Paediatric
Blue	22G	Small, fragile veins
Pink	20G	Regular IV drugs and fluid administration
Green	18G	Blood transfusions and fluids
White	17G	As above
Grey	16G	Rapid fluid administration, GI bleeds
Brown/Orange	14G	Major bleeds, usually placed prophylactically in theatre

between needle tip and plastic sheath is longer in larger cannulae.

6 Holding the cannula in the arm very still and the vein still tethered, advance the plastic cannulae into the vein – ideally with one hand – in effect covering the tip of the needle; *only then* when the plastic is in the vein withdraw the metal stylet. Quickly attach a vacutainer system or syringe to take blood or a bung.

7 Undo the tourniquet and secure the cannula with a dressing. It is a good idea to secure the cannula with a covering bandage to prevent it catching on bedclothes.

8 Tidy up, especially sharps. Beware that although many cannula have a safety sheath that deploys once the needle is fully withdrawn, these are typically absent on the smallest needles.

Choosing a vein

1 Ask the patient for his or her preferred arm. Usually the left arm is best for right-handed patients. Remember that the dorsum of the hand is more convenient for you, but less so for the patient. Obvious forearm veins are good (in dialysis patients, never use their AV fistula arm).

2 Avoid sites where two vein joins are tethered. While these can be easier to cannulate, the drip is more likely to tissue as a result of poor flexibility.

3 Avoid foot veins except as a last resort. They thrombose more readily and are prone to infection.

4 Avoid crossing joints.

5 Shave hairy arms for ease of cannulation and to reduce pain when removing the drip.

6 Palpate the vein and visualizing which way the needle will run along it.

7 If you can't find*a vein, see Venepuncture, above p. 169.

Hints

■ Emla anaesthetic cream is extremely useful for squeamish patients. Keep a tube handy. Apply over selected veins and cover with an occlusive dressing. Simply wipe off in 30 minutes to 1 hour and site the drip as usual. Injection of local anaesthetic is less useful as it often obscures the vein. This is not such a problem when you are more experi-

enced and is essential when putting in large cannulae in conscious patients.

■ It is helpful to take blood at the same time as putting in the cannula. This must not be done with 'precious' veins. Once the cannula is secured, elevate the arm above the level of the left atrium. Remove the cap and place a syringe into the back of the cannula. Lower the arm (sometimes you need to reinflate the cuff gently) and *very gently* aspirate the required amount of blood (rapid aspiration causes the vein to collapse down into the cannula). You may need to withdraw the cannula slightly, or lift the wings of the Venflon away from the skin a little way to initiate the flow of blood into the syringe (it is not unusual for blood to fail to flow because the tip of the cannula sits against a valve).

■ Pink, rather than green, cannulae are adequate for most routine purposes, such as saline infusions or IV drugs.

Saving a dying drip or cannula

When asked to resite a cannula because it has tissued:

1 Ask whether or not it is still really necessary and check the cannula yourself; it is not unusual for an inexperienced nurse to mistake a fully functioning cannula for one that has 'tissued' because of a loose connection, three-way tap in an off position or infusion pump problem. Many cannulae are also 'positional' and work perfectly well provided the limb is kept in a certain, usually neutral, position.

2 Many lines can be flushed gently with 5 ml of heparinized saline that clears any minor blockage. Small syringes (2 ml) are most effective at clearing minor blocks.

3 Always remove the cannula if the site is inflamed. Phlebitis is not to be ignored!

Times when a cannula MUST be in place, even at night

■ In the acutely ill or unstable patient, it is often essential to secure peripheral access before removing central lines in post-operative patients. The day you don't do this is the day you'll regret.

■ Hypovolaemia or poor oral intake.

■ Serious danger of blood or fluid loss.

■ Certain IV drug infusions – antibiotics, cardiac infusions, heparin, etc.

Central lines

Ensure that you are supervised for your first attempts; this procedure has the potential for some major complications. The two most commonly used veins are the internal jugular and, now rarely, sub-clavian. The right side is usually chosen. Other under-used approaches include the femoral vein and the median basilic vein, both of which are technically easier but don't last as long. The same principles apply to all CVP lines. The jugular approach should be attempted first, as it has fewer complications, and it is easy to stop any bleeding, including arterial bleeding, should you miss. Having said that, the artery is palpable next to the vein, and therefore more easily avoided than with the subclavian approach. Unless you feel very confident with central lines, it is better to call for help than to attempt subclavian access yourself. NICE guidance recommends ultrasound guidance for all central lines and it is now the gold-standard. Learn to use this early and save yourself trouble in the future.

Indications for CVP lines

■ Measurement of CVP.

■ Infusing certain drugs and TPN.

■ Inserting Swan–Ganz catheters or pacing wires.

Insertion of central lines

When it is more important to use the jugular approach

1 Clotting problems, typically when the INR is greater than 5 or the platelet count is less than $100 \times 10^9/l$.

2 Respiratory disease where a pneumothorax might be life-threatening; although they can still occur with this approach, it is less likely than the subclavian approach.

Have ready

1 Central line set.

2 Standard dressing pack.

3 Betadine.

4 Sterile gown and gloves.

5 One large sterile drape.

6 1 ml 1% lidocaine.

7 Two 10-ml syringes.

8 Heparinized saline (Hepsal) to flush lines.

9 25G (orange) and 21G (green) needles.

10 Suturing material (2–0 or 3–0 silk or prolene).

11 Scalpel blade.

12 Two adhesive dressings.

13 500-ml bag of saline and giving set.

14 CVP manometer.

The procedure
(see Fig. 13.4)

1 Have the trolley ready (sterile contents laid out). Remove all pillows. Tilt the bed to lower the patient's head to fill the neck veins; this is commonly called the Trendelenburg position. Tell the patient what you are about to do and why. Reassure them that while it is

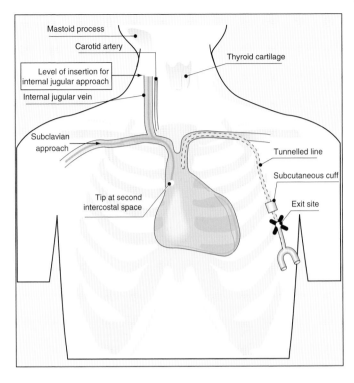

Fig. 13.4 Illustration of positions for insertion of central lines.

uncomfortable to lie still and backwards for about 20 minutes, the procedure is not painful.

2 Wash your hands well and put on gloves.

3 Flush the giving set and CVP manometer with heparin saline.

4 Clean a wide area of skin from the inside out around the puncture site and cover with the drape.

5 Flush the central venous cannula and connecting tubing with saline.

6 Check that the guide wire passes through the large-bore needle and

determine which is the soft, 'vessel-friendly' end.

Cannulating the right internal jugular vein

1 Feel for the pulse of the carotid artery with the left hand, alternatively locate the vessel with ultrasound. With the right hand, infiltrate local anaesthetic subcutaneously at the level of the thyroid cartilage (don't aim for this though!) and lateral to the carotid artery. Whenever you infiltrate with local anaesthetic, always aspirate while advancing to avoid injection into a blood vessel. Also remember that all vials look remarkably similar. Always take the time to check that you are drawing up the right stuff. (This may seem obvious, but it is easy to forget and regret!)

2 While guarding the carotid artery with the left hand, insert a green needle attached to a 10-ml syringe, at an angle of 45° to the neck, heading towards the right anterior superior iliac spine; the right nipple in males is also a good landmark. Some line kits come with a cannula that is fitted over a needle (a bit like a big Venflon). This contraption can be attached to a syringe and directly advanced in the same way as the green needle.

3 Advance slowly, aspirating for blood. The vein is superficial. Do not go more than a few centimetres. If you fail to get blood, withdraw slowly, you may have gone through the vein. If this doesn't work, try again, slightly more medially. If by mistake you do hit the carotid artery, don't panic; apply strong pressure for 5 minutes.

4 When you have found the vein, withdraw the needle. Take the large-bore needle with attached syringe and follow the line taken with the green needle. If using the cannula-over-needle supplied in the kit, then withdraw the needle alone once you have entered the vein, after advancing the cannula into the vein, as you would a Venflon. Aspirate to ensure that the cannula is sited in the vein. Cap or occlude its open end to prevent air entry, although this is unlikely to occur when the patient is in the Trendelenburg position. The cannula is now ready to accept the guide wire (see Inserting the guide wire, below). Once the guide wire is threaded, the cannula may be withdrawn over the wire (remember never to let go of the wire while doing this).

Inserting the guide wire

1 Before inserting the guide wire, ensure that you can aspirate blood freely through the needle.

2 Ask the patient to breathe out. As he or she is doing so, remove the syringe and place your thumb over the lumen to prevent air entry.

3 Insert the soft end of the guide wire. It should pass with minimal resistance. Never force it. If it won't pass, check if you can still aspirate blood and try again. If it still won't pass, change the angle of the needle slightly.

4 Pass about 50% of the length of the wire and remove the needle, holding the end of the wire firmly.

5 Nick the skin at the line's entry point with a scalpel blade. Thread the dilator and twist it down over the wire to the hilt. Remove the dilator, taking care not to pull out the wire, then thread the catheter. Remove the wire.

6 Check if you can aspirate blood from each lumen of the catheter. Flush with heparinized saline (Hepsal) before clamping each lumen.

7 Secure with two sutures and place two occlusive clear dressings like a sandwich over the cannula.

8 Do a CXR to check the line's position and to exclude a pneumothorax.

Hints

■ The breathless patient need only be flat or head down for cannulation of the vein and insertion of the guide wire. The rest can be done sitting up.

■ Always take the pulse following the procedure. Frequent ectopics suggest the catheter is in the right ventricle and should be pulled back into the vein.

■ If you hit the carotid or subclavian artery, apply firm pressure for a full 5 minutes (the latter is difficult to do because of the intervening clavicle).

■ Never attempt both subclavian veins without obtaining a CXR.

Problems with temporary and tunnelled central lines

You will often be called to sort out line problems. The commonest are:

■ *Sepsis*. If a patient with a central line develops a fever, take peripheral and central blood cultures. If the patient is clearly septic (temperature >38°C, tachycardia, pain/inflammation around entry site), discuss removing the line with your senior. Tunnelled lines can sometimes be treated with antibiotics if the patient is otherwise well, but this cannot be done for short-term lines when the track is much shorter. After removal of any central line, always cut the tip off with a sterile pair of scissors and send it for culture.

■ *Blocked lumen*. This is prevented by daily flushing with heparinized saline (available on most wards in prepared vials). If the line is blocked, flush using a 1–2-ml syringe with heparinized saline, applying moderate pressure. Remember to put in a heparin–saline lock after flushing. Lines near the lumen sometimes wind around on themselves; simple unwinding can sometimes alleviate apparently severe blocks. If still no luck, a dilute solution of urokinase can be instilled by repeated aspiration and injection. Leave it for 30 minutes, then try flushing again.

Hints

■ Taking blood from central lines should only be performed as a last resort. Phlebotomist should be counselled about refusing to bleed patients with central lines. There is a very real risk of infection. You need to discard the first 15ml of blood and use a good aseptic technique. Do not take samples for aminoglycoside levels from a central line as these drugs are absorbed by the cannula.

■ A 1–2-ml syringe is more effective for unblocking cannulae than a 5- or 10-ml syringe.

Using central lines

Hickman and Groschong lines are tunnelled lines intended for long-term use such as for chemotherapy or TPN. Groschong lines have a special two-way valve system at the tip of each lumen that prevents blockage after flushing and facilitates taking of blood samples. However, the valve excludes the use of the line for CVP measurements. It is extremely useful to know how to handle these lines. Infection is the major problem and most patients are trained in looking after their own line. They are very critical of sloppy technique. Therefore, before handling a line, ask a nurse or medical colleague to give you a quick tutorial. The basic technique outlined below is a guide only. Different units use different IV connectors, bungs, etc. For setting up an IV, giving drugs or taking blood via a tunnelled line, you will need to:

1 Open up:
   ● Dressing pack.
   ● Sterile gloves.
   ● One 5-ml syringe and heparin–saline or saline.
   ● One sterile bung (end plug for cannula).
   ● Four alcohol swabs.
   ● Cleaning solution, for example, betadine solution, and container.

2 Get an assistant (always handy).

3 Scrub up.

4 Keep one hand absolutely sterile.

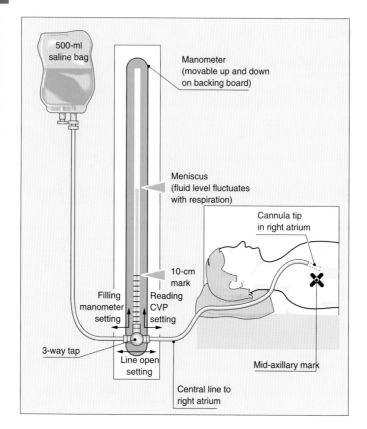

500-ml
saline bag

Manometer
(movable up and down
on backing board)

Meniscus
(fluid level fluctuates
with respiration)

Cannula tip
in right atrium

10-cm
mark

Filling
manometer
setting

Reading
CVP
setting

3-way tap

Line open
setting

Mid-axillary mark

Central line to
right atrium

Fig. 13.5 Diagrammatic illustration of CVP reading.

5 Handle the line with dry sterile gauze.

6 Remove the bung from the end of the line using a swab and discard.

7 Always open and shut the gate or clamp between procedures.

8 Attach drip or take bloods as appropriate.

Measuring the CVP
(see Fig. 13.5)

The CVP is measured with reference to a fixed point, either the mid-axillary line

or the manubriosternal angle. The pressures at the manubriosternal angle will be about 5–7 cm lower than those at the mid-axillary line. It does not matter which you use, as long as you remain consistent.

1 Lie the patient flat. Adjust the scale so that the 1-cm mark is opposite the chosen reference point (marked with an indelible pen). If you use the true '0-cm' level, you cannot measure negative values.

2 A three-way tap controls the flow of fluid between the IV bag, the CVP reading scale and the patient. Adjust the tap to run fluid from the bag up to the 30-cm mark on the manometer. Set the tap to connect the patient to the manometer. The manometer fluid level should swing with respiration and settle. The CVP is measured in cm of water.

Hints

1 Learn to measure the CVP yourself and take the time to ensure that nursing staff are familiar with doing CVP measurements. It is easy to get it wrong.

2 Normal values for CVP:

Using the 10-cm mark aligned with the manubriosternal angle: 7–14 cm. Using the 10-cm mark aligned with the mid-axillary line: 11–18 cm. (Subtract 10 cm if using the true 0-cm mark.)

3 The CVP reading should be regarded with suspicion if the right atrial pressure is likely to be abnormal:

- Raised   intrathoracic   pressure (pneumothorax).
- Altered intravascular volume (fluid overload or hypovolaemia).
- Abnormal venous tone (NB catecholamine release can maintain CVP readings despite significant blood loss). Other drugs can cause dramatic loss of tone and drops in CVP.
- Abnormal right ventricular function: CCF, pericardial tamponade/constriction, acute RVF. The CVP may be markedly raised following right-sided Myocardial Infarction or large PE. The CVP in these situations is an unreliable guide to fluid status. If called to see a patient with a rising or falling CVP, think of the above approach to guide you.

Chest drains

While you may be forgiven for being unfamiliar with inserting chest drains,

you will be expected to manage and remove them. The decision to remove a drain should be taken by your seniors. The following paragraphs give general guidelines for maintaining and removing drains (see Fig. 13.6).

Indications

Pneumothorax (A = Air = Apical drain) Haemothorax or empyema (B = Blood = Basal drain)

Managing a chest drain

Pneumothorax

1 Check for an air leak by asking the patient to cough. A bubbling drain implies an air leak from an unsealed hole, fistula or a leak in the tubing. You may need to apply suction to the drain if you suspect a hole or fistula. This should be done in consultation with a respiratory or cardiothoracic specialist, note that suction is not a panacea and can in fact hold open a pneumothorax. Exercise is difficult while on suction but a bedside exercise bike can help with lung inflation.

2 After the lung has re-expanded and the drain is no longer bubbling, clamp and re-X-ray. If there is no pneumothorax and the fluid is cleared, the drain can be removed. Never leave a drain clamped for any significant period or unsupervised – this can rapidly convert an open pneumothorax (with bubbling out into the drain) into a fatal tension pneumothorax!

3 If the pneumothorax is present after a surgical procedure like a pleurodesis, then avoid NSAIDs as they will inhibit inflammatory response and adhesion to the chest wall.

Effusion/haemothorax

1 Large effusions can drain over several days, up to a maximum of 1 l/hour and

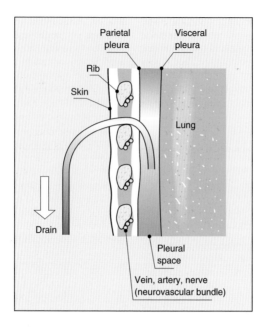

Fig. 13.6 Cross section through chest cage to illustrate chest drain.

not more than 4 l/day (otherwise there is a risk of 'reflex' pulmonary oedema). Remove the drain when the CXR reveals no further fluid.

2 For recurrent effusions you may consider talc/chemical pleurodesis; discuss with your team. This may be easily performed by injection down the chest drain itself.

3 Empyema drains require special consideration. Get a specialist opinion.

How to remove a drain

Have ready

1 Gloves.

2 Clamping forceps.

3 Pair of scissors.

4 One occlusive dressing.

The procedure

1 Clamp the tube with the forceps.

2 The entry point of the tube should have been secured with a purse-string suture that must be untied (not cut) and the ends firmly pulled to seal the hole as the tube slides out. Take your time the first few times you do this. It is easy to lose the stitching.

3 Withdraw the tube with positive intrathoracic pressure by asking the patient to blow hard against a closed nose and mouth ('make your ears pop'). Alternatively, ask the patient to take a deep breath and hold. Withdraw quickly and smoothly; do not dally. You should hear the hiss of the expulsion of the last bit of air as the end comes out. Quickly pull the purse string to seal the hole. Apply an occlusive dressing.

4 Do a CXR to assess the success of the drain and as a comparison for future X-rays.

Hint

Have a 4 × 4 cm gauze swab to hand to place over the hole in the event of a failed purse-string closure. Later, replace this with a large clear occlusive dressing over the hole.

DC cardioversion

As a junior doctor rotating through cardiology, you may be asked to do the elective cardioversion list for patients in stable atrial fibrillation. This may seem daunting, yet it is a straightforward procedure, providing the patient has been adequately prepared (see Chapter 11, Elective DC cardioversion). Similarly, you may be required to undertake this procedure in the emergency department if the patient is haemodynamically compromised.

1 Position the gel pads before the patient is anaesthetized. Anteroposterior position is more effective, but obviously can only be used if the defibrillator is a paddle-free one.

2 Once the patient has been anaesthetized, ask the anaesthetist whether he or she is happy for you to continue.

3 ENSURE THAT THE DEFIBRILLATOR IS SET TO 'SYNCHRONIZED'. Check that the defibrillator is sensing QRS complexes rather than T or P waves. You may need to adjust the gain to achieve this.

4 Set defibrillator to 100 J (sometimes different energies are used).

5 Warn all present that you are about to charge the paddles, and make sure everyone is standing clear (you will need to be particularly careful that the anaesthetist withdraws to a safe distance, taking the patient's oxygen mask with them).

6 Press the paddles firmly onto the pads on the patient, charge them up and deploy the shock. From the time you press the button to administer the shock, there may be some delay before the shock is deployed. This is because the defibrillator is waiting for the next QRS complex. During this delay, do not be tempted to think the paddles have not worked. It is sometimes the case that the machine cannot synchronize properly and so doesn't deliver a shock.

7 Replace the paddles and check the ECG or rhythm monitor. (Once the paddles have been replaced, the anaesthetist will continue ventilation.)

8 If the procedure has not worked, repeat at 200 J. If this too does not work, repeat at 360 J. Check the gel pads between each shock to make sure that they have not dried out, as this will lead to skin burns.

9 If, at 360 J, the procedure has not caused reversion to sinus rhythm, consider repositioning the paddles, with one at the left sternal border and one to the left of the spine at the same level, and administering another 360 J shock.

10 At the end of the procedure, do a formal 12-lead ECG, and ensure the patient is in the recovery position, and is self-ventilating well, with good oxygen saturation.

Hints

Do not be too hasty in judging whether a treatment cycle has been successful or unsuccessful on the basis of the rhythm monitor. It may take a few seconds for the rhythm to settle into sinus after a shock, and, likewise, the initial appearance of sinus rhythm may give way to atrial fibrillation within a minute or so.

Electrocardiogram

Many indications, especially history of IHD, DM, hypertension, SOB, chest pain, swollen leg and pre-op ECGs don't take much time and are harmless; if in doubt, just do one.

The procedure

1 Have the patient lie with their chest exposed. Explain to them what you are doing and reassure them that there is no way that they will get an electric shock.

2 Attach limb leads to the inner aspect of the forearm just below the wrist and the outer aspects of the leg above the ankle. The wires are usually labelled, but if not the colour code is most often as follows:

Red = right arm
Yellow = left arm
Green = left leg
Black = right leg

3 Ensure good contact.

4 For chest leads see Fig. 13.7.

Hints

Preventing spurious results

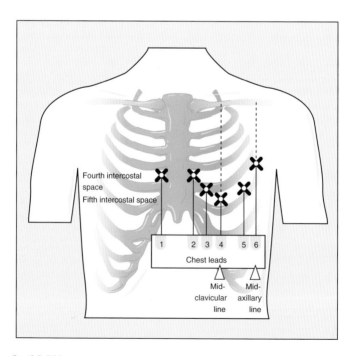

Fourth intercostal space
Fifth intercostal space

1   2 3 4   5 6
Chest leads

Mid-clavicular line   Mid-axillary line

Fig. 13.7 ECG chest lead placement.

■ The patient should be completely relaxed. Explain that the procedure is completely painless and harmless.

■ Make sure the chest lead electrodes do not overlap.

■ Lightly shave very hairy areas for proper contact.

■ If the patient has a hand tremor (e.g. Parkinson's), attach the leads higher up the arm.

■ The black (right leg) lead is an earth lead and can be attached to any part of the body. It has no bearing on the result.

■ For leg amputees, the green (left leg) lead can be placed on either leg. However, the arm leads must not be crossed. For an arm amputee, ensure that the arm electrodes are equidistant from the heart (they may be placed on the shoulders).

Reading ECGs
(see Chapter 7, Electrocardiograms)

Exercise stress test

Exercise (ECG) stress tests take approximately 20 minutes to perform. Your job is to encourage the patient to attain their peak heart rate if possible (= 220 − patient age), and to watch their ECG closely. Your aim is to detect and measure the severity of coronary artery disease, and to uncover arrhythmias.

Relative contraindications (discuss with senior)

Aortic stenosis
Hypertrophic obstructive cardiomyopathy
LBBB on ECG
Systolic BP > 200 mmHg; diastolic BP > 100 mmHg
Unstable angina
Uncontrolled arrhythmias
Note: Beta blockers should be stopped 2 days before the test.

The procedure

1 Make sure that there is resuscitation equipment immediately available. Approximately 1 per 4000 patients arrests during stress tests. Also have GTN ready.

2 Assess peak heart rate (about 220 − patient age).

3 Follow the instructions of the ECG technician, who has followed the protocol many times.

4 *Stop the test* if the patient complains of:

● Increasingly severe chest pain or other symptoms (such as faintness or dyspnoea). Consider administering GTN.
● A fall in systolic BP of more than 20 mmHg.
● A fall in heart rate.
● VT or VF.
● Progressive ST elevation.
● ST depression greater than or equal to 2 mm.
● Three or more consecutive ventricular ectopics.
● Peak heart rate is attained.

5 You must remain present at all times and monitor BP and pulse at regular intervals (ask the technician for local protocol). This includes the recovery period when the test may become positive, or (horrors) the patient may go into VT. (Be ready to resuscitate.)

Glucose tolerance test

Indications
Suspected diabetes mellitus.

Have ready

1 The patient should have fasted overnight.

2 75 g oral glucose dissolved in a glass of water.

3 Apparatus for taking blood with grey (glucose) tube.

The procedure

1 Take a fasting sample for blood glucose in a grey tube.

2 Give the patient the oral glucose with the water to drink over less than 5 minutes.

3 Take a second blood glucose sample after 2 hours.

Interpreting the results

1 *Normal result*: a fasting glucose level <6.1 mmol (in this case a glucose tolerance test is not indicated).

2 *Diabetes confirmed*: a fasting glucose level >7.0 (in this case a glucose tolerance test is not indicated). If the level is >6.1 but <7.0 mmol, then the patient has 'Impaired Fasting Glucose' and should undergo the glucose tolerance test.

3 *Impaired Glucose Tolerance*: fasting plasma level less than 7.0 mmol and the 2-hour level between 7.8 and 11.1 mmol (note that if the 2-hour result is <7.8, the diagnosis is still *IFG*).

4 *Diabetes confirmed*: a 2-hour level greater than 11.1 mmol.

Injections

Subcutaneous

Have ready

1 23–25G needle.

2 Alcohol swab.

The procedure

1 Choose a fatty site and use the smallest possible needle.

2 Clean site with an alcohol swab and allow to dry.

3 Gently pinch a wad of skin and fat between your thumb and index finger.

4 Place the needle on the skin for 3 seconds at an angle of about 60° before pushing through the skin. This reduces the sensation of pain. Release the skin.

5 Aspirate to ensure you do not inject into a blood vessel.

6 Slowly depress the plunger. Rapid injection will cause pain.

7 If you aspirate blood, remove and replace the needle and explain to the patient the need to repeat the injection.

Intramuscular

Have ready
As for SC.

The procedure

1 The deltoid muscle is usually good for small injections. If the patient is thin or wasted, use the gluteal muscles – choose the upper and outer quadrant below the iliac crest to avoid the sciatic nerve by drawing an imaginary line between the anterior superior iliac spine and the greater trochanter of the femur, and injecting posteriorly to and above this line (see Fig. 13.8).

2 Pull the skin taut and inject at 90° to the skin (pulling the skin ensures that the injection doesn't leak after you pull the needle out).

3 Aspirate to ensure that you do not inject into a blood vessel. Inject slowly.

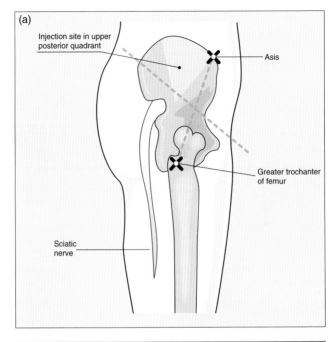

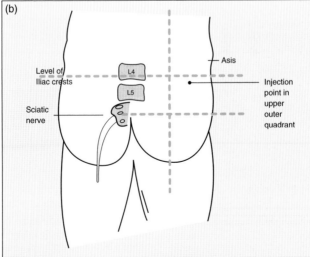

Fig. 13.8 Site for intramuscular injections (a) lateral view, (b) posterior view.

Intercostal block

Indications

Very effective for severe, localized, pleuritic chest pain (e.g. localized pleuritis, metastases, fractured ribs). Intercostal blocks usually abolish pain and surprisingly the relief lasts longer than the action of the anaesthetic.

Have ready

1 Dressing pack and sterile gloves.

2 Betadine.

3 One 10-ml syringe.

4 One 23G needle.

5 One 21G needle.

6 5–10 ml 2% lidocaine or 0.5% bupivacaine (preferred, because it is longer acting).

The procedure

1 Identify the interspace(s) where the pain is arising and the spaces above and below. Prepare the skin just anterior to the mid-axillary line. Anaesthetize the skin using a 23G needle just below the inferior margin of the rib with lidocaine. You need to deliver the drug close to the nerve (which is also close to the vessels that you want to avoid injecting into!).

2 Change needle to 21G (green). Going through the same puncture site, advance at an upward angle again towards the inferior margin of the rib. The nerve lies inferiorly in the groove. If you hit bone, withdraw slightly and try again, slightly more inferiorly. Aspirate to ensure the needle is not in a vessel and slowly inject 1–2 ml of bupivacaine.

3 Repeat the procedure for the interspaces above and below.

Joint aspiration/ injection

This is a useful procedure to learn from an expert, especially if you are an aspiring GP (or GP with special interest). Superb aseptic technique is vital as is a sound knowledge of the anatomy. Each joint requires a slightly different approach but the basic technique is the same.

Aspiration

Indications

Diagnostic:
■ Recent onset arthritis.
■ To rule out infection (acute and chronic).
■ Joint effusion – particularly a traumatic haemarthroses with pain.
Therapeutic:
■ Steroid injections.
■ Drainage of septic arthritis.

Have ready

1 Three syringes (5, 10 and 50 ml).

2 Two needles (25G and 21G).

3 Lidocaine 2%.

4 Sterile gloves.

5 Sterile dressing pack.

6 Betadine solution.

7 Three specimen containers and a fluoride tube (grey top) for infections.

The procedure

1 Written consent is advisable.

2 Find the site of maximal effusion and mark this point with indelible ink.

3 Scrub up and clean the area with betadine. Allow it to dry and wipe over the site of aspiration with an alcohol swab. Allow it to dry completely. Even

small amounts of betadine will ruin your culture results.

4 Anaesthetize the area, being careful to avoid injecting local anaesthetic into the joint – lidocaine is also bactericidal so will mess up cultures.

5 Insert the aspiration needle and advance it slowly while maintaining slight negative pressure. When you hit the effusion, tap it completely.

6 Never inject steroids if joint infection is a possibility. To inject steroids after tapping an effusion, disconnect the syringe leaving the needle in place. Attach the syringe containing the steroid. Aspirate to ensure you are not in a vessel, then inject. There should be minimal resistance. Stop if you feel you are in the tissues and try again.

7 Remove the needle and apply pressure for a minute. Dress the wound.

Hints

■ Phone microbiology to request urgent microscopy on the joint fluid. Some labs insist on special transport media when certain infections are suspected – get advice from the microbiologist.

■ The subtalar joint (below the ankle joint) is notoriously difficult to aspirate – get expert help.

Injecting joints

Many rheumatology departments teach a simple no-touch technique. The risk of infection following this method is no worse than that outlined above.

Have ready

1 Two 5-ml syringes – one for lidocaine (to anaesthetize the skin) if deemed necessary, and one for the steroid, ± lidocaine.

2 Two alcohol swabs.

3 A small plaster.

4 Triamcinolone (5–20 mg) or methylprednisolone (10–40 mg) for steroid injections. The dose will depend on the size of the joint.

The procedure

1 Inform the patient of the small risk of infection (see above).

2 Draw up the lidocaine (if required) and the steroid for injection. The latter is now available with lidocaine added. This limits the potentially painful response to the injection and lasts for about 2–3 hours. Note that the lidocaine for skin anaesthesia is still advisable for squeamish patients.

3 Locate the site for injection; clean with an alcohol swab and allow to dry. Without touching the site again, push through the skin and anaesthetize the skin down to the joint. Remember to aspirate to ensure you are not in a vessel. Remove and allow a minute for the local anaesthetic to work.

4 Repeat (3) except this time inject the joint with steroid. There should be minimal resistance to the injection.

5 Remove the needle and apply pressure for a minute. Dress the wound.

Hints

■ Tell the patient that mild pain and redness can occur after steroid injections and may persist for up to 24 hours. They are due to a reaction to the crystalline suspension used in long-acting steroids, but be wary of iatrogenic infection.

■ Never inject steroids if joint infection is a possibility.

Local anaesthesia (for any procedure)

Have ready

1 21G and 23G needle.

2 5–10-ml syringe.

3 Alcohol swabs.

4 1–2% lidocaine ampoules.

The procedure

1 Start with a 23–25G needle. Infiltrate the skin and SC tissues raising a small bleb. If deeper anaesthesia is required, switch to a larger needle (21G), wait 1 minute, then pass through the same puncture site.

2 Aspirate for blood before injecting anything. If you hit blood, withdraw a little and try again.

3 Alternatively, inject as you move the needle. This requires continuous movement so that any injection into a vessel would only occur transiently.

4 Wait at least 2 minutes for effect.

Hints

■ Lidocaine lasts approximately 2 hours. Marcain and bupivacaine are longer acting (8 hours) and useful for intercostal blocks.

■ Use lidocaine with adrenaline for very vascular sites where you need to incise skin, as adrenaline causes vasoconstriction, for example, the scalp. Never use adrenaline for a nerve block of an extremity, for example, a finger ring block or nose, or you will cause disastrous ischaemia.

■ To work out the dose of lidocaine in mg/ml, multiply the percentage concentration by 10. Maximum dose of lidocaine within 24 hours:

○ Without adrenaline: 3 mg/kg (i.e. 20 ml of 1% lidocaine for a 70-kg adult).

○ With adrenaline: 7 mg/kg.

Lumbar puncture

Lumbar punctures (aka spinal taps) are actually pretty easy once you get the hang of them. The thing to do is to reassure the patient that it is an uncomfortable but relatively painless procedure, and that it might take up to 30 minutes – so you don't feel rushed. Of all procedures, this one requires a slow, methodical approach for success.

Indications

Diagnostic:

■ Meningitis, SAH, rarities.

Therapeutic:

■ Intrathecal drugs (never to be given by junior doctors unless formally trained).

Contraindications (get help)

1 Local sepsis.

2 Raised ICP (vomiting, bradycardia, drowsiness, papilloedema).

3 Suspicion of a cord or posterior fossa mass.

4 Coagulopathy or platelet count <40.

If patient is drowsy, unconscious or has evidence of raised ICP, request an urgent CT scan before doing an LP.

Have ready

1 LP pack or, if none available:

2 Two sterile drapes.

3 One gallipot.

4 One pack gauze swabs.

5 One pack of cotton wool balls.

6 Two LP needles (an 18G (yellow) or a 20G (black); open one).

7 One sterile, disposable manometer.

8 Three sterile, 20-ml specimen containers.

9 Antiseptic (povidone/betadine solution or equivalent).

10 5–10 ml lidocaine 2%.

11 10-ml syringe.

12 23G and 21G needles.

13 Sterile gloves.

The procedure
(see Fig. 13.9)

1 Obtain consent. Explain to the patient what you are doing, that the procedure may take some time but that it is not very painful – just uncomfortable.

2 Ask the patient to lie as indicated in Fig. 13.9a – with knees tucked up under the chin as much as possible (to draw the spinal cord out of the way of the needle). Ensure the vertebral column is parallel to the bed (the hips are exactly perpendicular to the edge of the bed).

3 Get an LP pack ready on a trolley with plenty of room to manoeuvre. Make room for sharps and dirty items.

4 Scrub up as for a sterile technique.

5 Prepare skin with betadine and cover with a sterile drape.

6 Unscrew the tops of the three sterile sample containers.

7 Locate the puncture site L3–L4 or L4–L5 by drawing two imaginary lines, one joining the top of the iliac crests and the other running down the spine. These intersect at L3–L4. The spinal cord ends at L1–L2, so the L2–L3 interspace is safe if you cannot use the lower interspaces for some reason, but ensure the patient is properly curled up.

8 Anaesthetize using a 23G needle for superficial skin and SC infiltration. Switch

to a 21G needle for deeper infiltration into the interspinous ligament. Inject slowly waiting at least 2 minutes for effect.

9 Assemble the LP equipment, check that the stylet moves freely within the needle, and check how to use the manometer taps.

10 Insert the needle in the midline between the two spinous processes. Advance towards the patient's umbilicus (slightly towards the head). Resistance increases as the needle passes through the interspinous ligament. A small 'give' is felt as the needle punctures the ligamentum flavum. Withdraw the stylet to check for a flashback of CSF. If there is no CSF, advance the needle a few millimetres and check again.

11 Attach the manometer, allow the patient to relax and measure the pressure (recorded in cmH_2O; normal range 6–15 cm). The level will fluctuate with respiration.

12 Disconnect the manometer. From the open end of the needle collect:

- 2–5 drops for biochemistry.
- 5–10 drops for bacteriology (microscopy, culture and sensitivity).
- Up to 5–10 drops for cytology.

13 Withdraw the needle slowly, taking care not to spill too many drops of CSF (causing a severe headache afterwards). Dress the wound.

14 The patient should lie flat for 4 hours; this is usually done on the basis of convention as the evidence base does not actually support this. They may have a moderate headache afterwards. If they experience a severe headache they should inform the nurses or doctors. Severe low pressure headaches sometimes require an epidural blood patch which can be extremely effective.

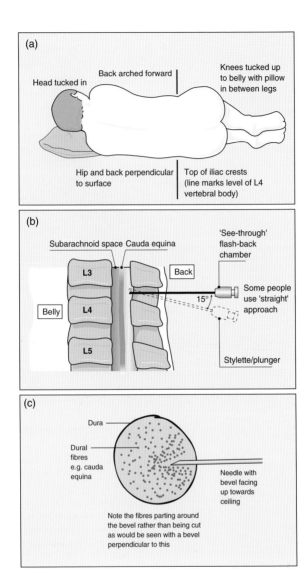

Fig. 13.9 (a) Patient position for lumbar puncture, (b) approaches for lumbar puncture, (c) close-up of lumbar puncture.

If you fail

■ Correct positioning is the key to success. If you fail, recheck the patient's position. Try another interspace if necessary.

■ If the patient is anatomically 'difficult' (e.g. very large or has an abnormal spinal column), ask a more experienced senior or enlist the help of a radiologist who can do the LP under X-ray screening.

■ If you feel you are in the right place but there is no CSF, then lightly rotate the needle through 90°; the bevel may be lying against a nerve root.

Hints

■ Sedate the patient if required: 2.5–5 mg diazepam orally 30 minutes before the procedure. The patient needs to remain horizontal for at least 4 hours post-LP to reduce the incidence of severe headache. Warn the patient that headaches can occur up to 3 days after an LP.

■ *Never* apply suction to a CSF needle.

■ Subarachnoid haemorrhage is easily distinguishable from a bloody tap by uniform blood staining of the three consecutive samples and xanthochromia in the supernatant (12 hours after the headache onset). The samples from a bloody tap gradually clear. Send samples for a cell count.

Normal values

● Opening pressure	8–22 mmHg
● Red cells	<5/mm^3
● Lymphocytes (WBC)	<5/mm^3
● Neutrophils	Nil
● Protein	<0.4 g/l
● Glucose	>50% of plasma level

● Colour Clear (if no vessels are hit you may obtain a 'Champagne Tap'; if this clear coloured CSF is obtained on your first ever attempt, then custom dictates

that your senior should buy you a bottle!)

Mantoux test

Indication

A Mantoux tests for a delayed-type hypersensitivity reaction to a partially purified protein derivative from *Mycobacterium tuberculosis*. For routine Pre-'Bacillus Calmetle Germain' (BCG) skin testing the 10-unit dose of tuberculin PPD (purified protein derivative) is used.

Have ready

1 Order PPD from pharmacy.

2 1 ml diabetic syringe (26G 1-cm needle).

3 Alcohol swab.

The procedure

1 Dilute PPD to a concentration of 100 TU/ml.

2 Draw up 0.1 ml (10 TU) into a diabetic syringe.

3 Clean a small area on the left forearm (convention).

4 Indicate the area to be injected with a marker pen.

5 Keeping the needle almost horizontal to the skin, carefully insert the needle intra-dermally and inject 0.1 ml so that a small bleb is raised.

6 A negative reaction at 48 hours indicates a negative response (either no infection or immunization, *or* overwhelming infection).

7 Read at 72 hours. Measure the diameter of induration, not the erythema:

● >10 mm = positive; suggestive of previous or current infection, not necessarily disease.

- >20 mm = strongly positive, highly suggestive of active disease.

Nasogastric tubes

Nurses are usually experienced at inserting NG tubes; you are usually called only if they fail. Therefore it is a good idea to do a few before such a call. They are usually straightforward.

Have ready

1 An apron and non-sterile gloves.

2 Fresh NG tube – size 10 (small) to 16 (large).

3 Kidney bowl and catheter drainage bag.

4 KY jelly.

5 Glass of water.

The procedure

1 Sit the patient upright with chin on chest.

2 Tell the patient what you are doing and ask for their help in swallowing the tube.

3 Lubricate the tube with jelly and insert into a nostril. Gently advance the tube towards the occiput (not upwards). Ask the patient to swallow when they feel the tube at the back of their throat and advance the tube as they swallow. They may find swallowing the water simultaneously to be helpful.

4 To assess position: aspirate some contents using a small syringe and test with blue litmus paper to check that the contents are gastric (blue litmus paper turns red on contact with acidic gastric juices); or, with a syringe, blow air down the tube while listening with a stethoscope over the stomach.

5 Attach the drainage bag.

If you fail

- Try the other nostril.

- Try oral insertion – ask the patient to swallow the tube. Sometimes keeping tubes in the fridge stiffens them and can help.

- Sometimes NG tubes have two lumens. If you don't block off one lumen when syringing air through the other to check the position of the NG tube, it will appear (falsely) as if the tube is not in the stomach.

- Get help from a senior.

- Consider endoscopic placement under mild sedation.

Hints

- NG tubes are uncomfortable and predispose to sinusitis. Remove as soon as possible.

- Use fine-bore tubes for enteral feeding and large-bore ones (Ryles) for drainage.

Peritoneal tap (paracentesis)

Like pleural aspiration, paracentesis is remarkably straightforward and can even be quite fun! The procedure is identical to pleural aspiration except for the position of the patient and puncture site.

The procedure

1 Ask the patient to empty their bladder. Explain what you are doing and why. Stress that the procedure is painless except for initial anaesthesia.

2 Lie the patient as flat as possible.

3 Percuss out the ascites.

4 Scrub up, prepare the skin and drape. Give local anaesthetic in the sites indicated in Fig. 13.10.

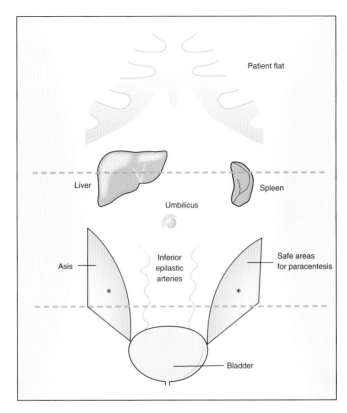

Patient flat

Liver

Spleen

Umbilicus

Asis

Inferior
epilastic
arteries

Safe areas
for paracentesis

*

*

Bladder

Fig. 13.10 Site for tapping ascites.

5 Follow the same procedure as for pleural aspiration (see Pleural aspiration, below).

6 For therapeutic taps, use a suprapubic or peritoneal dialysis catheter. These are usually supplied with drainage bags.

7 Send samples for biochemistry (protein, glucose, LDH), bacteriology (MC&S, ZN stain and TB culture) and cytology.

Hints

• Do not remove more than 500 ml in the first 10 minutes and no more than 1200 ml in 24 hours. Removing more fluid risks hypotension but may be appropriate for some patients; check with your senior.

• Avoid going too close to old surgical scars as bowel may be attached to the abdominal wall.

• You may need to reposition the catheter or 'jiggle' the patient to maintain the flow.

• Bizarre cells on cytology often represent reactive mesothelial cells not malignancy (mesothelial cells *do not* mean a mesothelioma!). Always get a formal report before embarking on a hunt for a tumour. If it is unclear, then you can always call the pathologist for an explanation; you would be extremely unlucky to meet criticism for this.

• Complications are rare but include perforated bowel, peritonitis, intra-abdominal haemorrhage and perforated bladder.

• Paracentesis is essential to rule out peritonitis in patients with cirrhosis and long-standing ascites who decompensate.

Pleural aspiration

Pleural aspiration is straightforward, although the idea of plunging tubing into someone's chest sounds daunting. Ask a senior nurse or medical colleague to supervise your first one.

Indications
Diagnostic:
■ Infection.
■ Malignancy.
Therapeutic:
■ Large effusions for relief of dyspnoea.

Have ready

1 Dressing pack (some hospitals have a prepared pleural aspiration pack).

2 Sterile gloves.

3 One 10-ml syringe.

4 One blue needle.

5 One yellow needle.

6 One green needle.

7 10 ml 2% lidocaine.

8 Three specimen jars (sterile).
For therapeutic taps add:

9 One large-bore IV cannula (brown or grey Venflon).

10 One three-way tap.

11 IV giving set and an empty, sterile bowl or saline bag.

The procedure

1 Confirm the size and extent of the effusion on the most recent CXR or CT. Scrub up. Tell the patient what you are doing and how long it will take.

2 Sit the patient upright in bed or sit them on a stool leaning slightly forward over the side of the bed or on a bedside table, resting their elbows on a pillow.

3 Select the insertion site by tapping out the effusion. The best sites are usually two to three spaces below the lowest point (angle) of the scapula or at the same level in the posterior axillary line. Avoid the mid-clavicular line on the left (and so the heart!).

4 Scrub up and drape as for a sterile procedure. Ensure you have a sterile, flat surface on which to put things.

5 Anaesthetize the skin first with a 23G (blue) needle for superficial infiltration and then again with an 18G (yellow) needle for deeper infiltration. The track of the needle should hug the upper border of the rib to avoid the neurovascular bundle (Fig. 13.11). Always withdraw before injecting local anaesthetic to make sure you are not in a blood vessel. In the average person, you should aspirate pleural fluid at the full depth of a green needle; obviously if the patient is thinner or fluid flows at a shallow depth, you don't need to push the needle deeper.

6 Attach a 20-ml syringe to the end of a green needle and insert the needle through the area already anaesthetized. Aspirate as you push forward. The flashback of fluid indicates that you have reached the effusion.

7 Gently aspirate 20 ml of fluid for analysis. Send for:

• Bacteriology: MC&S, ZN stains and TB culture.

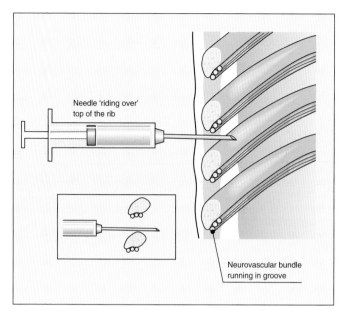

Needle 'riding over'
top of the rib

Neurovascular bundle
running in groove

Fig. 13.11 Pleural aspiration (diagram shows an oblique section).

• Chemistry: protein, glucose, LDH and amylase.

• Cytology – the more fluid the better (up to 10 ml) as the sample is spun down to concentrate the cells.

8 For therapeutic taps, attach a large (white/brown/grey) cannula to a 50-ml syringe; and after the flashback of fluid, advance the Venflon slightly and withdraw the needle, leaving the flexible cannula in place. As you do this, ask the patient to breathe out, placing your thumb over the cannula lumen to prevent air being sucked in. Again, ask the patient to breathe out as you attach the three-way tap. Secure the cannula with tape if you are aspirating a large effusion.

9 Aspirate 50 ml at a time, switching the tap settings to empty the syringe contents into the bowl or saline bag. Do not remove more than 1000 ml at one sitting; more than this can lead to reflex pulmonary oedema.

10 Withdraw the cannula, asking the patient to breathe out as you do so. Apply an occlusive dressing.

11 CXR is usually only necessary if you have removed a large volume of fluid (>500 ml) or you are concerned about a pneumothorax. However, prudence dictates you should err on the side of caution.

12 Document the procedure, including the macroscopic appearance of the fluid (straw-coloured, blood-stained, containing pus), the volume aspirated and if you have done (and checked) a CXR.

If you fail

A dry tap indicates a possible loculated effusion or empyema. Try redirecting the needle. If no luck, ask for help from a colleague or radiologist. In many hospitals, it is now fairly routine to ask a radiologist to ultrasound and mark the effusions pre-procedure.

Hints

■ Ask the patient to cough as you reach the end; this aids in expelling fluid. They usually cough reflexly as the visceral pleura touches the end of the cannula.
■ Have a vial of atropine to hand for vasovagals (1 ampoule (0.6 mg) IV stat).
■ A 'pre-med' of pethidine (50 mg) IM and prochlorperazine (12.5 mg) IM is very useful for anxious patients.

Pulsus paradoxus

Not a procedure per se but worth knowing about! During inspiration, intrathoracic pressure falls, which reduces the systolic ejection volume and therefore the systolic pressure. Normally, the difference in the systolic pressure during inspiration and expiration is less than 10 mmHg. This pressure difference is exaggerated by a large drop in intrathoracic pressure that occurs during inhalation in serious conditions, including severe asthma and cardiac tamponade. Pulsus paradoxus is defined by a difference in systolic BP between inspiration and expiration of more than 10 mmHg.

Have ready

A stethoscope and a sphygmomanometer.

The procedure

1 Inflate the cuff above systolic pressure, then slowly deflate until the first, inter-mittent sounds are heard (during expiration). Note the pressure.

2 Continue to deflate the cuff slowly until the sounds are continuous (i.e. heard during inspiration and expiration). The drop in mmHg between when the first sound is heard (intermittent) and when it becomes continuous represents the degree of paradox.

Respiratory function tests

Spirometry

Have ready

A spirometer, vitalograph paper and a disposable mouthpiece.

The procedure

1 Explain the procedure to the patient and that you need their cooperation.

2 Plug the machine in. Place the vitalograph paper in position on the spirometer. Make sure the spirometer's needle is set to zero. Place the disposable mouthpiece in the end of the spirometer's hosepipe.

3 Ask the patient to take a couple of deep breaths. When ready, ask them to breathe in as deeply as possible and then to breathe all the way out as quickly as possible into the mouthpiece. They should breathe out until the needle reaches the end of the graph paper.

4 Depending on how automated the machine is, you may need to push the record button while the patient is exhaling.

5 Repeat a few times, particularly if the first attempt(s) is feeble.

Table 13.4 Expected values for FEV$_1$ (litre).

Age (years)	Height (m) 1.5	1.6	1.7	1.8	1.9
(a) Males					
15–20	2.80	3.30	3.55	3.90	4.30
20–25	3.25	3.60	3.95	4.35	4.70
25–35	3.10	3.45	3.80	4.20	4.55
35–45	2.80	3.15	3.50	3.90	4.25
45–55	2.50	2.85	3.20	3.60	3.90
55–65	2.15	2.50	2.90	3.25	3.60
65–75	1.85	2.20	2.60	2.95	3.30
75–85	1.55	1.90	2.25	2.65	3.00
85+	1.40	1.75	2.10	2.50	2.85
(b) Females					
15–25	2.45	2.80	3.15	3.45	3.75
25–35	2.35	2.65	2.95	3.30	3.65
35–45	2.05	2.35	2.65	3.05	3.35
45–55	1.75	2.05	2.35	2.75	3.05
55–65	1.45	1.75	2.10	2.45	2.75
65–75	1.15	1.45	1.85	2.15	2.45
75–85	0.85	1.20	1.55	1.85	2.15
85+	0.75	1.05	1.35	1.70	2.05

Table 13.5 Expected normal values for FVC (litre).

Age (years)	Height (m) 1.5	1.6	1.7	1.8	1.9
(a) Males					
15–20	3.45	4.00	4.50	5.05	5.55
20–25	3.65	4.15	4.70	5.20	5.75
25–35	3.55	4.05	4.60	5.10	5.60
35–45	3.30	3.85	4.35	4.90	5.40
45–55	3.10	3.60	4.15	4.65	5.20
55–65	2.85	3.40	3.95	4.45	4.95
65–75	2.65	3.15	3.70	4.20	4.75
75–85	2.45	2.95	3.45	4.00	4.50
85+	2.35	2.85	3.35	3.90	4.40
(b) Females					
15–25	2.90	3.40	3.85	4.35	4.75
25–35	2.75	3.25	3.70	4.15	4.65
35–45	2.45	2.95	3.45	3.90	4.35
45–55	2.20	2.65	3.15	3.60	4.05
55–65	1.90	2.35	2.85	3.30	3.75
65–75	1.60	2.10	2.55	3.00	3.45
75–85	1.30	1.80	2.25	2.70	3.20
85+	1.20	1.65	2.10	2.60	3.05

6 Record the best FEV$_1$ and FVC in the notes, with expected values for the patient (see Tables 13.4 and 13.5):

The patient has a restrictive picture if FVC is reduced and FEV$_1$/FVC > 75%.

The patient has an obstructive picture if FEV$_1$/FVC < 75%.

Peak expiratory flow rate

Measures the maximum expiratory flow rate in the first 2 ms of expiration, and is useful for assessing the respiratory status of patients with asthma, COAD and other respiratory conditions, especially before surgery.

Have ready

A peak flow meter and disposable mouthpiece.

The procedure

1 Put the disposable mouthpiece into the peak flow meter.

2 Ask the patient to breathe in as deeply as possible.

3 With their lips tightly sealed around the mouthpiece, ask them to blow out

Table 13.6 Predicted values for PEFR (l/minute).

Age (years)	Height (m)				
	1.5	1.6	1.7	1.8	1.9
(a) Males					
15–20	440	475	510	545	580
20–25	535	570	610	645	680
25–35	525	560	595	630	665
35–45	500	535	570	605	635
45–55	480	510	545	575	610
55–65	455	490	520	550	580
65–75	435	465	495	525	550
75–85	410	440	465	495	525
85+	410	430	455	480	510
(b) Females					
15–25	360	395	435	470	510
25–35	350	385	420	460	495
35–45	325	365	400	440	475
45–55	305	345	380	420	455
55–65	285	320	360	395	435
65–75	265	300	340	375	415
75–85	245	280	315	355	390
85+	235	270	305	345	380

forcefully and quickly. Note the value attained.

4 Have them repeat it at least three times.

5 Record the best value in the notes, with the expected value (Table 13.6).

Sutures

As a qualified doctor you are expected to do simple suturing; this is a skill that should not be restricted to surgeons. The method is best learnt in A&E or in theatre. Ask someone to teach you how to tie a basic, non-slip knot as soon as

Table 13.7 When to remove sutures.

Area sutured	When to remove sutures
Face and neck	3–5 days
Scalp	5–7 days
Abdomen and chest	5–10 days
If impaired wound healing (e.g. steroids, cachexia, severe infection)	14 or more days

you can. Table 13.7 discusses times for suture removal.

Materials

1 Non-absorbable:
- Nylon (ethilon).
- Ethibond.
- Prolene.*
- Silk.*

2 Absorbable:
- Plain cat gut (5–10 days).
- Chromic gut (10–20 days).
- Vicryl (60–90 days).*
- Dexon (60–90 days).*

3 Sizes:

- Very coarse – 2, 1, 0, 1/0, 2/0, etc. Very fine – 6/0, 5/0, etc. (think of 2/0 as two zeros after the point i.e. 0.001).
- 3/0 and 4/0 are suitable for skin on arms and legs.
- 5/0 and 6/0 for face and back of the hand.
- 2/0 is most often used for securing lines and 1/0 for chest drains.

4 Needles:
Either use a cutting needle (with a bevelled edge) for suturing skin or a non-cutting needle (with a rounded end) for adipose and other soft tissues.

Hints

■ Nylon is less comfortable for patients. Use softer, non-absorbable material (silk or prolene) for securing lines and chest drains.

■ Some synthetic sutures are made as mono- or polyfilament. Monofilament sutures are more slippery, but are better if there is a high risk of infection. Polyfilament sutures facilitate tracking of fluid down the suture, leading to infection.

*Most commonly used for normal ward procedures.

Chapter 14
RADIOLOGY

Radiologists can help you manage patients if you give them enough information. Most of the following guidelines come from the Royal College of Radiologists. Your hospital may also have its own.

Requesting investigations

The task of requesting investigations is often delegated to junior doctors. You will receive no end of grilling from over-stretched radiology staff as to why this scan or that unusual view is needed. Take this as a learning exercise and a challenging opportunity to flex your communication skills, the ability to charm a scan an apparently unobtainable scan out of radiology is a rite of passage! It saves a lot of time and hassle if you can supply cogent answers, so don't be shy to ask your seniors why *precisely* the investigation is needed, if it isn't clear to you then it probably won't be clear to radiology either. Besides which, you may learn something from asking.

1 Always book procedures as early as possible. Most radiological departments are overbooked. This is particularly true for contrast studies, CTs and MRIs. In one of my previous jobs I just dropped the card into the department straight after my ward round and the scans were always done without fail without even talking to anyone face-to-face, I saw other juniors (with arguably more urgent requests) struggle against brick walls to get their scans done just because they

always asked later in the day. Do not underestimate the influence of getting your patient's name down first. If a scan needs to be done and you cannot persuade anyone to do it then *do not* ignore the problem. Let your seniors know as soon as possible or you will get it in the neck. It is not unusual for a consultant's '*vital*' scan to become suddenly less important when you inform them that it will not be done without consultant to consultant referral. That said most urgent scans are so called for good reason.

2 Include lots of information on the X-ray form, such as:

- Patient ID.
- Whether pregnant or not. Any reactions to contrast media.
- Whether patient is *Clostridium difficile* or MRSA positive.
- A specific question to be answered. Imagine being the radiologist reporting these scans without the benefit of patient history, examination or indeed notes. This is why writing a misleading request card to get a scan done more urgently is completely unacceptable.
- Clinical features (not just suspected diagnosis).
- Any factors which may complicate the procedure (e.g. diabetes, epilepsy).
- *Please* and *Thank you* go a long way.

3 Ask the radiographers about how to prepare patients for investigations if you are unsure, such as barium enemas. Often the radiographer will liaise directly with the ward nurse, in which case you don't have to do anything except prescribe preparations, such as enemas. It can be good, however, to find out about the different preparations so that you can tell patients in advance what they are letting themselves in for. Better still, try them yourself – you will never order a barium meal lightly again!

Minimizing radiation

■ 27% of the radiation we are exposed to comes from human generated radiological sources.

■ In terms of radiation, different procedures are ranked as indicated in Table 14.1.

Table 14.1 Radiation doses of radiological investigations.

Investigation	Radiation dose (mSv)	Number of CXRs equivalent
Abdomen	1.5	75
Barium–oesophagus study	2	100
Barium–small bowel study	6	300
Barium–stomach study	5	250
Biliary tract	1.3	65
Cervical spine	0.1	5
Chest film	0.02	1
CT chest/abdomen	8	400
CT head	2	100
Dorsal spine	1.0	50
Extremities (e.g. knee)	0.01	0.5
Hip (one)	0.3	15
IVU	4.6	230
Large bowel study	9	450
Lumbar spine	2.4	120
Nuclear study bone	3.8	190
Nuclear study liver/kidney	0.7	35
Nuclear study lung	1.2	60
Nuclear study myocardium	18	900
Nuclear study thyroid	1	50
Pelvic plain film	1	50

RCR Working Party. (1998) *Making the Best Use of a Department of Clinical Radiology: Guidelines for Doctors,* 4th edn. The Royal College of Radiologists, London.

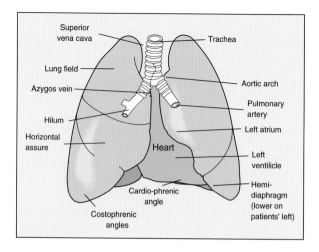

Fig. 14.1 Anatomy of a chest X-ray.

Common concerns about X-rays

Patients are usually concerned about being X-rayed. It is much kinder to address their likely concerns outright. Therefore, wherever possible, tell the patient:

1 What is about to happen to them.

2 Why they are having this done.

3 How long it might take.

4 Whether or not they will be sedated or have a general anaesthetic.

5 The amount and type of pain and discomfort to expect.

6 What to do if they have pain or other symptoms after the procedure.

7 When they can eat/drink/drive/talk/have sex.

8 Whether they will have any scars or permanent after effects.

9 Who is doing the procedure.

Pregnancy

■ Referring clinicians (i.e. you) are responsible for informing the radiologist if a patient is pregnant. Notify the radiologist clearly on the X-ray form. It is negligent not to do this. Where possible tell the radiologist yourself.

■ If you need to X-ray a pregnant patient, ask the radiologist for advice; they may suggest an alternative.

Plain films

Chest X-rays before surgery

If we are to be semantically pedantic, an X-ray is the beam of energy that penetrates the patient and film while the picture that it produces is a radiograph. This is why some more traditional clinicians refer to 'chest X-rays' as 'chest radiographs'. Whether you choose to follow this convention is up to you.

'Routine' CXRs are warranted pre-operatively if the patient has:

- Chronic heart or lung disease and no CXR within 12 months.
- Acute respiratory symptoms.
- Known/suspected malignant disease.
- Possible TB.

Age, smoking and mild hypertension are *not* reasons for routine chest X-rays (although surgeon/anaesthetic preference effectively *is*).

In terms of general 'non-surgical' indications, a CXR is best practice when the patient has any symptoms of dyspnoea or suspected respiratory disease including haemoptysis, chest pain including cardiac disease or thoracic dissection, or suspected perforation of intra-abdominal viscus (erect film). They do not generally change management in simple rib fractures or minor thoracic trauma and are not necessary in clinically unchanged COPD, atypical chest pain or simple Upper Respiratory Tract Infection (URTI). In children CXR are more difficult to interpret and should not be performed routinely unless there is a specific clinical indication.

Checking the CXR: the bare bones

1 Patient's name and the date of the film.

2 Trace the diaphragm and the lateral outline of the rib cage (look for pleural effusions, air under the diaphragm, raised hemi-diaphragm, pneumothorax).

3 Check the size and shape of the heart (look for enlarged heart, atrial shadows, calcified valve rings). Also look 'through' the heart for lesions that it partially obscures.

4 Check the position of trachea and heart (look for displaced or is the film rotated).

5 Look at the mediastinum (look for air, widened, lymphadenopathy).

6 Examine the hilar shadows (look for enlarged pulmonary arteries and veins).

7 Examine the lungs (look for opacities – consolidation, fluid or nodules). For interstitial oedema, look for straight lines (normal interstitial shadows are 'never' straight).

8 Check the bony structures (ribs, clavicles, spine) and the soft tissues (fractures, densities or lucencies, air in the tissues). The anatomy of a chest XR is demonstrated in Figure 14.1.

Skull X-rays

You rarely need to X-ray someone's skull after a head injury. A CT is the investigation of choice. The Royal College's guidelines are shown in Table 14.2. To differentiate CSF from normal nasal or aural discharge in a patient with head injury, speak to your biochemistry lab to test for tau protein or beta-trace protein. A bedside test is filter paper: the halos that CSF produce are fairly unique and show a 'double ring' where the blood separates from CSF.

Abdominal films

Radiation dose equivalent: 75 CXRs
Preparation:
None.
Tell the radiologist:
- Presenting symptoms.
- Past surgery.
- Erect films to check fluid levels.
Tell the patient:
- Quick, minimal irradiation.

Checking an abdominal plain film

1 Patient's name and date of the film; whether erect, supine or lateral decubitus.

Table 14.2 NICE guidelines regarding CT head *in adults*

CT head essential with reporting in *under 1 hour*

Any of the following:

- GCS <13 when first assessed in the emergency department
- GCS <15 when assessed in the emergency department 2 hours after injury
- Suspected open or closed skull fracture
- Signs of fracture at base of skull
- Post-traumatic seizure
- Focal neurological deficit
- >1 episode of vomiting
- None of the above but some amnesia or loss of consciousness since injury *and* a coagulopathy

CT head essential with reporting in *under 8 hours*

Any of the following:

- Amnesia of events >30 minutes before impact
- No indications for a scan in <1 hour *plus* any amnesia or loss of consciousness *and* age >65 *or* dangerous mechanism of injury (i.e. fall from >1 metre, ejection from motor vehicle or pedestrian/cyclist struck by vehicle)

Although not in the guidelines per se, common sense states that it is wise to err on the side of caution as scan risks, although real, are less than missing a significant bleed. This is particularly so with the elderly or alcoholics. If you don't pick up any abnormalities on scans within a year of emergency medicine, don't be too proud of your frugality – statistically you probably aren't scanning enough to catch them!

NICE (2007) Head injuries guidance.

2 Gas pattern; intestinal diameter (small bowel >2.5 cm, colon >6 cm indicates obstruction).

3 Look for ascites and soft tissue masses.

4 Identify the liver and spleen.

5 Check the borders of the kidneys, bladder and psoas muscles if possible.

6 Calculi (gall stones, renal and pancreatic calculi, aortic calcification).

7 Sub-diaphragmatic gas (or clear outline of organ) indicates perforation or recent surgery. (Note: sub-diaphragmatic gas is best seen on an erect CXR. The absence of free gas under the diaphragm does not rule out perforation.) A decubitus film is an alternative if the patient is too ill to sit up.

Contrast studies

Intravenous urography

Radiation dose equivalent: 230 CXRs
Preparation:
- Picolax (1 sachet) 12–24 hours before the procedure (not essential).

- Preferably NBM 6 hours before.
- Keep well hydrated before and after, to minimize contrast nephro-toxicity. IV fluids or N-acetylcysteine can be given.

Tell the radiologist:
- If the patient has renal damage, diabetes or myeloma.
- Contrast allergy or pregnancy.

Tell the patient:
- Warn about preparation.

IBD, PR bleeding); get radiologist's advice.

Tell the radiologist:
- Past surgery.
- Contrast allergy or pregnancy.

Tell the patient:
- Warn them about diet and laxative.
- Takes at least half an hour; may take 2 hours.
- Uncomfortable; requires upper GI intubation.

Barium swallow

Radiation dose equivalent: 100 CXRs
Preparation:
- NBM 6 hours before.

Tell the radiologist:
- Oesophageal disease or surgery.
- Contrast allergy or pregnancy.

Tell the patient:
- Quick, painless but tastes horrible!

Barium meal

Radiation dose equivalent: 250 CXRs
Preparation:
- NBM 6 hou rs before.

Tell the radiologist:
- Upper GI disease or surgery.
- Contrast allergy or pregnancy.

Tell the patient:
- Painless but tastes awful.

Small bowel enema

Radiation dose equivalent: 300 CXRs
Preparation:
- 24 hours low residue diet.
- Laxative (e.g. 1 sachet of Picolax) 24 and 12 hours prior to procedure *unless* contraindicated (e.g.

Barium enema

Radiation dose equivalent: 450 CXRs
Contraindication:
- Severe colonic inflammation (e.g. IBD, severe diverticulitis) and toxic megacolon.

Preparation:
- Do not perform immediately prior to CT abdomen/chest (barium hides detail on CT for at least 72 hours). Do the CT first or consider using gastrograffin.
- Book >72 hours after rectal biopsy and rigid sigmoidoscopy to avoid perforation.
- Strong laxative 24 and 12 hours before procedure *unless* acute IBD; ask radiologist for advice.

Tell the radiologist:
- Previous surgery.
- Contrast allergy or pregnancy.
- Results of sigmoidoscopy, rectal biopsy or rectal exam.

Tell the patient:
- Warn them of diet and laxative.
- Procedure takes 20–30 minutes.
- Pictures will be taken every 10–15 minutes while the patient is turned around on a platform. The procedure is very undignified, uncomfortable and often upsetting.

Ultrasound

> Radiation dose equivalent: No radiation or contraindications!
> Preparation:
> ■ Abdominal US: NBM 6 hours before.
> ■ Pelvic US: Requires full bladder.
> ■ The patient should start drinking a few hours before the procedure.
> Tell the radiologist:
> ■ For Doppler ultrasound of legs, make sure you identify which leg is the problem.
> Tell the patient:
> ■ No radiation dose or known hazards, painless, relatively quick.

Computed tomography

> Radiation dose equivalents:
> 400 CXRs for abdomen and chest CTs
> 100 CXRs for head CTs
> Preparation:
> ■ Nil; IV access needed if contrast is needed – ask the radiologist.
> Tell the radiologist:
> ■ Any metalwork in situ. These may be difficult to interpret due to metalwork induced streaking artefacts.
> Tell the patient:
> ■ Painless; will be told what to do by the doctor and nurse.

General

■ Usually hospital CTs are overbooked, so book your patient in as early as possible.

■ Do CTs *before* requesting barium studies. Barium hides detail on CT and takes at least 3 days to clear. Gastrograffin (water-soluble) can be used instead of barium if this is a problem.

■ Patients may require sedation before CT; 1–2mg lorazepam 30 minutes before the procedure is usually adequate.

CT head – some emergency indications

In strokes: to differentiate haemorrhage from infarct. May have poor sensitivity if done too early but this is not a reason to delay.

In subarachnoid haemorrhage: for diagnosis (but misses 10–15% of subarachnoid haemorrhages); to exclude a raised ICP before doing an LP; to assess the cause of deterioration (re-bleed, hydrocephalus, vasospasm).

In head injury: indicated if there is skull fracture and serious scalp injury, impaired consciousness, focal neurology, epilepsy, persistent confusion, deteriorating conscious level, depressed skull fracture, open skull fracture of vault or base. The NICE guidelines clearly outline which scans need to be done and reported within 1 hour, 8 hours or not at all. See the quick reference guide at www.nice.org.uk/CG056. It also includes guidance on management of suspected cervical spine injuries. Some examples of common CT head findings associated with traumatic mechanisms of injury are demonstrated in Figure 14.2.

Arteriography

> Preparation:
> ■ Nothing to eat for 6 hours before; nothing to drink 3 hours before.

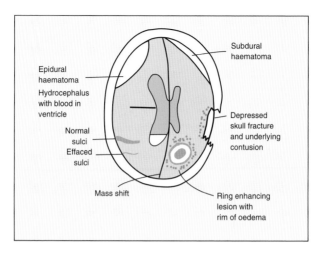

Fig. 14.2 CT head pathology.

Subdural
haematoma

Epidural
haematoma

Hydrocephalus
with blood in
ventricle

Normal
sulci

Effaced
sulci

Depressed
skull fracture
and underlying
contusion

Mass shift

Ring enhancing
lesion with
rim of oedema

■ G&S, FBC (specifically platelets), INR, find both femoral pulses.
■ Keep well hydrated before and after to minimize contrast nephro-toxicity; give IV fluids or N-acetyl-cysteine if necessary.
■ If patient has renal damage, diabetes or myeloma, discuss with radiologist.
Tell the radiologist:
■ Contrast allergy or pregnancy.
Tell the patient:
■ The radiologist will numb the skin in the groin and then inject some dye into the artery. They will probably suffer a bruise.

Risks:

1 3% chance of femoral puncture site damage.

2 0.5% risk of occlusion of the artery or pseudoaneurysm.

3 2% risk of unintended occlusion of selected vessel.

4 0.5% risk of distal embolism.

5 0.1% risk of arteriovenous fistulae.
If there is angioplasty and/or stenting, risks of the above all increase slightly.

Magnetic resonance imaging

■ MRI does not emit ionizing radiation but scans are expensive and the waiting list is often long. Does your patient really need one?
■ Book your patient in as early as possible and discuss with radiologist.
■ Inform the radiologist and get his or her advice if the patient has a pacemaker, metal heart valves or other metallic implants. Many modern implants are now 'MRI-safe', although you will need to check the make with the radiologist.
■ T1-weighted images give good anatomical detail. Fat is white, flowing blood is black.

■ T2-weighted images are good at showing abnormal tissue pathology but have poorer anatomical detail (though often still excellent). Fat and fluid are bright.

■ There are numerous newer MRI modalities with specific clinical and research applications, for example, functional MRI, diffusion-weighted imaging and tractography.

Preparation:
■ Sedation may be necessary (usually given by the radiologist).
■ The first time you enter an MRI scanner you *must* complete a safety questionnaire. This is not bureaucracy but is very important for your safety. You may find yourself surprised by the contraindications! On subsequent visits, always remove any metal and magnetic cards, etc., before entering as they will be wiped by the field. You can always spot an MRI aficionado as they start taking off their metalwork before entering a CT scanner!
Tell the radiologist:
■ If the patient is pregnant.
■ Discuss with the radiologist if the patient has any metal implants. **Do not allow the patient to be scanned unless you are certain that any implants are MRI-safe.**
■ Even non-ferrous (i.e. non magnetic) implants are subjected to 'eddy currents' that can cause heating effects in the metal work that

may have severe consequences. Often the scan sequences need to be individualized in these patients.
■ Warn the radiographers about any tattoos the patient has. These can also undergo significant heating. Tell the patient:
■ No irradiation is used.
■ The procedure is painless.
■ The patient will be in a very noisy, confined space for approximately 25 minutes, although it may seem longer.

Radioisotope scanning

Used to detect:

1 Bony metastases and sites of inflammation – technetium (Tm) scanning.

• Radioisotope scanning delivers variable radiation doses. Ensure that the patient is not pregnant.

• Most scanning does not require preparation, but as usual, book early.

2 Pulmonary embolism – ventilation perfusion (VQ) scans.

• There is no preparation for a VQ scan. These may only be available on certain days of the week, so make sure you book one well in advance.

• A d-dimer blood test may be useful in screening out those in which this test is not needed.

Chapter 15
SURGERY

With contributions from Sophia Opel

Looking after surgical patients is not intrinsically difficult, but it does involve a lot of running around. You will accompany surgeons on many rapid ward rounds. Have a piece of paper ready for the tasks that will be fired at you from all directions. You must know your patients well, and overall, the essential thing is timing – if nothing else, make sure you have patients and results ready for theatre.

Clerking: pre-admission clinic

You may be expected to run your own pre-admission clinic. These clinics are designed to ensure the patient is fit for surgery and to alleviate stress by providing an opportunity for patients to ask questions and discuss their concerns. While clerking routine surgical patients can be mundane, it is important to bear in mind that you may be the only one able to detect medical problems before the patient goes to theatre.

Before you see the patient:
■ Flick through the notes (summaries are particularly useful) to give yourself an idea of what has happened previously. This will reassure the patient and enables you to fill in the gaps in their medical history, saving time.

■ Clerking patients before nurses have finished their admission routine is sure to create havoc. Ask the nurse to let you know when they have finished.

■ While you are waiting, fill in any forms you can, for example, blood forms.

■ You will also need to prepare a drug chart for the patient. If there is a pharmacist present in the clinic you may just have to check and sign the chart or add any medications. If there is no pharmacist, then you should fill the drug chart with the patient's regular medications (omitting any that are contraindicated) and any additional medications they may require (see Perioperative prescribing, below).

■ The outpatient phlebotomy clinic and the outpatient ECG service will save you a lot of time. However, do not forget to check on the results the day after, to pre-empt any problems before the admission date.

■ Check the admission date and the date of the operation, and ensure that any cross-matched blood is available for the patient. If not, they will still need a blood sample for cross-matching on admission.

When the patient arrives:
Remember to be polite and friendly. You may be in a rush to finish your busy clinic, but most patients are likely to be anxious for their upcoming operation.

The Hands-on Guide for Junior Doctors, Fourth Edition. Anna Donald, Michael Stein and Ciaran Scott Hill.
© 2011 Anna Donald, Michael Stein and Ciaran Scott Hill. Published 2011 by Blackwell Publishing Ltd.

Important points:

1 Details: Name, Age, Planned operation.

2 History of presenting complaint.

3 Past surgical history.

4 Past medical history.

a. MJ THREADS

i. MI, Jaundice, TB/Thyroid, Rheumatoid, Epilepsy, Asthma/arrhythmia, Diabetes, Sickle cell or stroke

b. HASH CREDIT

i. Hypertension, Asthma/COAD, Sickle cell, Hepatitis, CVA, AF, Epilepsy, Diabetes, Ischaemic Heart Disease, TB.

5 Medications and CASES.

a. Contraception, Anticoagulants, Steroids, Etoh/alcohol, Smoking.

6 In women of child-bearing age, ask for the date of their last menstrual period and whether they may be pregnant.

7 *Allergies* (very important – especially latex allergies, antibiotics and past drug reactions to anaesthesia).

8 Home care (lives with, home help, family diseases, mobility).

9 Functional enquiry: CVS, RS, GI, GU, CNS, MSK.

10 Examination.

11 Impression.

12 Differential diagnoses.

13 Plan.

■ You can make your own custom-designed protocol clerking sheet, but these days you are likely to be provided with a pro forma (see Fig. 15.1). Consider including a pre-op anaesthetist checklist.

■ If you have literally 3 minutes to clerk a patient, at least make sure that:

(a) the patient has the problem that they are supposed to have and you have checked the side

(b) the patient is fit for surgery

(c) you know when the patient last ate and if he has any allergies

■ You may be the only person that checks them for cardiovascular and respiratory problems. Listen carefully for cardiac murmurs or abnormal breath sounds. Be prepared to take responsibility for their medical fitness. Check the patient's ECG and CXR. This may be the first time they are having one.

Check the patient's observations, especially their blood pressure. Again, it may be the first time they are having it checked.

■ G&S or cross-match patients ahead of time. It is wise to routinely G&S all patients on admission if you have not already cross-matched them. If necessary you can then phone the blood bank to cross-match them quickly (in 30 minutes). Unless you ask the lab to hold onto it for longer, G&S blood is usually thrown out after a period of time and may need to be repeated (see Table 15.1).

■ Check local transfusion requirements for specific operations.

■ ITU can be a frightening place. Try to organize for patients undergoing major operations to meet ITU staff or visit the ITU before theatre in preparation for their post-op stay. Nurses will often organize this for you.

■ Do a sickle cell test on black patients if their haematological status is unknown.

■ Patients must be NBM for solids for at least 6 hours before going to theatre, and 3 hours for sips of liquid. This is a

Name: .... DOB: .... Occupation: ....

Admitted for: ....

HPC: ....
....
....
....

☐ Weight loss   ☐ Past PU
☐ Change in bowel habit   ☐ Alcohol intake
☐ Blood in stool   ☐ Smoking
☐ Abdominal pain

Last meal:.................... Last menstrual period: ....

PMH ....
....
....
....
....

☐ H/T   ☐ RF
☐ Asthma/COAD   ☐ Epil.
☐ Sickle   ☐ DM
☐ HIV/HEP   ☐ IHD
☐ CVA   ☐ TB

Drugs:....................   **Allergies:** ....
....

F/SHx: ....
....

☐ Lives with   ☐ Family diseases
☐ Home help   ☐ Mobility

F/E ....

R/CVs
☐ Chest pain
☐ SOB
☐ Dysuria
GU ☐ Urgency
☐ Froth in urine
CNS ☐ Fits/faints/funny turns
D/MSK ☐ Joint pain
Other ....

☐ Cough w/y/g/sputum
☐ PND
☐ Frequency
☐ Stream

☐ Change in vision/speech
☐ Rash

☐ Palps
☐ Pillows
☐ Incontinence
☐ Haematuria

☐ Weakness

Examination   P = ...   Reg/irreg ....   BP = .../......
   T = ...   RR = ...

General	R/CVS	Abdomen	Legs
☐ Jaundice	☐ JVP	☐ Bowel sounds	☐ SOA
☐ Pallor	☐ Apex	☐ Tender	☐ Ulcers
☐ Cyanosis	☐ Bruit	☐ Mass	☐ Skin changes
☐ Lymphadenopathy	☐ Expansion	☐ Bruit	
☐ Pitting oedema	☐ Breath sounds	☐ Shifting dullness	
☐ Clubbing	☐ PN	**CNS**	
☐ Rash	☐ SOA	☐ Reflexes ☐ Plantars ☐ Strength	
☐ Arcus	☐ HS	☐ Coordination ☐ Sensation	

Impression ....

Differential diagnosis ....

Plan ....

Fig. 15.1 Surgical protocol clerking sheet.

Table 15.1 Preparations for different operations.

Operation	G&S/ cross-match	Special needs
Abdominoperineal repair/ Abdominoperineal Resection	4	Prepare for stoma
Amputation, minor	G&S	Pain ± grief
Amputation, major	2	Fentanyl-clonidine infusion works; gabapentin reduces neurogenic pain
Aneurysm repair (elective)	6	Post-op ITU
Aneurysm repair (emergency)	10	Post-op ITU
Aortobifemoral repair	6	
Appendicectomy	G&S	Metronidazole post-op saves a drip
Arthroscopy	Nil	
Carotid endarterectomy	2	Aspirin post-op
Cholecystectomy	G&S	
Colectomy	2	Prepare for stoma
Craniotomy/Burr hole	2	Be alert to any changes in GCS
Dynamic hip screw	2	Be alert to post-op infection
ERCP	G&S	Pre-op abdominal US, post-op amylase
Femoropopliteal repair	2	
Gastrectomy	2	Bad pain post-op, try continuous morphine infusion
Hemi-arthroplasty	2	
Hernia repair	2	
Ileal reservoir	2	
Laparotomy	2	Consent for colostomy/ileostomy
Liver biopsy	G&S	Pre-op INR (see preoperative prescribing, p. 213)
Liver/pancreatic surgery	6	Post-op amylase
Mastectomy	G&S	Prepare for grief over loss of breasts and body image. Get a prosthesis nurse to talk to patient. Drains remain in until it stops discharging
Oesophagectomy	4	
Prostactectomy (TURP)	2–4	Watch for post-op haemorrhage (i.e. haematuria). May need to cross-match more blood post-op
Splenectomy	2	Pre-op pneumococcal ± HiB ± meningococcal vaccines

Table 15.1 *Cont'd*

Operation	G&S/ cross-match	Special needs
Thyroidectomy	2–4	Pre-op vocal cord assessment, post-op Ca^{2+} check
Total hip replacement	4	Watch for DVT/PE and infection
TURT	G&S	Pre-op MSU
Varicose veins	G&S	

strict rule. In a real emergency, when patients may have eaten or drunk fluids, anaesthetists do 'crash induction' aka 'rapid sequence' where the patient is paralysed and cricoid pressure is maintained to reduce aspiration risk. Discuss this if necessary with the anaesthetist.

■ Remember, when the patient turns up, to check that nothing has changed since the pre-admission clinic. Make sure the relevant scans and results (e.g. CT scans and blood results) are available on the ward.

After the clinic:

■ Check the results of any investigations that you have requested.

■ If you think that a patient needs anaesthetic review, request it. The nursing staff will typically be able to advise you how to do this. It may involve simply faxing a letter to the anaesthetist, calling them or going to find them.

Perioperative prescribing

■ Prescribe as much as possible during the clerking, as it saves time later: regular drugs, pre-medication, anti-emetics, prophylactic antibiotics, prophylactic heparin, analgesia, routine post-op antibiotics, extra steroids if the patient takes them already (to cover post-op stress).

■ Check the firm's use of prophylactic antibiotics and anticoagulants. If in doubt, ask a member of the team.

■ Diabetics may need to stop their regular anti-hyperglycaemics, and be placed on an insulin sliding scale. The hospital pharmacist can advise you about this (see Table 15.2).

■ 20 mg temazepam orally with a small sip of water can be used as a pre-med if necessary. This should be given 3 hours before surgery but can sometimes be given within an hour of theatre. Check with the anaesthetist if in doubt.

■ A fentanyl infusion can be effective pain relief (less side effects than morphine but more expensive; problems appear within the first 10–15 minutes).

■ Patients should stop taking anticoagulants at least a week (preferably a month) before surgery unless they have a condition that requires continuous anticoagulation such as patients with artificial heart valves. If they have not stopped taking their anticoagulants, ask your senior or anaesthetist for your firm's policy on how to proceed. The effects of anticoagulants fall within days of stopping them and usually you can cover patients with FFP. Patients with artificial heart valves or other conditions requiring continuous anticoagulation should be switched over to intravenous heparin – consult your seniors.

Table 15.2 Surgical protocols for people with diabetes.

	Minor surgery (eating same day)	Major surgery (not eating for several days)
Type II diabetes mellitus on oral agents	Omit morning hypoglycaemic drugs	Omit hypoglycaemic drugs
		Monitor blood glucose Four Times a Day (QDS)
		Insulin sliding scale if uncontrolled glucose levels
Type I and II diabetes mellitus on insulin	Omit morning insulin	Needs an insulin sliding scale until eating
	Monitor blood glucose	Return to usual insulin regime as soon as eating

■ Some surgeons prefer not to operate on patients on aspirin. If aspirin needs to be stopped, it should be 5 days preoperatively so remind the patient at any pre-admission clinic.

■ The *BNF* recommends that people stop taking the oral contraceptive pill at least 4 weeks before major surgery. If the patient has not done this, consider IV or SC heparin before surgery, but check with the anaesthetist or surgeon first. The pill does not need to be stopped for minor surgery such as laparoscopic sterilization. Progestagen-only pills do not need to be stopped. In people who have stopped or have not been using contraception, exclude pregnancy. Consider a formal pregnancy test.

Consent

Criteria for valid consent[1]

1 No coercion
2 Patient informed
3 Patient competent

---

[1] Hope R.A. et al. (1994) *Oxford Practice Skills Project: Sample Teaching Materials*. Oxford Medical School, Oxford.

■ However rushed you are, patients must understand major and common hazards and discomforts of the procedure they are about to undergo. Note: GMC guidelines state that you can obtain consent for a procedure if you are familiar with the indications and complications, even if you have never performed it yourself. However, it really is the responsibility of the operator that adequate consent is obtained; so if you are uncertain, just give the patient information in advance of the operator getting informed consent (to make their job easier). Consent is usually obtained by the operator in clinic, or the day of or day before the operation.

■ If you will perform the procedure yourself, never get consent if you do not know all the risks or logistics of the procedure. Whenever in doubt, ask your senior.

■ While taking consent, you should spend a few minutes improving the patient's understanding of their overall course of management and alternatives (not just the procedure). This is a good opportunity to develop a relationship with the patient.

■ NB: a signature alone does not stand in a court of law as adequate proof of consent. The patient must understand the procedure.

■ Get parental consent for minors while the parents are on the ward, or you will have to call them in from home. Remember that minors require a different consent form from adults: the form has place for the guardian as well as the child if the child wishes to do so. ('Minors' are people under 16 years of age.) Occasionally it may be lawful to treat a child under 16 without parental consent, but you must be sure that he or she fully understands the treatment, that his or her health would be likely to suffer without treatment, that you have attempted to persuade the child to involve their parents and that you are sure it is in the child's best interest to proceed without informing the parents. You must get senior advice in these situations. Rarely, parents refuse consent for their child's treatment. Unless it is an acute situation, an application will be necessary through the hospital's solicitors or Social Services.

■ In patients who are unable to consent due to their illness (e.g. unconscious, confusion, dementia), there are special consent forms for these situations that only require a doctor's signature. However, it is always good practice to speak to any relatives or next of kin before proceeding.

■ Diagrams can save many words. If you are in a specialty where you need consent for a particular procedure many times, a well-constructed diagram can save you a lot of time in the long run. Photocopy it and leave it with the patient.

■ Remember that while you may understand anatomical diagrams, the patient may not. Sometimes a conceptual diagram is more useful, if not as accurate.

■ Check with nurses to see whether your department has approved patient information leaflets to give to your patient.

■ Always consent patients undergoing laparoscopic surgery for open surgery. (For example, 5–10% of patients undergoing laparoscopic cholecystectomy end up having open surgery.)

■ Always consider consenting patients undergoing bowel resection or laparoscopy for a colostomy or ileostomy in case they need one. (Write '± colostomy/ileostomy' on the consent form.) Warn them that this may happen and arrange with the nurses for a stoma nurse to see them.

In all cases of surgery, it is important to inform patients of:

■ Fatigue. Tell patients that they can expect to feel quite low and very tired for several weeks post-op (1–3 months for major surgery).

■ Anaesthetic risk. Although the anaesthetist will need consent for the anaesthetic, it is a good idea to ask whether or not the patient has had any previous adverse reactions.

■ Bleeding. Reassure patients that major bleeding is very uncommon (they often fear it the most). However, it is a risk they should be aware of.

■ Infection.

■ Advise about the likelihood of waking up with an O_2 mask, drains from the wound and NGT. These may be in place for several days. Advise also that post-op nausea from the anaesthetic is possible and that post-op pain will be treated.

NB – it is a good idea to check the actual risks (e.g. bleeding, infection etc.) for the procedure in question with your senior. (Note: some hospitals collect and publish the complications of surgery and procedures on a regular basis.)

Common or important expected side effects after specific surgical procedures

Amputation. Sloughing; cramps; phantom pain; psychological distress; need for revision.

Aortic aneurysm repair. Bleeding; thromboembolism; ureteric damage; paraplegia (from anterior spinal artery damage); gut ischaemia; ARDS; renal failure; aortoenteric fistula. Also fatigue and feeling low. These patients usually go to ITU post-op.

Biliary surgery. Jaundice; damage to the bile ducts causing strictures or a bile leak requiring further intervention (radiological or open surgery); pancreatitis; hepatorenal syndrome; bleeding; drainage tubes in place.

Abdominal/colonic surgery. Constipation (ileus); fistulae; anastomotic leaks; obstruction; trauma to ureters. The patient will need counselling about a stoma; contact your stoma nurse to arrange this if the nurses have not already done so. Always consent patients undergoing colonic surgery for ileostomy/ colostomy and warn them that they may have one when they wake up.

Genito-urinary surgery. Ureteral and renal damage causing strictures or leaks requiring further intervention. Infection.

Mastectomy. Arm oedema; anxiety/ depression.

Splenectomy. Infection (pneumococcal septicaemia); thrombocytosis. The patient should have been given pneumococcal, HiB ± meningococcal vaccines at least 1 week prior to surgery; if not, consult immediately with seniors. Splenectomized patients need prophylactic antibiotics (penicillin V 250–500 mgbd) probably for the rest of their lives (people have died of pneumococcal sepsis 20 years post-op). In addition, give advice about coping with the side effects of antibiotics (diarrhoea, candidiasis, particularly vaginal thrush); and they should carry a card and preferably a medical bracelet to alert others that they have no spleen.

Thyroid surgery. Bleeding; hoarseness (laryngeal nerve palsy); requirement for replacement therapy depending on the nature of the surgery.

Tracheostomy. Stenosis; mediastinitis; surgical emphysema.

Prostatectomy. Urinary retention post-op; urethral stricture and incontinence; bleeding; retrograde ejaculation (usually asymptomatic but important to mention and can cause infertility!).

Haemorrhoidectomy. Bleeding and anal stricture.

Anaesthetics

■ Anaesthetists usually come to see patients (and you) the evening before theatre. It is important they trust you as a member of the team so make friends with them and have everything ready; have an anaesthetic/surgical checklist for each patient (see Pre-op checklist, below).

■ Get the rota from the anaesthetic department. This saves time when you need to find the anaesthetist to warn them of late changes or patient complications.

■ Inform your anaesthetist about (a) late changes to a patient or procedure, and (b) high-risk patients.

■ Check whether you or the anaesthetist needs to prescribe the premedication.

■ Arrange for ECGs to be done on admission for anyone older than 50.

■ Arrange for CXRs well in time for theatre according to local protocols (routine pre-op CXRs are not recommended by the Royal College of

Radiologists; see Chapter 14, Requesting investigations).

■ Arrange for neck X-rays for patients with rheumatoid arthritis.

■ Write a checklist in the notes for patients going to theatre. The following is routine, but add or subtract lines depending on your specialty.

Pre-op checklist

Premed	Prescribed/Given
NBM	X hours
FBC	Result
U&E	Result
ECG	Done/NA
CXR	Report
Any sickle cell disease, liver disease, COAD, CVS disease, renal failure?	Details
Allergies?	Details
Special needs?	Details

■ Have the anaesthetist insert cannulae if you have trouble pre-op. It is much less stressful putting them into unconscious patients.

■ Ask the anaesthetist to teach you how to intubate patients.

Note: The National Patient Safety Agency (UK) recommends that surgical teams use the WHO Surgical Checklist (adapted for local use) within the operating theatre before the start of the procedure. This is proven to reduce surgical complications. Current versions are available at http://www.nrls.npsa.nhs.uk/resources/clinical-specialty/surgery/?entryid45=59860. It is well worth reading up about this resource to impress (and sometimes inform) your seniors!

Drawing up theatre lists

Some hospitals require junior doctors to do this.

■ Include: Name of the surgeon to do each case, name of the theatre, date and time the list is supposed to start, name, sex, age, hospital number and ward of each patient, procedure, special information (e.g. high-risk status).

■ Put children and diabetics first.

■ Put 'dirty' (bowel) surgery and high-risk patients last.

■ Let theatre staff know that a patient is high risk so they can get prepared.

Marking patients for surgery

■ Use an indelible pen and mark boldly. Double-check the site (side and position). Ask the patient and check the notes carefully if in any doubt.

■ Discuss varicose vein marking with the surgeon.

Post-operative care

Be alert to post-op emergencies as well as slow onset complications. PEs, stress-induced heart failure, MI, haemorrhage, anaesthetic and steroid reactions, as well as terrible pain, all require urgent action. It is vital to remember emergency routines for these problems, even if you do not use them much during your surgical rotation. Nursing staff on surgical convalescent wards may not know much about medical emergencies and it may be up to you to start rapid treatment. Most of all, remember to seek senior help after stabilization of your patient.

1 It is a good idea to conduct your own daily ward round, particularly as surgical ward rounds are fast paced. *Dunn and Rawlinson*[2] provide a useful ward round checklist that enables you to manage your ward efficiently:

- Ask the patient about pain, breathing, eating, bowels and bladder output.
- Examine the chest, abdomen, wound, legs, mental state.
- Check drains, lines and catheters for drainage and local infection. Are they still necessary?
- Look at the charts for pyrexia, tachycardia, changes in BP and fluid balance.
- Make sure the patient is written up for adequate analgesia, night sedation, antibiotics and fluids. Are they all still necessary?
- Check FBC and U&E post-op.
- Check U&E daily for as long as the patient is on a drip.
- Check other tests for specific complications of different operations.

2 Remember to look for the '4W' complications: wound, walking, wind, water (i.e. wound infection, DVT, chest infection/PE and poor urine output). Ileus is also a common problem typically but not always limited to post-abdominal surgery.

Complicated patients

Jaundice

Problems: excessive bleeding and dehydration, hepatorenal syndrome
Do:
■ Pre- and post-op liver function tests, INR and APTT.

[2] Dunn D.C., Rawlinson N. (1999) *Surgical Diagnosis and Management: A Guide to General Surgical Care*. Blackwell Science, Oxford.

■ Avoid morphine in pre-medication.
■ Ensure adequate IV fluids. Hydrate pre-op if necessary (be wary of heart failure, ascites or low albumin). Use 5% dextrose, not saline.
Consider:
■ Pre-op vitamin K.
■ Post-op 2-hourly urine output check.
■ Post-op IV fluids to match fluid losses (urine, NGT, stool).
■ Measure U&E daily.
■ Avoid saline if the person is in liver failure and has ascites.

Diabetes

Problems: hypoglycaemia, ketoacidosis precipitated by stress and dehydration, post-op infection. Also, this group has a high percentage of silent MIs. For surgical protocol see Table 15.2.

For all diabetics
■ Consider ECG.
■ Check local protocols.

For well-controlled NIDDM
■ Do pre-op fasting glucose (preferably the day before surgery).
■ If pre-op fasting glucose is less than 11 mmol/l, halve the oral hypoglycaemic dose the day before surgery and omit the oral hypoglycaemic on the day of surgery.
■ If pre-op fasting glucose is greater than 11 mmol/l, follow the IDDM regime in Table 15.2.
■ For minor procedures and even larger procedures, if the patient is eating on the same day, simply omit the morning hypoglycaemic. Institute IV insulin sliding scale or the alternative PIG regime (Table 15.3) if uncontrolled (capillary blood glucose > 10 mmol/l).
■ If the patient is undergoing major surgery, follow the PIG and omit the oral hypoglycaemic agent on the day of surgery.

Table 15.3 The alternative PIG (potassium, insulin, glucose) insulin sliding scale – as used in Newcastle.

500 ml of 10% dextrose with 10 mmol KCl and 12–16 units Actrapid. Infuse at 80 ml/hour
If blood glucose >10 and rising, put up a new bag containing 4 more units of insulin
If blood glucose 7–10, continue on same regime
If blood glucose <7, use a new bag with 4 units less insulin
If blood glucose <3, give 200 ml 10% dextrose and recheck the blood glucose
The rationale of this regime is that it provides both insulin and dextrose. It thus suppresses ketone production and avoids problems that might occur with separate insulin and glucose infusions, such as the glucose drip finishing or blocking while the insulin drip carries on, potentially causing hypoglycaemia

For IDDM and poorly controlled NIDDM

■ Put the patient first on the list and tell the surgeon (or theatre sister) that the patient is diabetic.

■ Pre-op fasting glucose, U&E, FBC (at least).

■ Ensure good IV access pre-op.

■ If the operation is in the morning, omit all insulin or hypoglycaemic drugs.

■ Use the PIG regime (see Table 15.3).

Insulin infusion

■ Draw up 50 units of short-acting insulin (e.g. Actrapid) in a 50 ml syringe and then fill the syringe with 50 ml of normal saline. This means that there is 1 unit of insulin per ml, allowing easy adjustment on the sliding scale shown in Table 15.4.

■ Label the syringe.

■ Set up an infusion pump (Chapter 9, To make up an infusion) or put the syringe in the fridge and let the nurses know where it is.

■ To convert this scale to a SC scale, give four times the IV dose. This is because SC insulin is given every 4 hours instead of every hour.

■ Work out how much insulin the patient normally receives, in whatever form. For example, if he or she gets a total of 100 units/24 hours as a mixture of long- and short-acting insulin, then adjust the sliding scale so that roughly 100 units of short-acting insulin is given over 24 hours. However, you will need to reduce the normal dose while the patient is not eating.

■ Make sure you check U&E at least once daily while the patient is on a sliding scale of insulin and a K^+ infusion. Adjust K^+ accordingly. Remember that K^+ comes out of cells as blood glucose rises and so can suddenly drop if the patient's glucose comes under control.

■ Measure blood glucose regularly (depending on the sliding scale being used). If the capillary blood glucose is persistently >10 or constantly <4.0 mmol/l, modify the sliding scale.

Steroid-dependent patients

(see Chapter 10, The patient on steroids)

Problem: Addisonian crisis. These patients need extra steroid cover for surgical stress.

■ Ensure good IV access.

Table 15.4 A sample insulin sliding scale.

Capillary blood		Modifying the scale	
Glucose (mmol/l)	IV insulin (units/hour)	If constantly >10	If constantly <3
<2	Stop, give 50 ml 50% glucose	No change	No change
4.0–6.4	0.5	No change	−0.5
6.5–9.0	1.0	No change	−0.5
9.1–11.0	2.0	+1	−1
11.1–17.0	3.0	+1	−1
17.1–28.0	4.0	+1 to +2	−1
>28	Call doctor	No change	No change

■ Major surgery: 100 mg hydrocortisone IV with pre-med, then 6-hourly for 3 days.
■ Minor surgery: as above, but only give post-op hydrocortisone for 24 hours.

Thyroid surgery

Problems: vocal chord damage, post-op thyroid storm, bleeding.
■ Have vocal chords checked by ENT pre-op.
■ Cross-match at least 2–4 units pre-op and G&S post-op.
■ Ensure good IV access.
■ Measure Ca^{2+} post-op.
■ Patients who have undergone thyroid surgery should have clip removers at the bedside. If they bleed suddenly the surgical clips should be removed to prevent suffocation and to allow the bleeding to be controlled directly with pressure.

Pituitary surgery

Problems: deterioration of vision, CSF leak post-op, diabetes insipidus, Addisonian crisis.

■ Have visual fields checked formally by ophthamology pre-op.
■ Ensure good steroid cover (see Steroid-dependent patients, above).
■ Measure urine output, U&E and serum osmolality daily post-op.

Day surgery

More and more operations are being done as day surgery; the Royal College of Surgeons' target is 50%.
■ Don't spend too much time clerking day surgery patients (usually 10 minutes). They typically will have been checked over at least twice already, but if not spend more time with them. You need to ensure they have no obvious CVS or respiratory problems (like a recent cold), and if necessary, to send them home.
■ Develop a protocol clerking sheet for your day patients (see p. 211).
■ Prescribe adequate take-home analgesia. Poor pain relief is a very common problem for patients – and for GPs who have to prescribe it. A few paracetamol are not adequate postoperatively.

Co-dydramol (2 tabs) 4–6-hourly is standard, but check with your surgeons and the nursing staff.

■ Tell patients what to expect, especially within the first 24 hours. For instance, fatigue and wound-related discomfort are normal. Tell patients that you are giving them painkillers to take home with them and that they should use them!

■ Tell patients: they can't drive home, they can eat and drink and they should have a contact number for the hospital and their GP should any problems arise (it is helpful to give the hospital day surgery contact number to patients and their relatives). You should advise patients that they should not drive until they feel comfortable performing an emergency stop.

■ Your senior is responsible for discharging patients from day surgery. Legally you may not sign discharge forms for patients until you have full medical registration.

Oro-facio-maxillary surgery

Being a junior doctor for the oro-facio-maxillary surgeons usually involves rapid clerking of patients who are going to have their teeth pulled, usually their wisdom teeth. These patients are often teenagers and rarely present problems.

■ Make sure you get under-16 parental consent while the parents are on ward; otherwise you will have to bring them in from home to sign the consent form.

■ Try writing and photocopying a prototype clerking sheet for these patients.

■ Always ask about heart lesions and blood clotting disorders. Listen for murmurs. Have a list of antibiotics for prophylactic cover to fill into the drug chart.

■ Know how to read dental shorthand for teeth:

(European version)

Adults

R $\dfrac{8+7+6+5+4+3+2+1+|+1+2+3+4+5+6+7+8}{8-7-6-5-4-3-2-1-|-1-2-3-4-5-6-7-8}$ L

Children

R $\dfrac{5+4+3+2+1+|+1+2+3+4+5}{5-4-3-2-1-|-1-2-3-4-5}$ L

■ Examples of teeth notation:
The upper and lower right wisdom teeth are $\underline{8}+/\bar{8}-$

The upper left wisdom tooth is $+\underline{8}$.
The lower left wisdom tooth is $-\bar{8}$.

Surgical protocol clerking sheet

Figure 15.1 is a condensed example of a surgical protocol clerking sheet that you might want to reproduce to ensure comprehensive, legible clerking. You may need to modify it to suit your particular specialty. It is also a good idea to leave plenty of space for additional comments for patients whose details are not covered by the protocol. It is easy to photocopy the protocol directly onto your hospital's clerking forms, but you first need to make a template to photocopy from. Use a word processor and adjust the page margins to fit the hospital forms – typically size A4. Type out the protocol so that it 'lines up' with the hospital form. Repeat for the second (and maybe third) page of the protocol. Print out the form/s and then load a photocopier's tray with hospital forms and photocopy the protocol onto them.

Chapter 16
GENERAL PRACTICE

With contributions from Dr Nicole Corriette

General practice is a wonderful experience. You will meet many new people, encounter all sorts of conditions and never know what is coming next. At the same time, you may be unsure of a lot of what you see: strange skin rashes, lumps and bumps, aches and sprains, odd-sounding symptoms, to name a few. Do not be afraid to ask. The GP partners know you are in training and are more than happy to review patients if you are unsure. Use the opportunity to learn – general practice is one of the few times where you have the privilege of being the sole trainee to several tutors.

What you can and cannot do

You can:

■ Run your own surgeries and decide patient management independently (one of the partners can sign 'outside' prescriptions you have written if you are in the first foundation year).

■ Write and sign referral letters, but always write the name of the GP in charge of the patient underneath your name.

■ Perform any duty expected of a doctor that you are trained for and feel comfortable doing, for example, smear tests, minor surgery, adjusting medication, etc.

You cannot:

■ Sign legal documents, for example, prescriptions, sick notes, abortion certificates while you are still 'pre-registration', that is, in your first year of work while provisionally registered with the GMC.

Referral letters and note keeping

The most important thing is to write referral letters as soon as possible after seeing patients. Practice notes are much briefer than hospital notes, so may not provide sufficient detail for referral letters weeks later.

General points

■ Keep both referral letters and notes brief. Write the presenting complaint and any salient positive findings from the history and examination. This should only take 1 to 2 lines.

■ Write clearly the diagnosis and any treatment you have given. It is important to document the full details of any prescriptions, including the dose and the amount you supplied the patient with.

■ Stick to a simple format:

○ The first line should tell the consultant exactly what is wrong, for example,

---

The Hands-on Guide for Junior Doctors, Fourth Edition. Anna Donald, Michael Stein and Ciaran Scott Hill.

'Thank you for seeing 17-year-old girl with recurrent bouts of tonsillitis'.

○ The next line/s should provide a brief summary of the history and a summary of any relevant examination findings.

○ The last paragraph should clearly state what you would like the consultant to do, for example, 'I would be grateful if you could therefore consider this woman for tonsillectomy'. Note the wording; you can *ask* but never *tell* another professional what to do. In other cases you may simply be seeking their specialist opinion 'I would be grateful if you could give me your opinion about…'.

Public health and health promotion

Do not hesitate to seek advice about public health and health promotion from colleagues and from the local Primary Care Trust (the practice will have its phone number). Here are the most common public health and health promotion matters you are likely to encounter:

■ *Contraception*. You need to be able to discuss the pros and cons of the different kinds of contraception in detail with any woman over the age of 16 and any Gillick[1] – competent female below 16 who asks for advice, especially the oral contraceptive pill (one of the most common consultations).

■ *Smoking*. Actively encourage patients to stop smoking and offer them as much advice and support as you can. Research

[1] Gillick v West Norfolk and Wisbech Area Health Authority [1985] 3 All ER 402 (HL) states parental right to determine whether or not their minor child below the age of 16 will have medical treatment terminated if and when the child achieves sufficient understanding and intelligence to enable him or her to understand fully what is proposed.

finds that GP encouragement *does* make a big difference to cessation rates. This may include patches, gum or just a friendly chat when willpower is fading. Be aware of smoking cessation clinics and other local services available (ask your colleagues for details).

■ *Lifestyle advice*. This is important, particularly for preventing coronary heart disease. In addition to offering smoking cessation advice to smokers, you can offer advice about diet, alcohol and exercise. Even 30 minutes of exercise a day can make a big difference to a patient with cardiovascular risk factors. Encourage overweight patients to lose weight and explain the potential long-term health problems. (Ask colleagues or the Trust for detailed information and patient leaflets.)

■ *Notifiable diseases*. Ask practice staff for a form if you think a patient has a notifiable disease. The form lists notifiable diseases. The most common is food poisoning. The important thing to remember when filling out these forms is the person's work address, or name and address of any school or institution they are attending. This helps keep track of outbreaks.

■ *Vaccinations*: Flu jabs should be offered to all people 65 years old or older, as well as those with immunosuppression (check with colleagues) or chronic illness such as heart failure, asthma, COPD. Pneumococcal vaccines are currently offered for people older than 75 and those with chronic illnesses such as COPD and heart failure, but are not used routinely for people with asthma (the eligible age for free vaccination may be lowered in future). Immunizations for children are usually performed by the practice nurse or health visitors, but you may need to give them too, if you are confident.

■ *Breast screening*. You are rarely involved in routine screening. You do, however, need to be confident in breast examination and be aware of the local facilities offered, for example, breast clinics. Between age 50 and 70, a mammogram screening test is offered every 3 years. The government plan is to extend this to ages 47–73 by 2012. However, current NICE guidance states that those with a moderate to severe family history should be tested from their 40's. The evidence for women picking up breast lumps on self examination is poor so if there is an indication you should perform the examination or refer to a one-stop breast clinic (where they will receive triple investigation with history, examination and Ultrasound scan (USS)/mammogram).

■ *Cervical screening* is common in general practice. Women eligible are those between 25 and 64 and should have a routine letter from the local health authority reminding them that they are due for a smear. However, it is your job to encourage any women who are overdue their smear to book an appointment (you will usually be prompted by the desktop computer). Cervical smears are repeated every 3 years between ages 25 and 49 then every 5 years between ages 50 and 64. Smears in the eligible age range are free. Women outside this range can pay for a private smear test but it is best to discuss this with seniors first.

■ *Sexual health*. With the numerous GUM clinics around, you may not encounter many people with sexual health issues. However, you should remember to promote safe sex and remind anyone who is considering non-barrier contraception that it will not protect them from STIs. You should also be prepared to take swabs from people presenting with symptoms of an STI, or tell them how to contact the closest GUM clinic.

The hidden agenda and health beliefs

What a patient presents with may not be what is really bothering them. The most common example is depression. Depression can manifest as a variety of physical conditions. Be alert to people who keep returning with seemingly minor physical ailments. To give people the opportunity to reveal their real underlying concern, try:

■ Asking if there is anything more they would like to tell you.

■ Asking why they feel they are not getting better if they are attending with the same issues.

■ Allowing for a longer consultation (many GPs operate on a 7–10-minute appointment slot although trainees should be allocated more time).

You will also encounter people from different social and cultural backgrounds with different health beliefs to yours. To avoid mistrust and dissatisfaction with your care, try:

■ Explaining clearly your diagnosis and why you are treating them as you are.

■ Asking what the person expects or would like, for example, do they believe they need treatment, do they think they need referring and explaining why you agree or disagree with their expectations.

■ Providing leaflets and information explaining their condition and what they should expect. This is more realistic, as time is not always sufficient for a verbal explanation and people rarely remember everything you tell them. NHS Choices (www.nhs.uk) has a fairly comprehensive and well-written encyclopaedia (Health A–Z) for most conditions.

The key to dealing with both issues is being alert to people with repeat attendances or strange symptoms, and to allow people to talk. Ask open questions and let them lead the consultation. And seek advice from seniors.

Follow-up

One of the main differences, and perhaps one of the beauties about general practice, is that you get to follow up most patients. Always tell people to come back if things do not improve. People may present with symptoms that you don't have an immediate answer for. Sometimes the only way to realise that trivial symptoms are part of a bigger illness is when those symptoms persist. There are some people, however, whom you should insist return for a follow-up appointment. These include:

■ Depressed or anxious people who are starting medication. At first, you should only give them 28 days of antidepressants and follow them up 2 weeks after starting treatment to see if their symptoms are improving. You should follow them up again 2 weeks after this, at the end of the 28 days, before issuing a repeat prescription. Further follow-ups can then be monthly or less frequent if you feel they are stable enough on their current medications.

■ Women on the OCP who should always have their blood pressure checked every 6 months before offering a repeat prescription. Some specialist family planning clinics may extend this to 12 months if the patient has been taking the pill without concern for several repeats. Also remember that when starting somebody on the OCP for the first time or when changing to a different brand, they should only be given 3 months' supply and reviewed before a further prescription is given.

■ Hypertension. Any person with a single high BP reading should have at least two further readings before being diagnosed as hypertensive. Give lifestyle advice and tests for end organ damage. Any confirmed hypertensive patients started on medications should have their BP checked monthly unless the hypertension is more severe, when more regular monitoring may be needed.

■ Diabetics. Because BP, lipid and arterial risk factor checks are performed annually, you will probably not follow these patients up during a short(ish) stint in general practice. However, if the BP or lipid profile is abnormal you will probably need to bring the person back for earlier repeat testing or intervention.

Home visits

Most home visits will either be to people who are housebound, in residential/ nursing homes and/or with chronic illnesses. They can be a bit daunting at first. Try reading the person's notes beforehand to get a feel for what s/he is normally like and the problems they face. If possible, discuss with their regular GP. You may occasionally be asked to see a patient who was previously fit and well. This is rare, as most patients will usually go straight to A&E rather than the local surgery.

■ Make sure the home visit is warranted before setting out. Find out what the problem is and why they cannot come to the surgery. Some diagnoses might be clear cut from the phone and warrant hospital admission, for example, suspicion of an MI, or some visits may simply be for prescriptions which can be done and left at the reception for a relative to pick up.

■ Don't forget your equipment. You never know what you are going to face on a home visit so be prepared with your kit, for example, thermometer, stethoscope, emergency meds, oto-scope, etc. These should all be provided by the practice.

■ Be safe. As you will be travelling alone and going into people's homes, make sure that the surgery knows where you are and you have a mobile phone in case of an emergency. If at all concerned, seek advice from seniors.

Chapter 17
SELF-CARE

How are doctors supposed to take care of patients if they don't take care of themselves? If you grind yourself down to the bone to provide for your patients, at the expense of yourself, sooner or later you will begin resenting them. Most of us are not taught much about self-care in medical school. Look after yourself and become a more humane doctor in the process.

Accommodation

Sadly, the days of doctors being provided with free on-site accommodation is at an end. This is because doctors used to be obliged to be resident on site for long periods of time. However, many hospitals still offer accommodation. This is often (but not always) at favourable rates. You should probably try and see your accommodation before signing a contract but one of the benefits of this type of housing is that you can usually terminate it with very little notice if required. If a hospital offers accommodation it must comply with national regulations governing minimum acceptable standards. This is certainly not negotiable given that you are paying for it directly!

■ Your room should contain a 3-by-6 foot bed, telephone, cupboards, drawers, desk, chair, armchair, washbasin, be carpeted and have curtains. It should be heated and regularly cleaned.

■ There should be a nearby bathroom and toilet, cooking facilities, a common room and on-site laundry facilities. Common areas should be regularly cleaned.

■ On-call rooms (if they still exist in your hospital) *should* be clean and have clean sheets and a phone. Call the Domestic Supervisor if there is a problem.

If you have a specific problem with your quarters, contact the designated 'Accommodation officer' or equivalent through switchboard. This person will also supply you with replacement light bulbs, toilet paper, etc. If the quarters en bloc are below standard, involve your doctors' mess and the junior doctors' committee. If the rooms are truly substandard then refuse to stay there – do not give them your money.

Alternative careers

What if you have come all this way and you find that you don't want to be a doctor? Or you like it, but not enough to dedicate your life to it? Little known to many medics, having a medical degree opens many great doors. Chekhov, JPR Williams, Harry Hill, Che Guevara and Keats were all once doctors – to name a few.

■ Medical training gives you all sorts of skills that you probably never even noticed. These include leadership, managerial, communicating and observational skills; interviewing, analytic, mechanical, adversarial skills; and the ability to work within a hierarchy and still get what you

The Hands-on Guide for Junior Doctors, Fourth Edition. Anna Donald, Michael Stein and Ciaran Scott Hill.
© 2011 Anna Donald, Michael Stein and Ciaran Scott Hill. Published 2011 by Blackwell Publishing Ltd.

want. Sheer endurance and persistence (much prized in the workforce), experience of the human condition at its most vulnerable and many other talents can be developed through medicine. Never think that these are wasted in a 'non-medical' career. Having medical training will enable you to bring something special to whatever you do.

■ Having said that, *in general* we would advise completing at least your Foundation programme before saying good-bye to medicine. Many people find that they enjoy working much more than being a student. Without working, it is hard to assess what it is all about. In any case, having full registration is useful if you ever wish to work in the future.

■ Do not underestimate the breadth of careers available in medicine. Within the 8 years or so you have spent at medical school and foundation training, you are unlikely to have even skimmed the surface of what is possible, both from a specialty and a location point of view. You can do helicopter mountain rescue in France, research anticancer drugs for pharmaceutical companies in Australia, enjoy office-based occupational health in Dubai, cash-in with disability assessments for the UK government, be a sports physician for Olympic athletes or work at the cutting edge of forensic pathology in New York. These and countless other careers are all within your grasp if you have the imagination and motivation to achieve them. A good book for inspiration is the *Medic's Guide to Work and Electives Around the World* by Mark Wilson.

Bleep

■ Pick up your bleep from switchboard. They will replace the batteries.

■ If your bleep is too loud, cover the speaker with masking tape (or just turn it down).

■ Leave your bleep on the ward (or switch it off) if you are not on call, as switchboard may call you even when you are off-duty.

British Medical Association (BMA)

Becoming a member of the BMA not only brings you the *BMJ* with all the job adverts for the next year (not particularly relevant at foundation level but interesting nonetheless) and professional courses, but provides advice and support in all areas of your work, leave, contracts, tax and financial planning. It is also a negotiating body on behalf of all doctors. The *BMJ* is a reasonable journal in its own right, it is one of the easiest to browse with its almost magazine-like approach but it also has the odd gem of research. Arguably, the *NEJM* (*New England Journal of Medicine*) is scientifically more robust but the two are probably fairly seen as a good complementary introduction to general medical journals. The BMA receive a lot of criticism for their apparent under-representation of junior doctors during the troubled times of Medical Training Application Service (MTAS), but many doctors who are returning now seem more in line with the opinions of the masses. Specific benefits of membership include:

1 Personal advice on contracts and terms of service.

2 Assistance and representation in disagreements with hospital management. This is becoming more important as Trusts and management try to change contracts and reduce pay. For example, the BMA has threatened court action against Trust management which has tried to cut pay,

now protected under the New Deal terms. The BMA can assist with claims for overtime and additional hours.

3 Independent financial advice by salaried representatives on pensions, income protection, etc.

4 Insurance services. The personal contents policy is particularly useful.

5 The fee is tax deductible.

Car and insurance

You may buy your first car during your first year. While you may need to purchase it in July just prior to moving to your new job, cars are most expensive around July–August. Also, it is worth asking your hospital for moving expenses, in the current climate this is not an obligation for foundation trainees but it may be worth enquiring.

Car insurance varies a lot. The BMA offers insurance for doctors, but it may be more expensive than you need, particularly if you have bought an old car. Probably the best thing to do is to ring local brokers who deal with many different insurance firms and who can get you the best deal for the cover you need. Alternatively, a good internet search is a good way forward. Many firms give a discount for female drivers. Be aware that you can purchase third-party insurance, fire and theft, if your car is not valuable although this may not build your 'no-claims' discount, an important factor in reducing the eventual costs of insurance.

Clothes (laundry/ stains)

■ Smart clothes are often touted as helping maintain professional demeanour; this is particularly so since white coats and suits have been vilified in the name of infection control. Clothing is too personal a choice to be lectured about here but it is something that certainly deserves some sober thought. If your trust has a policy on their professional dress code, be careful not to fall foul of it; these things are rarely worth getting into hot water about.

■ Remove blood from washable items by soaking them in warm (not hot), soapy water with added salt and then washing them regularly. Sponging the item as soon as possible helps too. For old stains, soak or wash the item in a soapy solution containing a few drops of ammonia or hydrogen peroxide.

■ Remove blood from non-washable items by sponging with cold water. Cover silk with a paste of starch and water; allow to dry and brush off.

■ Alternatively, *Stain Devils* remove most stains. You can buy them in large supermarkets or at dry-cleaning outlets. Make sure you buy the right one for the stain you have. These are particularly useful for ink and ball-point stains.

■ Finally, most stains can be removed with dry-cleaning. Hospitals should reimburse you for dry-cleaning costs if you got the stain at work. Whether they will or not is another matter; contact Personnel through the switchboard to find out how to apply for reimbursement. Apathy in such maters is how doctors have ended up losing out in the past.

Contacting medical colleagues

After graduation, all doctors are entered into the UK *Medical Directory*. This is a reasonably reliable way of tracking down friends from medical school and beyond. The *Directory* is available in hospital libraries and also from the General Medical Council nearest you. You can search the register at the GMC web site, www.gmc-uk.org. There are now internet services dedicated to doctors which can supply doctors with contact details of colleagues who have also subscribed.

Contract and conditions of service

Doctors' working conditions are negotiated by the Junior Doctors' Committee. More recently, the Junior Doctors' agreement has altered the rates at which overtime is paid, and stipulated the maximum hours for which you can be contracted to work. All hospitals, including Trusts, have to abide by these nationally agreed guidelines.

What you need to know about your contract

Your contract is a binding agreement, regulating your hours and conditions of service, pay, holiday and notice. It cannot be altered unilaterally by either you or your employer. In particular, pay protection means that your pay cannot be cut from the time of accepting the job, even if the banding of the job changes. Also note that you will need to sign a new contract for each post you rotate through in your Foundation programme.

1 Rotas

Virtually all junior doctors now work a full-shift rota with additional duty periods every few days (e.g. 1 in 5), meaning that they work a 40-hour working week and are also on duty every fifth night and/or every fifth weekend. They do stipulate the maximum number of hours you work, the amount and type of rest breaks

you are entitled to during your working day and the amount of time you must have off.

■ It is important not to get confused by colloquial use of the term 'on call' for full-shift duty periods. This is erroneous as it implies you are entitled to sleep during the duty periods. As a junior doctor you are now unlikely to find a job where you are 'allowed' to sleep in your contract.

■ Prospective cover means that when colleagues are away on holiday, the remaining junior doctors cover the duty periods the missing colleague would have done. This works out equitably if everyone takes the same amount of holiday. Virtually all contracts stipulate that you cover your colleagues if they are sick. This provision does not give authorities the power to force you to cover foreseen and notified absences such as annual leave. See Table 17.1 for information of the New Deal for Doctors regarding shift patterns.

2 Working time monitoring

This is a mandatory obligation of your contract. At least twice a year, your medical personnel department will run a monitoring exercise over the period of 2–4 weeks, where the junior doctors on the same rota will be required to document what they do in 15-minute time slots. This is to ascertain whether the post meets European Working Time Directive requirements and also to determine the amount of pay you get. That alone should be an incentive to take part! The European Working Time Directive did stipulate a maximum of 56 working hours per week that was cut down to 48 in 2008 (see Table 17.2).

■ Monitoring exercises should not be viewed as 'checking up' on you. They are your chance to demonstrate the commitments of your job and get the remuneration you deserve. Never allow yourself

Table 17.1 New Deal hours.

Rotation pattern	Maximum period of continuous work	Minimum period off-duty between work periods	Minimum continuous period of duty
Full shift	14 hours	8 hours	48 hours + 62 hours in 28 days
Partial shift	16 hours	8 hours	48 hours + 62 hours in 28 days
On-call rota	32 hours (56 hours at weekend)	12 hours	48 hours + 62 hours in 21 days

Table 17.2 European Working Time Directive.

Maximum working time per week of 56 hours:

■ Working time is defined as any period during which doctors are working, at their employers' disposal and carrying out their activity or duties, and any period during which they are receiving relevant training. This includes time when resident in hospital on call (even if asleep).

The rest requirements which came into effect in August 2004 are as follows:

■ A minimum daily consecutive period of 11 hours.

■ A minimum rest break of 20 minutes when the working day exceeds 6 hours.

■ A minimum rest period of 24 hours in each 7-day period (this can be averaged to be a 48-hour rest period in 14 days).

■ For occasions when working time is in excess, compensatory rest must be taken immediately following the period of work which it is supposed to counteract (i.e. before commencing the next period of work).

A minimum of 4 weeks' paid annual leave.

to be pressurized into lying on them; you must stand up for what you deserve.

■ There is no need to document exactly what you are doing in each 15-minute period, just simply whether you are working, resting, eating or studying. Documentation substantially reinforces pay claims. Answering a bleep is considered work.

■ It is not your individual working time in a particular week that needs to be in line with the European Working Time Directive. It is the average weekly working time for all the junior doctors on the same rota.

■ Monitoring exercises need not be initiated by the medical personnel department. This is significant if there is a dispute over working time arrangements or the running of the exercise. All you need to do is print diary sheets and distribute one to every doctor on the same rota and get them to fill it in. You can request monitoring at any time.

Table 17.3 Banding.

Banding	Pay multiple	Description
'Debanded'	0	<48 hours per week, sociable hours.
1A	1.5	<48 hours per week, high proportion of antisocial hours
1B	1.4	<48 hours per week, low proportion of antisocial hours
1C	1.2	<48 hours per week, non-resident on calls
2A	1.8	48–56 hours per week, high proportion of antisocial hours
2B	1.5	48–56 hours per week, low proportion of antisocial hours
3	2.0	>56 hours per week, insufficient rest (few of these jobs now remain)

Note: Pay protection does not protect Band 3 pay, it only protects up to Band 2A.

3 Pay

NHS doctors' rates of pay are agreed nationally by the Doctors and Dentists' Review Body, which negotiates the annual pay increase each April. Your pay is calculated on the basis of a banding system. The banding system takes into consideration the type of rota worked and the duration and intensity of out-of-hours work. Your band dictates the supplement received for out-of-hours work as a multiple of your basic salary. Junior doctors in general practice who have an out-of-hours commitment receive an additional 22.5% over and above basic salary regardless of the duration or frequency of that commitment. The BMA web site (bma.org.uk) features a band calculator, allowing you to check that your employer is complying with national requirements (see Table 17.3).

■ Your band is specified in your contract. The band allocation is based on the previous working time monitoring exercise, which should be done twice yearly.

■ Overtime for early starts and late finishes can (in theory) be paid retrospectively. It requires your consultant to sign the appropriate claim form, confirming your extra work. In practice it can be difficult to achieve. Consultants and management may not look kindly on such claims, although this varies considerably from hospital to hospital.

■ While the odd hour here or there probably does not warrant special overtime claims, if you are systematically working extra hours (e.g. by starting at 8 a.m. instead of 9 and finishing at 7 p.m. instead of 5), then do not feel ashamed to ask for pay for honest work that you have done. This is best achieved through a working time monitoring exercise rather than an individual claim.

■ Your salary is protected such that even if your banding changes during the time you are working, your monthly salary cannot drop below the banding when you signed your contract. The only exception is Band 3, which is only protected to Band 2A should the job be down-banded by a monitoring exercise.

4 Holiday

Junior doctors are entitled to 5 weeks' holiday/year, or roughly 2½ weeks/6-month job, excluding bank holidays.

■ Try to avoid carrying leave forward. In theory, up to 4 days' leave can be carried forward from the first job to the second, but this is often hard to achieve. Contact Personnel both at your current hospital and your future place of work to try to ensure you are granted the extra leave.

■ Leave can be supplemented by 'in-lieu' days. Over the year you are likely to work several bank holidays and statutory hospital holidays. You can take a day off 'in lieu' of each holiday worked or if you work overnight beyond 9 a.m. on the holiday morning.

■ Find out the procedure for booking leave early. It may involve simply inform-ing your consultant and his or her secre-tary, or there may be specific forms to be filled in and signed by your consultant (more likely).

5 Notice

Junior doctors only need to give 2 weeks' notice of their intention to leave their post. However, to be eligible for full GMC registration you need to have completed 12 months as a FY1 doctor. Although rare, it is not unheard of for trainees to be given notice if the employ-ing hospital is cutting back staff. In this unfortunate circumstance, you will need to discuss the situation with your educa-tional supervision, the deanery and your representative union, for example, the BMA. You may be able to find good job vacancies at short notice; it is often worth phoning individual trusts even if they have nothing formally advertised. Talk to the dean's office of your founda-tion school or your educational supervi-sor and look in the *BMJ Classifieds*.

6 Leave

Compassionate leave

In the event of family or personal bereavement, paid leave will usually be given. Tell your consultant. If there is any difficulty, talk to your clinical tutor and Personnel.

Maternity (and paternity) leave

Regulations and rates of parental leave are complex, depending on how long you have worked and whether you intend to return to work. New female doctors are unlikely to have worked for more than 1 year and, therefore, are allowed only 18 weeks' unpaid leave. By comparison, doctors who have worked for longer than 1 year are entitled to 8 weeks' full pay, 10 weeks' half pay and up to 34 weeks of additional leave, to a total absence of 52 weeks. Doctors who have not declared intention to return to work receive fewer benefits.

■ If you or your partner is pregnant or considering it, discuss the options for leave fully with your personnel depart-ment or the BMA.

■ The UK now has up to 2 weeks paid paternity leave as an entitlement for employees. However, if you are an expectant father and need more time off, it is worth discussing with your employer and the BMA.

Study leave

Pre-registration (F1) doctors are not usu-ally allocated study leave other than time during the working day to attend clinical and pathology meetings. Post-registration doctors are entitled to 30 days of study leave per year. Note that in many trusts this is not the actual time you can take off though. For example, 10 days may be automatically allocated to 'generic teaching' during bleep-free time on a given afternoon. A further 10 days may be allocated as 'taster weeks' that can be spent gaining experience in specialties you are interested in. The final 10 days are in theory for you to use as you wish (courses, conferences, etc.) – however, many foundation schools will not have allocated study leave for activities that fall outside of the rather narrow range of appointed 'foundation competencies'. The author has personal experience of being refused time for an APLS (advanced paediatric life support) course while working in A + E where he frequently saw children because 'paediatrics is not in your core curriculum'. This is likely to be something you will have to battle out at a local level. If you feel unfairly treated you must be prepared to fight your corner, ideally with the support of your BMA or foundation year representative and a sympathetic consultant.

Sick leave

Physical illness: It is still the case in most hospitals that if you are sick, your colleagues must cover for you in addition to doing their own jobs. Because of this very few doctors will tell you to go home. Therefore, you *must* take control of the situation and go home if you need to. You may not be at death's door, but if you are struggling to keep up with your tasks *just go home*. It rarely impresses anyone and the ward will cope. They might even celebrate. You are doing nobody any favours by lurking around shedding your virus and bad temper. That said, sick leave for hangovers and the like is always unacceptable and painfully unfair to your colleagues.

Mental illness: If you are struggling with mental burnout (depression, serious anxiety, grief, whatever) it is more important

that you get help and rest. Mental fatigue and illness is common among doctors yet so little spoken about. It is also a cause of long-term absence and loss of self-esteem which could be avoided with a bit of self-care.

Prolonged illness: Even if you fall ill on the first day of work and cannot work again, you are still entitled to sick pay equal to your full salary for 1 month. After this you will receive the usual state benefits. After completing 4 months full-time work, a junior doctor is entitled to 1 month of full pay and 2 months of half pay. If you fall ill towards the end of the contract and the illness continues after the time when you would have finished, you are entitled to continued sick pay as long as the illness lasts or until you have had all the sick pay you are entitled to.

If you have trouble with illness of any kind, consider doing the following:

■ Tell someone who loves you that you're sick/in trouble. They can help you summon up the courage to take time off and get help.

■ See the hospital staff's doctor or nurse or your GP. They can help you medically and psychologically. They will give you any documentation you need (e.g. sick notes) and may be able to speak with your seniors if necessary. You are obliged to tell your consultant that you're sick (after 3 days of absence). Unlike more junior colleagues, your consultant won't suffer directly if you take time off and will probably be sympathetic.

■ Tell your immediate senior and the nurses on your wards so they can make arrangements for cover as soon as possible.

■ Learn to care for yourself now and it will serve you throughout your life. This is preferable to a heart attack or chronic martyrdom syndrome when you're 45 (it does happen!).

7 Occupational health requirements

■ Hospitals recommend that you register with a local GP, although in practice your notes will barely have caught up with you when you have to move on.

■ On arrival at the hospital, the Occupational Health Department will ask about your immunization record. They may take nose or take swabs, particularly if you have worked in a different region or where there has been an MRSA (methicillin-resistant *Staphylococcus aureus*) outbreak. Try and keep a copy of this in a memorable place; you will change jobs a lot and life will be simpler.

■ Ask Occupational Health to check your Hepatitis B immunity, which may have dramatically declined since immunization as a student. It should be around '100%' although a portion of the population will always be 'non-responders'. If you do become infected with active Hepatitis B, you cannot be a surgeon or a specialist who does invasive work. See below for needlestick injuries.

■ Contact the Occupational Health Department if you are ill for longer than 3 days. They will clear you for sick leave and may well give you some TLC in the meantime.

Doctors' mess

The doctors' mess may be a scruffy room strewn with old newspapers and coffee cups or a comfortable lounge with a coffee machine, satellite TV and a PlayStation. Most messes run with a Mess President, Secretary and Treasurer and a variable number of committee members. If there is not much going on, organize an event and take command!

Making money for the mess

■ Have regular drug lunches and charge the reps £100 to talk while you provide the catering at £50 per session.

■ Organize with your colleagues and the financial people handling cremation fees for a part of each cremation fee to be given to the mess (e.g. £3).

■ Hold a party. Have free drinks before 8.30 p.m. to make sure everyone arrives early, or no one will come until the pubs close.

■ Ask doctors to make a regular deduction from their salary and arrange this with Personnel. Many now have an automatic contribution taken from doctors' wage slip although people may opt out. The mess president should keep a list of 'members' and those that do not contribute should not enjoy the privileges (harsh but fair!).

Drug representatives

Drug company representatives will approach you from time to time to try to influence your prescribing policy. You need to decide for yourself how you deal with them and their practice of bribing doctors with items and services (ranging from pens to dinners at local restaurants). Just a few tips:

■ You are not obliged to spend time with drug reps. You can tell them politely that you do not have time to see them, or that you are not interested in discussing their products.

■ On the other hand, you can influence drug availability by talking with representatives. For instance, you can point out that X antibiotic would be more practical if it could be made up and left in the fridge (like metronidazole) for a few hours, rather than needing to be given stat.

■ Be wary of drug company literature. While some is reliable, much of it is misleading. To learn about drugs, you'd be better off reading a pharmacology textbook: the *BNF* or the *Drug and Therapeutics Bulletin* which you receive free as an junior doctor.

European Working Time Directive

See what you need to know about your contract, p. 230.

Insurance (room contents)

Probably the best room contents' insurance against theft and damage is BMA-arranged insurance, because it is designed specifically for junior doctors. Other policies may not have plans appropriate for your unusual living situation and generally cost much more. If you have time you can shop around online.

Jobs

■ Foundation year programmes are the newest form of general training which aims to consolidate house officer and the first year of senior house officer training into a structured 2-year programme (see Chapter 5). This is to prevent the need for constant 6-monthly application for jobs, to ensure all junior doctors get the essential generic skills and to provide a structured career path towards general training and then higher specialist training. They are an inevitable phenomenon as the Royal Colleges modernize the training structure.

■ Your F2 post is where the big divide begins: surgery/medicine/primary care or a specialist run-through post. Confer with your consultants, friends and older colleagues about which jobs are good for your career goal. Do not feel limited by what posts you end up being allocated to as Foundation programmes are designed to provide good all-round experience.

■ Network. Tell your consultant what you're hoping to do next. If you are set on a particular job or hospital, ask the consultant if he or she knows anyone there. The days of 'jobs for the boys' may be gone but do not underestimate the importance of getting your face known and having a good reputation. Regardless of the objectivity of the assessment centres, if you are being marked by a consultant who knows and likes you already you are unlikely to score badly. Such brownie-points are also valuable for the future.

■ Choose your referees carefully. One is usually the consultant you are currently working for. Well-known professors and consultants add a little weight to your list – provided you actually know them well enough for them to write about you, and you are sure that they will say nice things! Do not be afraid to ask to see your reference before it is sent. This is not easy but is very important. Apparently, helpful consultants are not beyond sabotaging a bright young trainee's prospects for no apparent reasons. Keep a healthy suspicion about your encounters.

■ Application form. Make sure you get the basics right. If it asks to be typed or printed in green ink, do it. Include photographs or whatever else is requested. Don't jeopardize your chances at this early stage. Consider using recorded or registered delivery.

■ I cannot overemphasize the importance of planning ahead when you decide on your specialty. Many a sorry soul has spent their foundation years compiling what they believe to be a shining CV only to discover that the application form gives no credit to their endeavours. See the form at least 6 months before you apply and go tick those boxes.

Trust and other non-training posts

All Foundation programme jobs are mandatory training posts. Upon completing a Foundation programme, it is planned that junior doctors move seamlessly into specialist training. Under the current scheme, new doctors have only 2 years of generic training prior to specialist training. The Foundation programme is good at providing more general training on your way to being whatever you want to be. Alternatively, if you want experience at a junior level of a particular specialty before enrolling for specialist training it can sometimes be achieved but lack of jobs in many specialist areas can make this task insurmountable. There are a whole plethora of posts out there, for example, 'Clinical fellow', 'Trust-grade doctor', 'SHO-equivalent doctor'.

The crucial thing at all times is to check whether a post is recognized by the regional deanery as a training post. Training posts are partially funded by the regional deanery and count towards your general professional training. Non-training posts are fully funded by the hospital and require and receive no recognition from the deanery. They are also known as 'service' posts as they were created purely for providing a service to the hospital. A few important points about non-training posts:

■ The pay scale will often follow the pay scale and working time arrangements of training posts, but this is not always the case. Check in the job description.

■ Check the contract or job description for any time limits. These often do not follow clear 4-, 6- or 12-month patterns as for training posts. They also often start immediately.

■ Job contracts are much more negotiable than in training posts, especially since there is only one party to negotiate with.

■ They are often less competitive than training posts and they account for the largest increase in number of posts in the last few years as a result of the European Working Time Directive.

■ There may be an element of stigma against non-training posts. However, many doctors take on a non-training post at some point in their career as they are more flexible, so there should not be any prejudice.

Curriculum vitae

It is probably easiest to type out your CV yourself so you can make small changes as necessary. Use high-quality paper. Your consultant's secretary might oblige.

■ Make sure you meticulously spell-check and proofread your CV. Misspellings are unlikely to be forgiven. Read your CV aloud to make sure that it does not contain any disastrous sentences or factual errors. Never write anything on your CV that is not true. Beware of bending the truth, the consequences might well be disastrous.

■ Try to be concrete about what you want to do. People love hearing concrete plans that are easy for them to imagine. If you know what your planned career is, say so. Put 'Career objective: chest medicine' at the top of your CV under your name. You should always be able to answer the question 'where do you see yourself in 5 (or 10) years' time?'. If you can't answer this question, it is probably the time to sit down and think about it.

■ Make the most of your experience, listing skills you have acquired and responsibilities you have taken. Don't forget skills such as computing and languages. Make sure you include honours or prizes; depending on your stage and CV this may include those from school. That said, do not overload your CV with 'filler' if it is already strong. Your best achievements may be lost among the rest.

■ Avoid one-word interests such as 'Reading'. Try to be concrete in demonstrating what you have done. For example, instead of saying 'Running', you might specify your running activities: 'Participation in Anglia regional running events, club secretary'.

■ Create your CV so it shows you as you want to be seen. CVs are not shopping lists, nor are they confessions. If you did badly one year you can minimize the fact in how you present your CV. Just make sure that you don't say things that are blatantly untrue, and that you include certain professional details (see later).

■ When applying for a post-registration job, it also helps to sell yourself and your clinical experience. You may feel fairly inexperienced compared to the consultant reading your CV, but think in terms of clinical skills that you have that they would appreciate you having when working for them (e.g. done three assisted and one unassisted pleural aspirations, etc.). The demonstration of experience is now largely displayed by logbooks and DOPS (direct observation of procedural skills) but there is still a place for this on most CVs.

■ When asking for a reference, supply your referee with a current CV and a brief outline of achievements you want them to mention. A wise consultant once told me to always ensure you see the reference you have asked for before it is sent. If someone is unhappy to see what they have written about you, then it may not be what you want.

■ Show your CV to your family or a close friend to make sure that you haven't left anything important out. Consider showing it to your present colleagues, registrars or consultant who have probably seen many CVs and can give you good advice on both content and style. The reviewer need not be medical.

■ If the form you are given for your CV is inadequate, consider stapling your CV to it, unless the instructions strictly state otherwise (which is often the case for specialist trainee posts, but less so for service provision jobs).

A CV should include:

1 *Personal*: name, address and phone number/email, date of birth, relevant memberships, brief general education, and employment history (if any).

2 *Medical*: undergraduate education including medical school, date of entry and graduation, qualifications, honours or prizes, previous and present appointments, career plans, publications and presentations, leadership and teaching experience, society memberships, referee names and contact details (you do not always need to provide these but resist the temptation to state '*References available on request*'; this is frighteningly obvious).

The interview

■ Try to visit the hospital before the interview, see the department and meet the consultants. If you have already met some of the interview panel you may be more relaxed. DO not underestimate how important this is. It is increasingly expected as you progress up the career ladder.

■ Follow the basics: clean suit, hair and shoes, be punctual and courteous.

■ Find out from the person coordinating the interview what you can expect inside the interview room, such as how many interviewers you will face and the expected length of the interview.

■ Early questions are likely to focus on why you want the job, your CV and experience. Be prepared to discuss and expand on anything you have mentioned. At this level you may be asked general clinical questions but these will be basic ones regarding safe general care and should not be revised for. Be prepared for questions about your career plans. Try to say something concrete, even if you are unsure about your future career. At all costs avoid looking aimless. BE ENTHUSIASTIC! If you don't sound like you really want the job you will be unlikely to get it. Ethical issues may be discussed. Issues such as quality control, audit and clinical governance are also very likely to arise.

■ Listen attentively to the interviewers' questions and take care to answer them directly rather than blurring the issue. Don't ramble.

■ While remaining relatively formal, don't be afraid to be yourself. If the interviewer doesn't like you as you really are, you probably don't want to work for them anyway.

■ Write thank-you letters to your referees for their help and support. You may need them again in the future!

Consultant career prospects

The medical and dental staffing prospects are published annually in the journal *Health Trends*, published by the Department of Health. The prospects include the current number of SpRs, consultants, likely consultant vacancies and future consultant numbers, by specialty. The journal should be in your medical library; if not, ring the Department of Health in London. The Modernising Medical Careers web site may also give some indication of plans for specialty expansion in the future.

Locums

Locums pay well if you can bear working through your holidays and weekends. Get registered with one or more locum agencies. These may be much better than the basic 'NHS (National Health Service) locum' rate you will get if unregistered and doing a locum shift in your current hospital. Agencies are advertised in the *BMJ Classifieds*. Medical personnel at your hospital will know the name of local agencies. Note that different agencies pay very different rates. Shop around. You can register with more than one. Try to negotiate travel expenses with the agency. If you secure a locum at a hospital you don't know, the following is a checklist of things to do when you arrive:

1 Sign in at the switchboard. Sign-in registers what time you arrive at the hospital – the locum agency may check when working out your pay.

2 From switchboard and reception, pick up: bleep, keys, map of the hospital, identification (if necessary) and essential telephone numbers:

- A&E.
- Admissions.
- Biochemistry (and on-call bleep number).
- Haematology (and on-call bleep number).
- Porters.
- Wards.
- Radiology department (and on-call bleep number).

3 Find out (on the hospital map) where these are:

- Blood gas machines.
- Canteen.
- Doctors' residence.
- Drinks machine.
- ITU.
- Radiology department.
- Wards.

4 Bleep your senior and arrange to meet.

5 Dump your overnight bag in the doctors' residence.

6 Go to the wards and introduce yourself.

7 On the wards, stuff a folder (see Chapter 2, Personal folder and the lists) with: blood forms, history sheets, consents, fluid charts, drug charts, X-ray forms. Clip the phone numbers to the front of the folder.

8 Locate IV equipment, catheters, drug cupboard, resuscitation equipment.

9 Find out:

- Who gives IV drugs.
- If there is a phlebotomist in the morning and where to leave requests.

10 If possible, speak to the person who usually carries your bleep about any useful information he or she may know about patients, staff and the hospital.

11 If you are required to attend a ward round when you should have finished the locum, you are entitled to extra hours' pay; contact the locum agency as soon as possible about this. If you have to leave on the dot, let your senior know this from the outset.

12 Hospitals that are desperate to fill locums will often negotiate terms with you, such as allowing you to arrive late or leave early if necessary.

13 On a professional note, try and perform to the same standards on your locum shift as you do at work normally. Locums have a poor reputation but if you work hard, you will build a good reputation that will not only get you more work but will also put you in favour with consultants and colleagues who you may work with in the future. Strive to maintain your professionalism at all times.

Meals

■ Try not to miss meals (easy to say and hard to do!). Twenty minutes for a hot evening meal makes little difference to patient care, but it will keep *you* going. If you think that missing a meal doesn't affect your performance or energy levels, then try going for a jog straight after a shift when you haven't eaten. I challenge you to say you feel as good as you otherwise would.

■ Don't forget to drink as much liquid as possible. It's easy to get dehydrated and even more tired when you're too busy to stop for tea breaks. Carry a flask – there is nothing wrong with keeping a hot drink in this. It is also a way to boost your caffeine intake without upsetting patients and infection control with dirty mugs.

■ If canteen food is awful, take in microwave meals. It's comforting to have a treat such as fruit or a chocolate bar.

■ Find out about local takeaways. Some may discount hospital staff. There are almost always people on the shift who will share a meal with you and cut down the delivery cost. A pizza late in the evening is a great morale booster.

Medical defence

Historically, it was compulsory to belong to a defence organization for representation and insurance against medico-legal complaints arising out of the care of patients. This changed in 1990 when Crown Indemnity came into force, so that the Crown, or rather the NHS employer, will pay the costs of investigation and damages for cases arising during your employment with them. This is sometimes called *vicarious liability* and means that you will not suffer directly so long as your actions were 'reasonable' and in line with your trusts' policy. However, protection under vicarious liability is limited and if the hospital is sued for a mistake you make, they have the option of then suing *you* directly to recoup costs. It does *not* cover incidents arising outside the hospital, such as 'good Samaritan' acts, nor private practice. Most importantly, Crown Indemnity may not support you if you have a conflict with your employer. The advantage of joining a medical defence organization is expert, round-the-clock advice with *your* interests at heart. Investigate the benefits offered by various organizations (e.g. MDU, MPS) and join whichever one suits your needs.

Money

For the first time, your bank account will be filling up with up to £2000 or so each month. Be a bit careful. It's not unusual for people to run up thousands of pounds of credit card debts – and to spend the next few years paying them off. You should be prepared to find that for the first year or two your lifestyle may not be much better than as a student.

Income protection if long-term sick or disabled

Various organizations offer income protection (also known as PHI or permanent health insurance). On payment of a monthly premium, you are covered for prolonged absence, even if you never work again. If you have a mortgage and family, sickness cover becomes more important. Research the various policy options carefully – some have limited payment durations. Others pay more from year to year in line with your expected career progression. Most do not. Perhaps most important is to check if you will be paid if you cannot work *as a doctor* or only if you cannot do *any type work* (the company is likely to find that this will very rarely be the case).

Student debt

Many experienced financial advisers have compiled good data to show that the best way to save money is to pay off all existing debt, as virtually all debt has an interest rate higher than the national savings rate. As medical students have 5–6 years to acquire a sizable debt, particularly with the introduction of increasingly expensive tuition fees, it is advisable to start chipping away at this as early as you can. Your governmental student loan will automatically be repaid with deductions from your pay cheque 6 months after starting work. This has a low interest rate (but NOT zero unless there are exceptional circumstances with a very low national base-rate). Because of this, it is usually best not to try and pay this off early but to just let it get chipped away at from month to month (just try and forget about it). Credit cards and personal loans are a different matter and these need to be paid off as soon as you can. That said, it is not the end of the world if you need a temporary personal loan so long as you are sensible about it and live within your limits. Avoid *negative equity*; this is just the financial term for more going out of your bank account each month than goes in! Setting up direct debits are a good way of making sure you are strict about repayments, they can be set up for credit cards also.

Mortgages

Some banks and building societies provide special mortgages for professionals such as doctors and solicitors, to account for the structured career path and salary increases. These often are willing to lend larger amounts of money (e.g. $4\times$ annual salary rather than $2.5\times$), but be aware that you should only borrow what you can afford to pay back on a monthly basis. As a rough guide try and avoid deductions of more than £200 a month when you start work. More than this and you may find repayments difficult (obviously this varies hugely depending on personal circumstances but for someone with average student debts and rent this is probably a fair ballpark figure).

Your hospital may have a relocation policy to help pay the expenses of moving or buying a house in the area as a result of working at the hospital. This is unlikely to be available at a trainee level (and is certainly not available for movement between F1 and F2 hospitals), but check with the medical personnel department if you think you might qualify.

Payslip deductions

National Insurance is a compulsory contribution which will pay for your future state pension, maternity pay and sick leave.

Superannuation is not compulsory but is essential for your pension. The national state pension is meagre. The NHS superannuation scheme is your employer's scheme to allow you to make additional pension contributions that the government will supplement.

■ You have to sign a form at the start of your job stating your intention to stay with or opt out of the superannuation scheme. The only people who might not want to contribute towards their own superannuation are those who are pretty sure that they will not be working for long in the NHS, such as foreign graduates. However, NHS superannuation can be accrued to other public sector positions in the UK such as the civil service and university posts.

■ You can reclaim superannuation contributions if you have worked for the NHS for *less than 2 years*. Otherwise your contributions will stay locked in the scheme.

■ Think long and hard before leaving the superannuation scheme to join a private pension plan. It is highly unlikely that you could ever match the security and returns of the NHS scheme. It is no barrier to joining an *additional* private scheme.

Pensions

As described above, the superannuation scheme provides the main pension for doctors. When you retire, your benefits are an annual pension of up to half your salary and a lump sum of three times your annual pension. The exact calculations are:

> **Pension = years of service/40 ×**
> **pensionable salary**
> Pensionable salary = highest annual
> salary earned in any of the 3 years
> prior to retirement

■ Few doctors complete the full 40 years of service that would allow them to receive the maximum possible pension. However, it is possible to make additional contributions to your future pension. The most cost-effective way is to make additional voluntary contributions (AVCs) into the NHS Group Scheme. This is a well-kept secret, with low commission and charges. You should contact your local BMA office. It is also possible to buy 'added years', as if you had worked for longer than you really have.

■ You will doubtless meet financial salesmen who will offer to sell you Free Standing AVCs, that is, a way of investing your contributions in their company's policies (and earning them a bonus). Be aware that your whole first year's contribution may disappear in the salesperson's commission.

■ Your expenses as a young doctor may be high – with a new house, a car and possibly a family. As long as you are aware that you should consider further pension contributions at some date, these need not be a priority in your first year of work (whatever financial advisers may say).

Tax

Earning a regular salary means paying serious tax. You will save time, trouble and money if you make an effort to keep basic records. Each month you should get a payslip giving details of your pay, national insurance and any other deductions you have authorized such as telephone bills or car parking charges. Check this to see you have not been overcharged – sadly this is not uncommon.

A P60 is sent to you at the end of the tax year (5 April). It is your record of how much income you have received and tax you have paid. A P45 is given to you when you leave the job, to take to the finance department at your next job to show how much tax you have been paying. If you lose it you will probably be taxed the wrong amount (usually overtaxed) until the tax office sorts it out – which may take months.

Understanding your tax

Doctors have tax deducted automatically from their pay before they receive it (known as PAYE – pay as you earn). The Inland Revenue works out how much tax you are likely to owe throughout the year and this is deducted monthly from your salary.

Junior doctors start work in August, part way through the tax year which runs from 6 April to 5 April. This means that your first ever pay cheque will be larger than any of the subsequent months. The tax year ends on 5 April. After this your tax office will send you a note stating how much tax you paid in the last year, and how much tax you ought to pay in the next year (P60). You could just leave it there. However, it is quite likely that you have been overtaxed and could claim money back on tax-deductible items. You also have a duty to declare untaxed income so that it can be taxed (this includes money paid for completion of cremation forms or certain psychiatric documentation relating to sections of the Mental Health Act). At the simplest, you could just write a letter declaring your tax-deductible items and untaxed income; alternatively contact your tax office for a full tax return form. Your personnel department will be able to give you full details of your tax office, which is usually determined by where you work.

Tax-deductible items (on which you can reclaim money you have paid in tax) include:

1 GMC fee (but only the renewal fee, not the initial joining-up fee).

2 Medical defence subscription.

3 BMA membership.

In later years, membership to the Royal Colleges is also tax deductible.

Untaxed income that must be declared

The main item here is cremation fees ('ash cash'), worth approximately £70, which you receive for completing part I of the cremation form. In recent years, the Inland Revenue has tightened up on this potential evasion. It is not unknown for them to investigate funeral directors' records and compare them with doctors' tax returns. Non-declaration constitutes tax evasion and is penalized accordingly. You should declare full cremation fees even if there is a deduction, for example, for mess expenses. Other untaxed cash payments such as the fees for completing other forms should also be declared. There has been recent public criticism of doctors being paid to complete these forms, as such some people choose to give this money to charity.

Tax allowances

Everyone has a personal allowance, that is, an amount of income they can earn before being taxed. In 2010–2011 you may earn £6,475 before paying tax. The rest of your earnings (above your personal allowance) up to £37,400 is taxed at 20%. The high bracket rate of 40% is paid on any income above this. Since 2010 there is a new tax bracket for over £150,000 set at 50%. See www.hmrc.gov.uk for more information.

Tax-free savings

Each person is allowed to save up to £10,020 each tax year in a tax-free savings account called an ISA (individual savings account). These accounts give high rates of tax-free interest, and are offered by most banks. There are various types of ISA on offer. Some (called 'cash' ISAs) guarantee growth of your savings (in effect a straightforward tax-free savings account). Alternatively, you may choose an ISA where the bank will invest in named stocks and shares on your behalf. These 'equity' ISAs are more risky, especially if you may need to withdraw the money in the short term, but may have much greater yield in the longer term, although they can't guarantee that you will get back everything that you put in. ISAs seldom have instant access, so don't use them instead of a current account. However, they are a good way of putting away savings for the future. Seek financial advice to help you choose between the ISA packages on offer.

Telephone and online banking

Consider switching to telephone or online banking, which allow 24-hour access to your account, in addition to all the other services provided by a high street account (including use of cash machines). *Which?* magazine regularly reviews banking services; so look out for the next *Which?* report. These accounts can offer a high rate of interest, although many exclusively online banks will offer these rates only as a promotion, with interest rates quickly falling back to more moderate (although often competitive) levels. Check to see that the online and other services offered fit your needs. Also be aware that exclusively online banks may not be covered by the banking ombudsman (the government watchdog for banks). High street banks with online 'branches' are covered.

Needlestick injuries

You should familiarize yourself with your occupational health or department's policy for needlesticks before you come across one. If you do encounter a needlestick, follow their advice, seek help from A + E/virology or do the following:

1 Go to a sink. Run the wound under fast running, lukewarm water.

2 See your occupational health consultant immediately (and inform your own consultant). You may need to take post-exposure anti-HIV prophylaxis (at present this consists of triple therapy) or anti-hepatitis immunoglobulin depending on your status.

3 Don't panic. Virtually all doctors needlestick themselves from time to time and very, very few have contracted anything undesirable, even from patients infected with HIV and hepatitis. Even if the patient is known HIV-positive, the chance of a full needlestick transmitting the virus to you is only around 1 in 250.

4 If they consent to it and are counselled about the implications of having an HIV test done, take one clotted (brown) tube of blood from the patient. This needs to be analysed immediately for HIV and hepatitis.

5 Alert your senior and/or the public health unit in the hospital. They will instruct you further. They will require you to do the following, depending on patient status.

6 If you can safely leave your current duties and have a colleague cover you, then consider having at least a few hours or the day off from work. The shock of a needlestick may not be immediately apparent to you but is quite likely to affect your immediate performance.

If the patient is known to be HIV-positive

Don't panic. Thousands of HIV needlestick injuries have resulted in only a handful of cases of HIV worldwide. The chances of your getting HIV are very small. On the other hand, don't give yourself a hard time if you do panic. Almost everyone does, and people who haven't stuck themselves with HIV-infected blood just don't understand what this is like. Seek help from a counsellor or GP if you are suffering from excessive anxiety about it.

1 Have one clotted tube of blood taken from yourself. Give it to the public health unit/GP for storage. This is to ascertain your hepatitis/HIV status at the time of injury. It will only be analysed in the unlikely event that you are later found to be positive.

2 You will need to take anti-retroviral triple therapy for post-exposure prophylaxis. Seek the advice of your occupational health service.

3 After 3 months (at least) have an HIV check. Over 95% of people who are going to seroconvert do so within 3 months. If this is negative, repeat it at 6 months and 1–2 years. The second test will give you peace of mind.

4 Use condoms at least until the 3-month check.

5 Having HIV tests does not usually pose a problem for getting life insurance (as it once did), if you explain that you are a health professional having a routine HIV check. However, if you are concerned, you can usually have your blood checked confidentially by your virology lab or the hospital's STD clinic (so it will not be recorded in your medical records). The latter is preferable, as you will get proper counselling for the test.

If the patient is known to be hepatitis-positive

1 Follow your doctor's instructions. Give the lab a clotted sample of your blood as soon as possible after injury to ascertain your hepatitis antibody status at the time of injury.

2 Find out what kind of hepatitis the patient has. They may have chronic hepatitis from lupus which is not infective. If they have Hep B, you may need instant immunoglobulin; if they have Hep C you may need interferon treatment.

3 You may need to be re-tested for hepatitis antigen after 6 months. In the meantime, it is advisable to practise safe sex.

Not coping

Coping is not about 'just getting a grip'. You may hear this from some colleagues, but most likely they are just putting on a mask to their peers. You are not alone. *Everyone* has disastrous days, weeks, months and even years. Almost everyone thinks about giving up medicine, sometimes frequently! If you feel like chucking it all in, this does not mean that you are less motivated or committed than anyone else. In fact the chances are that if you are feeling like that, so is everyone else, except that they'd rather die than admit it. Group studies suggest that when one person is feeling lonely, isolated, alienated and generally miserable, it is much more likely that others in the environment are too. Studies show that a substantial proportion of junior doctors become clinically depressed; most suffer depression and anxiety at least a few times during their career.

■ Confidential counselling services have been established which provide support for doctors who are not coping. The BMA can advise you where such services are and how to contact them.

■ Make sure that you do not blame yourself for structural problems in your workplace that have nothing to do with you. For instance, a bullying consultant or charge nurse will make anyone's life hell, not just yours. Consider talking to others – or even to your local representative – about such problems before taking it all upon yourself.

■ Everyone experiences considerable turbulence upon entering the workplace. Remember that feeling low or anxious may just be manifestations of adjusting to a completely new way of life, and will pass within a few months, however painful they seem at present. This may well reoccur with job changes.

■ Simple fatigue can greatly exacerbate mental distress; in difficult times don't be afraid to acknowledge this to yourself.

Part-time work (flexible training)

■ It is now possible to be a part-time junior doctor. At present, part-time jobs are individually negotiated and created by postgraduate tutors. Part-time usually means half-time, doing half the number of on-call nights. Unfortunately, the corollary of doing half-time is that you end up taking more time to complete your training and get paid proportionally.

■ It is possible to continue flexible part-time training as an SHO, up to and including consultant level. At Registrar level and above, national recognition and approval for part-time training is required. At SHO level, simple agreement with the Postgraduate Dean suffices.

Representation of junior doctors

You can get a great deal done if you and your colleagues work together on agreed goals. You can act as a body in several ways:

1 *Doctors mess, mess president and committee*. This may meet regularly or on an ad hoc basis. It usually has several roles: organization of social events, representation of junior doctors' interests to management, administration of mess funds, rooms, etc. Mess presidency is a good way to begin to develop leadership and management skills for your CV.

2 *Junior doctors' division*. This is usually a hospital committee which meets every few months to discuss issues relevant to junior doctors. The main frustration for junior doctor representatives is that you rarely work at the hospital long enough to see changes implemented.

3 *New Deal committee*. Hospitals should have convened this committee or something similar to consider and implement the issues arising from the Junior Doctors' New Deal, that is, reducing doctors' hours and delegating inappropriate duties.

4 *BMA*. Junior doctors may stand as representatives for local, regional and national committees like the *BMA*. You should be allowed a reasonable amount of time off to attend these activities; your consultant is not obliged to do so but it is a reasonable request if they can maintain the service effectively while you are away. In practice, it is usually doctors beyond the initial foundation year who have the career stability to embark upon medical politics.

Sleep and on-call rooms

Those who have not been sleep-deprived cannot understand what it's like to be obsessed by the thought of sleep. Admittedly, the situation has much improved since the 1980s. However, you can still get very run down if you don't take care of yourself.

■ If you've had little or no sleep the night before, a shower and breakfast go a long way to prevent the awful grey feeling of fatigue.

■ Ask someone else to hold your bleep for a few hours. Have a nap at lunch time in an on-call room.

■ After long shifts, go to bed, go directly to bed, do not pass Go, do not collect £200! You will be grateful the next morning.

■ Another trick is to sleep in a doctor's room while on call. This radically cuts down time getting up and travelling across car parks and long corridors to the ward, and rarely results in more calls. In the morning, you only have to get up minutes before the ward round. Always strip your own sheets in the morning. Be careful though, as in some trusts it is now a disciplinary matter to sleep while on duty even if it is an on call!

When things go wrong

The F1 year is one of the most challenging years you will ever experience due to the steep learning curve. Usually your problems are focused on matters like more sleep, not feeling experienced enough, etc. A feeling of being unsupported is a worryingly common concern and on the rare occasion, you may encounter more difficult complex problems.

Bullying and psychological stress

It is important to stress that this rarely ever happens, but when it does it can really ruin your working life. People who have never been bullied are unable to understand the feeling of powerlessness when being psychologically assaulted. This can be even more difficult when the person doing the bullying is senior to you or even your boss.

■ Talk to someone. There are many avenues of support available: your postgraduate tutor, your previous tutors in medical school, BMA support lines, your medical defence agency, even your non-medical friends. If you do not feel like divulging names, you don't have to, but it helps greatly to look at your problem outside the perspective of the victim.

■ Find a witness to any bullying. This may be a nurse, a colleague or anyone else also employed by the hospital. While patients under your care may be witness to bullying, it is considered unprofessional to enlist their help against a colleague.

■ Confrontation is one strategy for dealing with bullying but it may not be suited for a hierarchical structure like medicine. If you are being bullied by your direct senior, you should voice your concerns to the person senior to him or her (or at the least a sympathetic fellow consultant) as they may not be aware of your plight.

■ If intending to confront someone, have a witness present. Be as formal as possible. Start with an explanation of your feelings of being threatened and how you want to avoid the situation again. Do not launch into accusations.

■ Document incidents with date, time, details of conversation and those present.

■ Threats to leave a permanent blight on your career are empty ones. Careers are built on more than the word of a single individual no matter how illustrious.

Whistle-blowing

This has become a major issue in light of the number of high-profile medical scandals in the past decade. It is important to stress that these incidents are not scandals because they are medical disasters; they are scandalous because safeguards which should have been in place were not working. There are existing channels for voicing out problems, and these should be used when available. The term whistle-blowing still holds some stigma but in essence is a professional obligation to ensure high-quality care. It should be undertaken in accordance with trust and GMC policy. It is definitely NOT going to the press, something we would strongly counsel against doing!

■ Speak to your medical defence agency before taking any action.

■ Document everything (letters, memos, emails, conversations in the corridor) on paper with date, times, those present and details.

■ Before whistle-blowing, you should ensure that the person who is responsible for the problem is aware of the problem. It is unfair to whistle-blow on a problem which could easily be fixed with a phone call.

■ Whom to whistle-blow to is just as important as what to whistle-blow about. Depending on the scale of the problem, you should pick the appropriate agency to talk to. There is no point complaining to the General Medical Council about the state of cleanliness of the toilets. For hospital-scale problems or problems with doctors, the order of preference is: the hospital management, the General Medical Council, then finally in exceptional circumstances the media.

■ Check the GMC web site which has guidance on whistle-blowing: http://www.gmc-uk.org/guidance/ethical_guidance/raising_concerns.asp

Appendix
USEFUL TESTS, NUMBERS AND OTHER INFORMATION

Addresses

Diabetes UK (formerly The British Diabetic Association), 10 Queen Ann Street, London W1M 0BD (web: www.diabetes.org.uk; tel: 020-7323 1531)

British Medical Association (and BMJ), BMA House, Tavistock Square, London WC1H 9JP (web: www.bma.org.uk; tel: 020-7387 4499)

Central Public Health Lab, 61 Colindale Avenue, London NW9 5HT (web: http://www.phls.co.uk; tel: 020-8200 4400)

Communicable Disease Surveillance Centre (for notifying diseases), 61 Colindale Avenue, London NW9 5DF (web: http://www.phls.co.uk; tel: 020-8200 6868)

Disabled Living Foundation (for advice on equipment), 380–384 Harrow Road, London W9 2HU (web: http://www.dlf.org.uk; tel: 020-7289 6111)

Driving and Vehicle Licensing Authority (www.dvla.gov.uk)

General Medical Council, 178 Portland Street, London W1N 6JE (web: www.gmcuk.org; tel: 020-7580 7642)

Medical Defence Union, 230 Black-friars Rd, London SE1 8PJ (web: http://www.themdu.com; tel: 020-7202 1500)

Medical and Dental Defence Union of Scotland, Mackintosh House, 120 Blythwood Street, Glasgow G2 4EH (web: http://www.mddus.com; tel: 0141-221 5858)

Medical Protection Society, 33 Cavendish Square, London W1G 0PS (http://www.mps.org.uk; tel: 020-7399 1300)

Medical Sickness Society, Colmore Circus, Birmingham B4 6AR (web: http://www.medical-sickness.co.uk; tel: 0808-100 1884)

Multiple Sclerosis Society, 372 Edgeware Rd, London NW2 6ND (web: http://www.mssociety.org.uk; tel: 020-8438 0700)

NHS Direct, www.nhsdirect.nhs.uk (tel: 0845 4647)

Poisons information	
Belfast	028 9024 0503
Birmingham	0121 507 5588
	0121 507 5589
Cardiff	029 2070 9901
Dublin	+353 1 837 9964
	+353 1 837 9966
Edinburgh	0131 536 2300
London	020 7635 9191

Barthel score

The Barthel score helps you to assess quickly whether someone can manage at home. It is particularly useful at social rounds. A total score of 15 or more is 'good'.

Bathing

0 dependent

1 independent (bath and shower, in and out)

Bladder

0 incontinent or catheterized and unable to cope alone

The Hands-on Guide for Junior Doctors, Fourth Edition. Anna Donald, Michael Stein and Ciaran Scott Hill. © 2011 Anna Donald, Michael Stein and Ciaran Scott Hill. Published 2011 by Blackwell Publishing Ltd.

I   occasional incontinence (1/day)
2   fully continent

Bowels
0   incontinent
I   occasional incontinence (1/week)
2   fully continent

Dressing
0   dependent
I   needs some help (e.g. with buttons, laces)
2   independent

Feeding
0   dependent
I   needs some help (e.g. with cutting)
2   independent (food within reach)

Grooming
0   dependent (hair, teeth, shaving)
I   independent

Mobility
0   immobile without help
I   independent with wheelchair (includes turning)
2   walks with one person assisting
3   independent

Stairs
0   dependent
I   needs assistance (physical, verbal, mechanical)
2   independent (up and down)

Toilet
0   dependent
I   needs some help
2   independent (transfer, wiping, dressing)

Transfer
0   unable (cannot balance to sit)
I   needs major assistance (2 people) but can sit

2   needs minor assistance (physical or verbal)
3   independent

Glasgow Coma Scale (GCS)

Eyes open
4   spontaneously
3   to voice
2   to pain
I   none

Verbal response
5   oriented
4   confused
3   inappropriate words
2   incomprehensible words
I   none

Motor response
6   obeys command
5   localizes to pain
4   withdraws
3   flexes
2   extends
I   none

Total (out of 15)
Serious: <8
Moderate: 9–12
Mild: 13–15

Mental Health Act

I Always get senior advice before using the Mental Health Act.

2 Section 4 states that for an emergency admission, the nearest relative *or* an approved Senior Nurse *or* a social worker *or* a doctor *as well as* the medical recommendation of one doctor who must have seen the patient within the previous 24 hours can apply for 72 hours of compulsory admission on the grounds of:

- Urgent necessity.
- Mental disorder requiring hospital admission.
- Danger to him/herself or others.

3 Section 5(2) states that a patient already in hospital as a voluntary patient can be detained for 72 hours under the same conditions as Section 4, except that it only requires a single medical recommendation by the doctor in charge of the patient's care, or another doctor on the staff of the hospital who is nominated by the doctor in charge.

4 Sectioning a patient does not permit you to treat a concurrent physical condition unless it is life-threatening.

Mini-mental test score

There are several versions of the mini-mental test score. This is one of them. It gives you a quick, ballpark measure of someone's mental state. This can be very useful in casualty or in the middle of the night. Folstein's full mental test score is outlined in the *Oxford Handbook of Clinical Medicine*.

1 What month is it?

2 What year is it?

3 Where are you now?

4 Recall an address (have the person repeat this after you and then ask it from them at the end of the other questions).

5 Name three objects (e.g. pen, hand, watch).

6 What is your name?

7 Start of World War I (1914) or World War II (1939)?

8 Name of the current UK monarch.

9 Name of the Prime Minister.

10 Count backwards from 20 to 1 without an error.

- When giving the patient an address to recall, use one that you know so that you remember it. There is nothing more embarrassing than failing your own mini-mental test!
- Questions 7–9 are culturally specific. They can be substituted for questions the patient is likely to know.

Notifiable diseases

Doctors are legally required to report notifiable diseases to their local medical officer for environmental health. The microbiology department know who this is, as do people at the town hall. Alternatively you can contact the Communicable Disease Surveillance Centre: 61 Colindale Avenue, London NW9 5EQ (tel: 020-8200-6868).

Recognized notifiable diseases are those listed below:

Acute encephalitis
Acute poliomyelitis
Anthrax
Cholera
Diphtheria
Dysentery
Food poisoning
Leptospirosis
Malaria
Measles
Meningitis:
    meningococcal
    pneumococcal
    haemophilus influenzae
    viral
    other specified
    unspecified
Meningococcal septicaemia (without meningitis)
Mumps
Ophthalmia neonatorum
Paratyphoid fever

Plague
Rabies
Relapsing fever
Rubella
Scarlet fever
Smallpox
Tetanus
Tuberculosis
Typhoid fever
Typhus fever
Viral haemorrhagic fever
Viral hepatitis:
    Hepatitis A
    Hepatitis B
    Hepatitis C
    other
Whooping cough
Yellow fever

INR (factors I, II, VII, X) Normal INR is 1.0	(expressed as ratio versus control)
Lymphocytes	1.3–3.5 (20–45%) $\times 10^9$/l
MCV	76–96fl
Monocytes	0.2–0.8 (2–10%) $\times 10^9$/l
Neutrophils	2–7.5 (40–75%) $\times 10^9$/l
Platelets	150–400 $\times 10^9$/l
Prothrombin	10–14 seconds
RCC (female)	3.9–5.6 $\times 10^{12}$/l
RCC (male)	4.5–6.5 $\times 10^{12}$/l
Reticulocytes	0.8–2% (25–100 $\times 10^9$/l)
WCC	4–11 $\times 10^9$/l

Results

The following are normal ranges for results of tests. However, every lab is different; make sure that you use their values, particularly for unusual tests, which require local calibration of lab equipment.

Consider copying the normal ranges that are important for your job onto a single sheet, which you can stick at the back of a folder or Filofax for easy reference.

Haematology

APTT (factors VIII, IX, XI, XII)	35–45 seconds
Eosinophils	0.04–0.44 (1–6%) $\times 10^9$/l
ESR (female)	(Age + 10)/2
ESR (male)	Age/2
FDP	Lab-dependent
Hb (male)	13.5–18 g/dl
Hb (female)	11.5–16 g/dl

Biochemistry

Acid phosphatase (prostate)	0–1 IU/l
Acid phosphatase (total)	1–5 IU/l
ACTH	3.3–15.4 pmol/l
ADH	0.9–4.6 pmol/l
Albumin	35–50 g/l
Aldosterone	100–500 pmol/l
Alkaline phosphate	30–300 IU/l
Alpha fetoprotein	< 10 IU/l
ALT	5–35 IU/l
Amylase	0–18 0U
Angiotensin II	5–35 units
AST	5–35IU/l
Bicarbonate	24–30 mmol/l
Bilirubin	3–17 mmol/l
Ca (ionized)	1–1.25 mmol/l
Ca (total)	2.12–2.65 mmol/l
Chloride	95–105 mmol/l
Cholesterol	3.9–7.8 (>5 is high) mmol/l

Cortisol (am)	280–700 nmol/l
Cortisol (pm)	140–280 nmol/l
Creatine kinase (males)	25–195 IU/l
Creatine kinase (females)	25–170 IU/l
Creatinine	70–120 mmol/l
CSF glucose	>2/3 of plasma glucose
Ferritin	20–300 mmol/l
Folate	5–6.3 nmol/l
FSH	2–8 U/l
GGT (males)	11–51 IU
GGT (females)	7–33 IU
Glucose (fasting)	4–6 mmol/l
Glycosylated Hb	6–8.5%
Haptoglobin	20–125 mmol/l
Iron (male)	14–31 mmol/l
Iron (female)	11–30 mmol/l
LDH	240–545 IU/l
Magnesium	0.75–0.15 mmol/l
Osmolality	278–305 mOsm/kg
PTH	<0.1–0.7 mg/l
Phosphate	0.8–1.45 mmol/l
Potassium	3.5–5.0 mmol/l
Prolactin (males)	<450 units
Prolactin (females, non-pregnant)	<600 units
Protein (total)	60–80 g/l
Red cell folate	0.36–1.44 mmol/l
Sodium	135–145 mmol/l
Troponin	Lab-dependent
TSH	0.5–5.7 U/l
T_4	70–140 nmol/l
Thyroxine (free)	9–22 pmol/l
TIBC	54–75 mmol/l
Triglyceride	0.55–1.9 mmol/l
T_3	1.2–3.0 nmol/l
Urea	2.5–6.7 mmol/l
Uric acid (males)	210–480 mmol/l

Uric acid (females)	150–390 mmol/l
Vitamin B_{12}	0.13–0.68 nmol/l or >150 ng/l

Arterial blood gases

pH	7.35–7.45
PaO_2	>10.6 kPa
$PaCO_2$	4.7–6.0 kPa
Base excess	± 2 mmol/l
Bicarbonate	22–26 mmol/l
Type 1 respiratory failure	$Pao_2 < 8$ $Paco_2 < 6$
Type 2 respiratory failure	$Pao_2 < 8$ $Paco_2 > 6$

Useful biochemical formulae

- The anion gap is made up of ions such as phosphate, sulphate, lactate.

- It is high in any condition with reduced clearance or excess production of any unmeasured anions (e.g. DKA, lactic acidosis).

- It is low in hyperalbuminaemia, liver disease and paraproteinaemias.

Corrected calcium = reported total Ca + 0.2 × (40 − the actual albumin)

Creatinine clearance (males)

$$= \frac{1.23 \times (140 - age) \times weight(kg)}{creatinine}$$

Creatinine clearance (females)

$$= \frac{1.04 \times (140 - age) \times weight(kg)}{creatinine}$$

Fitness to drive

Condition	Normal licence	Notification of DVLA	Vocational licence
Anaesthetic	Avoid for 48 hours post general anaesthetic	No	
Angina, chronic and stable		No	Many restrictions; refer to DVLA
Angioplasty	1 month	No	Check with DVLA
Aortic aneurysm	No restrictions	Yes	Permanent ban
Arrhythmias	Avoid driving if symptomatic while driving. Driving may continue once symptoms are controlled	Yes	
Occasional ventricular premature beats	No restrictions	No	
Frequent or polymorphic premature beats	Stop driving, pending CVS investigation	Yes	Check with DVLA
Ventricular tachycardia	Stop driving, pending CVS investigation. Driving may continue once symptoms are controlled with annual review	Yes	
Implanted defibrillator	Avoid driving forever	Yes	
CNS disorders	Where definite diagnosis of progressive disability; refer to DVLC for specific advice with consent of patient	Yes	Check with DVLA
Complete heart block	Driving forbidden until 1 month after pacing	Yes	Forbidden

Fitness to drive *(cont'd)*

Condition	Normal licence	Notification of DVLA	Vocational licence
Conduction abnormalities	If symptomatic, avoid driving pending CVS investigation. Can drive when symptoms are controlled	Yes	Check with DVLA
Congenital heart anomalies	No restrictions unless arrhythmia, angina or syncope	No	Check with DVLA
Post-surgery	1 month	No	
Congenital heart block (usually bradycardia)	3-year licence after CVS investigation, including stress test and 24-hour ECG, repeated annually	Yes	Usually forbidden
Diabetes mellitus	Can hold licence for 1, 2 or 3 years depending on type and complications. Insulin-requiring patients need to demonstrate: ■ Understanding of disease ■ Reasonable control ■ No frequent or unexplained hypoglycaemic attacks Always carry sugar in car	Yes	Need to notify DVLC if becomes IDDM, with individual review. Established type I diabetes will not be granted new vocational licences
Drugs (if impairs consciousness or motor response)	Avoid driving while taking drug. Warn patient that alcohol potentiates side effects of many drugs	No	

Epilepsy	Can hold (renewable) licence for up to 3 years if:	Allowed if fit-free since 5 years of age or fit-free for 10 years and off medication and annual review to confirm fit-free
	■ Free of fits for 2 years	Yes
	■ Fits only while asleep for 3 years	Yes
	■ Avoid for 6 months during treatment changes	Yes
Single fit	■ Cannot drive until investigated	Yes	Fit-free for 10 years and off medication and annual review to confirm fit-free
	■ Possible 1-year ban		
Hypertension (uncomplicated)	No restriction	No	
Impaired locomotor system	Avoid driving. If permanent disability, refer to DVLA	Yes	Refer to DVLA
MI	Avoid driving for 1 month	No	Many restrictions; refer to DVLA
Pacemakers	Can hold licence for up to 3 years 1 month post-implantation if:	Yes	Refer to DVLA
	■ Followed up annually		
	■ Asymptomatic		
PVD	No restriction	No	
Syncope, TIA, LOC	Avoid driving until problem solved; 3-month ban	Yes	Permanent ban
Valvular heart disease	No restrictions if no arrhythmia, angina or syncope	No	Check with DVLA

From Raffel A. (ed.) (1985) Medical Aspects of Fitness to Drive: A Guide for Medical Practitioners. Medical Commission on Accident Prevention, London.

APPENDIX

Index

Page numbers in *italics* indicate figures and tables.

The Hands-on Guide for Junior Doctors, Fourth Edition. Anna Donald, Michael Stein and Ciaran Scott Hill.
© 2011 Anna Donald, Michael Stein and Ciaran Scott Hill. Published 2011 by Blackwell Publishing Ltd.

Further Resources

Books

Colledge NR, Walker, BR and Ralston SJ. *Davidson's Principle's and Practice of Medicine*, 21st ed. 2010. Churchill Livingstone, London.

Corne J. *The CXR Made Easy*, 3rd ed. 2009. Churchill Livingstone, London.

Douglas GD, Nicol F and Robertson C. *Macleod's Clinical Examination*, 12th ed. 2009. Churchill Livingstone, London.

Eccles S and Sanders S. *So You Want to Be a Brain Surgeon? (Success in Medicine)*, 3rd ed. 2008. Oxford University Press, Oxford.

Goldberg A and Stansby G. *Surgical Talk: Lecture Notes in Undergraduate Surgery*, 3rd ed. 2011. Imperial College Press, London.

Hampton JR. *The ECG Made Easy*, 7th ed. 2008. Churchill Livingstone, London.

Hill CS. *Pocket Examiner*. 2009. Wiley Blackwell, London.

Kumar P and Clark M. *Clinical Medicine*, 7th ed. 2009. Saunders Elsevier.

Longmore M, Wilkinson I, Davidson E and Foulkes A. *Oxford Handbook of Clinical Medicine*, 8th ed. 2010. Oxford University Press, Oxford.

Nicholson TRJ, Gunarethne A and Singer DRJ. *Pocket Prescriber*. 2010. Hodder Arnold, London.

Wilson M and Layne K. *The Medic's Guide to Work and Electives around the World*, 2nd ed. 2009. Hodder Arnold, London.

Websites

British National Formulary: www.bnf.org

General Medical Council: www.gmc-uk.org

General Practitioner's Notebook: www.gpnotebook.co.uk

Intercollegiate Surgical Curriculum Programme: www.iscp.ac.uk

Map of Medicine: www.mapofmedicine.com

Medical Specialist Training in England: www.mmc.nhs.uk

National Institute for Health and Clinical Excellence: www.nice.org.uk

NHS email: www.nhs.net

Pubmed: www.ncbi.nlm.nih.gov/sites/entrez

Resuscitation Council: www.resus.org.uk

Royal College of Anaesthetists: www.rcoa.ac.uk

Royal College of General Practitioners: www.rcgp.org.uk

Royal College of Physicians: www.rcplondon.ac.uk

Royal College of Surgeons: www.rcseng.ac.uk

Royal Society of Medicine: www.rsm.ac.uk/

The British Medical Journal: www.bmj.com

The New England Journal of Medicine: www.nejm.org

Toxbase: www.toxbase.org

Up to date: www.uptodate.com

The Hands-on Guide for Junior Doctors, Fourth Edition. Anna Donald, Michael Stein and Ciaran Scott Hill.
© 2011 Anna Donald, Michael Stein and Ciaran Scott Hill. Published 2011 by Blackwell Publishing Ltd.

Notes

NOTES